Praise for *The Long Fix*

"Deeply researched, clearly written, and with a wealth of examples and colorful anecdotes, *The Long Fix* is necessary reading for anyone seeking to understand—and, more importantly, repair—our ailing health care system. Few people have the breadth and depth of Vivian Lee's experience, and her pragmatic, results-oriented approach offers a compelling and convincing blueprint for doctors, health care professionals, patients, and legislators, on both sides of the aisle."

—Eric Schmidt, PhD, former CEO of Google

"Dr. Lee has drawn upon her extensive experience and a wide range of physician and administrator colleagues to provide a deep understanding of the ailments plaguing the US health care system, accompanied by practical suggestions for how to remedy them. An excellent overview of the problems and potential solutions."

—Robert S. Kaplan, PhD, senior fellow, Marvin Bower Professor of Leadership Development, emeritus, Harvard Business School

"In *The Long Fix*, Vivian Lee, MD, crisply diagnoses the imperative to repair America's health care system and offers understandable principles as a guide. She lights a path forward by applying lessons and observations from her unique experiences as a physician, health system leader, and now technology executive. This book matters to patients and their families. It matters to Americans who care about the economic future of our nation. It especially matters to the government leaders and health care executives we depend on to find strategies that work for everyone."

—Michael O. Leavitt, former governor of Utah and former secretary of Health and Human Services

"Dr. Lee's book is an insightful diagnostic look at what is not working in American medicine, and why, that is made compelling by her succinct, practical recommendations for what each of us—policy maker, consumer, physician/health professional, and payer—can do now to realize the person-centered, high-value health care system we all so long for."

—Karen DeSalvo, MD, chief health officer, Google Health, and former US national coordinator for health information technology

"This is a well-researched and thoughtful book from one of our nation's leaders in health care reform. Dr. Lee has written a practical guide with actionable solutions for policy makers, health care providers, and patients—a must-read!"

—Dr. Leana S. Wen, MD, visiting professor at George Washington University, former president and CEO of Planned Parenthood, and former Baltimore city health commissioner

"An essential and timely guide for students, faculty, clinicians, and policy makers—Dr. Lee has produced a highly readable, concise, and persuasive case for reinventing the business of health care in order to create a more efficient, safer system for all. This is the book to read if you want to understand how we can improve health care in America."

—David Cutler, PhD, Otto Eckstein Professor of Applied Economics, Harvard University

"*The Long Fix* is one of the books I ask Cornell students to read for the US Health Care System course that I teach. Dr. Lee concisely and persuasively documents why we're not getting our money's worth in health care and what patients, health professionals, and policy makers should do to improve our system."

—Sean Nicholson, PhD, professor, Policy Analysis and Management, director, Sloan Program in Health Administration, Cornell University

"As I read *The Long Fix*, I realized that I had finally found *the* book that I have long sought for my students. Vivian Lee's insightful and balanced analysis of the problems plaguing our health care system—and the actions we can take to address them—provides a coherent path toward lasting change and improvement."

—Robert S. Huckman, PhD, Albert J. Weatherhead III Professor of Business Administration, faculty chair, Health Care Initiative, Harvard Business School

"*The Long Fix* is a highly readable, brilliantly crafted playbook of solutions to America's ailing health care system. Dr. Lee has shown how the nation can achieve higher quality and safer care that will help keep its communities healthier and, in turn, lower costs. This book is an inspiring and practical call to action for patients, physicians, policy makers, and employers to engage in one of the most important issues of our time."

—Carolyn Clancy, MD, former director, Agency for Healthcare Research and Quality (AHRQ)

"An engaging and upbeat book, *The Long Fix* doesn't flinch from the challenges needed to overhaul the US health care system, but rather helps the reader envision what's necessary for every player—hospitals, doctors, pharmaceutical companies, patients, and technology companies, among others—to play their part. Weaving together diverse case studies with richly referenced explanations and analyses, Lee paints a picture of a brighter future where the right investments in prevention, public health, data, and technology can create a better health care system for all."

—Rainu Kaushal, MD, chair, Department of Population Health Sciences, Weill Cornell Medical College

THE LONG FIX

THE
LONG FIX

Solving America's Health
Care Crisis with Strategies
That Work for Everyone

VIVIAN S. LEE, MD

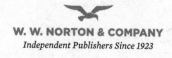

W. W. NORTON & COMPANY
Independent Publishers Since 1923

For information about permission to reproduce selections from this book, write to Permissions, W. W. Norton & Company, Inc., 500 Fifth Avenue, New York, NY 10110

For information about special discounts for bulk purchases, please contact W. W. Norton Special Sales at specialsales@wwnorton.com or 800-233-4830

Manufacturing by Lake Book
Book design by Dana Sloan
Production manager: Anna Oler

Library of Congress Cataloging-in-Publication Data

Names: Lee, Vivian S., 1966– author.
Title: The long fix : solving America's health care crisis with strategies that work for
everyone / Vivian S. Lee.
Description: First edition. | New York, N.Y. : W.W. Norton & Company, [2020] |
Includes bibliographical references and index.
Identifiers: LCCN 2020009618 | ISBN 9781324006671 (hardcover) |
ISBN 9781324006688 (epub)
Subjects: MESH: Health Care Costs | Health Care Reform | Quality of Health Care |
Delivery of Health Care—economics | United States
Classification: LCC RA971.3 | NLM W 74 AA1 | DDC 362.1068/1—dc23
LC record available at https://lccn.loc.gov/2020009618

ISBN 978-0-393-86744-2 pbk.

W. W. Norton & Company, Inc., 500 Fifth Avenue, New York, N.Y. 10110
www.wwnorton.com

W. W. Norton & Company Ltd., 15 Carlisle Street, London W1D 3BS

1 2 3 4 5 6 7 8 9 0

To my parents, Sam and Elisa Lee, and to my sister, Jennifer Lee, who have devoted their lives to improving the health of our communities through research, teaching, and innovation.

To my lifelong partner, Benedict Kingsbury, and to our four daughters, who bring immeasurable joy to our lives.

CONTENTS

THE LONG FIX

CHAPTER 1

A REVOLUTION OF COMMON SENSE

It was the best of times, it was the worst of times,
it was the age of wisdom, it was the age of foolish-
ness, it was the epoch of belief, it was the epoch of
incredulity . . .

—Charles Dickens, *A Tale of Two Cities*

The rumbling engine of the wood-paneled station wagon cut through the scorching Oklahoma summer heat as it pulled over to the curb. The radio, tuned as always to the local country station, blared Loretta Lynn's latest hit. As I slipped into the front seat, Hal Belknap leaned forward in the driver's seat to turn it down and shot me an apologetic look, as he always did.

Dr. Belknap—we all called him "Dr. B"—was a prominent internal medicine doctor in Norman, Oklahoma. In 1979, he had volunteered for a program that matched junior high students with community leaders, and I got lucky. For the next few years, I spent my Saturday mornings at Norman Regional Hospital, tagging along as he made his rounds and feeling rather like an extra on *Marcus Welby, M.D.*, that popular TV show from the 1970s.

On a typical morning, we would set out to find Mabel, Fred, Hank, Rosetta, and the other patients propped up in their hospital beds, eagerly awaiting us. (Well, mostly eagerly awaiting Dr. B.) After swinging their breakfast trays to the side—careful not to spill the small cartons of milk and bowls of cereal and canned fruit medley—Dr. B would sit on the side of their beds and listen to their hearts, their lungs, and their stories. He was always deeply attentive to their medical ailments, but he also wanted to find out what was on their minds. I could see him making mental notes as he asked after their families: the granddaughter's wedding (note: have Vicki—his nurse—send a card), the husband who had just been discharged from the hospital (note: set up home nursing visits), and the son who was moving back home (note: invite grandson to join Dr. B's Boy Scout troop).

After completing rounds, Dr. B scrawled his practically indecipherable notes in their charts, gave instructions to the nurses, and occasionally ordered a study or lab test. A naturally sharp diagnostician, he didn't request many studies or interventions, relying mostly on his intuition and judgment. He placed the most weight on what was best for the patient and often reminded me that less was more, even in medicine.

Caring for patients back then was less complicated, less bureaucratic, less expensive. Dr. B and his colleagues kept all their medical records on paper and carried tone-only pagers (no screens). CT (computed tomography, or "CAT") scans were new, and MRI (magnetic resonance imaging)—my future specialty—had not yet come into the picture. Drug prices were reasonable and rarely made the news. But not everything was better when it was simpler. Most patients who had strokes and heart attacks died or were debilitated by them. We hadn't imagined gene therapies or robotic surgeries or electronic medical records. I also never heard the words "health care reform."

I decided back then that I wanted to be a doctor. I was certain that Dr. B had improved the lives of his patients and that it was rewarding for him, too. I set off in pursuit of this noble profession with a determined optimism.

The Journey to MD and CEO

Fifteen years later—after college, graduate school, medical school, a surgical internship, radiology residency, and a fellowship in MRI—I emerged in 1998 ready for my first real job ("Finally!" my parents said). In the two decades since I had accompanied Dr. B, medicine had changed dramatically. For one, my field—magnetic resonance imaging—had been invented. MRI radiologists were spotting small cancers early enough to save patients' lives and sparing others from the poking and prodding of procedures such as angiograms, cholangiograms, and fistulograms. New medications like clot-busting drugs were saving patients with heart attacks and strokes. And deaths due to cancer were finally starting to decline, thanks to better prevention and new chemotherapies. As a researcher and later, as chief scientific officer at NYU Langone Medical Center in New York, I could see that the discoveries coming out of research laboratories—genomics, stem cell therapy, immunotherapy, the microbiome, and more—were offering new hope for many, even the possibility of curing the incurable.

At the same time, health care was also showing signs of changing for the worse. Doctoring involved a lot more negotiating with insurance companies than sitting at the bedside or thinking through hard-to-diagnose conditions. A series of widely cited reports from the Institute of Medicine (now the National Academy of Medicine) cast a deeply critical eye on safety and quality in the American health system. All the while, health costs were increasing so rapidly that it became clear that if we didn't reduce the costs of care and get our system back on track, all those scientific advances might be for naught.

These realizations were weighing heavily on me when I made a visit to Boston in 2010 that changed the trajectory of my career. I went to see an old friend of mine, Gregg Meyer, an internal medicine physician who at the time was the senior vice president for quality and safety at the Massachusetts General Hospital. I was there to learn about research administration from a hospital famous for its scientific excellence.

While there, Gregg introduced me to their sophisticated electronic health records system. He told me how it was completely changing the way his hospital was approaching care. When patients turned 50, for example, the computers automatically offered them a pamphlet or DVD (the latest technology then) that explained why they should undergo a colonoscopy to screen for colon cancer. No more relying on doctors to remember. For each doctor, the computer system also tracked which of their patients with high blood pressure were getting better with treatment and which needed more attention.

Instead of getting paid for every procedure or exam clinicians performed, the hospital proposed that it should get paid for keeping patients healthy. This could include making sure they had undergone colon cancer screening and effectively lowering blood pressure in patients with hypertension. The insurers agreed. Before long, thanks to its exceptional electronic records, the Massachusetts General Hospital successfully achieved its targets. Hypertensive patients had lower blood pressures, and the hospital was rewarded with higher payments. It was a win-win.

For me, this was an epiphany. With the right tools, leaders could reinvent health care and create a system where everyone would be paid to deliver better care. I wanted to help build that future.

During that visit to Boston, Gregg also unexpectedly introduced me to health care in a state I knew little about—Utah. He gave me a book written by his colleague, physician and Harvard Business School professor Richard Bohmer, called *Designing Care*. It featured Intermountain Healthcare, the eminent Salt Lake City–based hospital system that had similarly used its electronic health system to achieve superior care. Utah suddenly seemed to be everywhere. That year, according to the national rankings of university hospitals, NYU had been ranked #10 in quality and safety, while the University of Utah ranked #1. When I got back to NYU, I tried to persuade my colleagues to make a field trip to Utah. As if on cue, an executive search firm rang up, asking if I might like to visit Salt Lake City. The University of Utah was looking for a new leader of its health system and academic health sciences campus. I got my trip out West, and a new job to boot.

The Front Lines

In July 2011, I began my new role as CEO of University of Utah Health, a health system that serves a large swath of the western United States: Utah, Idaho, Wyoming, Montana, western Colorado, and also parts of Nevada. By the end of my six years there, we had grown into a $3.6 billion system that included four hospitals, 12 neighborhood health centers, numerous specialty clinics like cancer, dialysis, and urgent care, and an affiliate hospital network of over 18 hospitals in the region. We employed over 1,400 board-certified physicians and had 1.7 million patient visits per year. We also owned and operated a national reference laboratory company (where each day tens of thousands of specimens were sent to us for blood analyses, genetic studies, and other tests). University of Utah Health was recognized for its health care system innovations that enabled higher-quality care at lower costs, with higher patient and employee satisfaction. In 2016, the hospital was again ranked #1 in the nation in quality and safety among all university hospitals.

As CEO, I was also responsible for over 15,000 employees and trainees. We ran our own health plan (we were self-insured) to manage our employees' health benefits and those of many of the state's Medicaid beneficiaries. We transformed the plan into a commercial health insurance company to take care of the health benefits programs of other employers in our community and region.

Part of the CEO job entailed serving as the university's medical school dean and senior vice president. I oversaw scientific research and the training of the future workforce in medicine, nursing, pharmacy, dentistry, and allied health professionals. The vibrant academic enterprise gave us even more opportunities to innovate. We taught our students to work on interdisciplinary teams, connected patients with rare and undiagnosed diseases to genetic scientists, worked with our engineering colleagues to establish an innovation center that included videogames and apps for health, and learned valuable management lessons from our business school colleagues.

Over the course of these and other experiences, I have gained a deep understanding of the complexity of the US health care system—its great challenges and wealth of opportunities. And I have emerged profoundly optimistic that as a nation, we can provide affordable and high-quality health care for all. But what exactly are those challenges and opportunities? And what is the basis for that optimism?

The Maddening Paradox

By a few measures, the US health care system is one of the best in the world and, by some measures, it is one of the worst.

The United States leads the world in medical innovation, and its scientists are discovering new cures at an exhilarating pace. Patients with leukemia are being treated with their own immune cells, engineered to attack cancer cells. Cardiologists can replace the heart's aortic valve using catheters placed through arteries in the leg, without opening the chest. Patients with chronic hepatitis C can now be cured. At the same time, some of the most ordinary but vital care isn't being received. For example, 46% of US adults have high blood pressure, which is a risk factor for heart attack, stroke, and even dementia, but half of those affected aren't taking the life-saving pills that can cost just ten cents per day.

Hands down, the United States spends more on health care per capita than any other nation—nearly one-fifth of the US economy goes to pay for health. That's two to three times more than other high-income Organization for Economic Co-operation and Development (OECD) nations like the UK, Canada, Germany, Japan, and Australia, where health coverage is universal. Despite this, about 1 in 11 Americans don't have health insurance and can't afford care.

Cutting-edge operations and advanced treatments developed in America provide hope to patients all over the world, but here at home, we face an epidemic of diseases of despair. In 2017, while we performed 34,768 life-saving organ transplants, we lost more than 47,600 people to opioid overdoses and another 47,174 to suicide. As a result, while most of the rest of the world is getting healthier and living longer, life expectancy in the United

States is declining. Babies born in the United States in 2017 are expected to live 78.6 years, 5.6 years less than those born in Japan, which places us 26th out of 35 OECD nations in life expectancy.

The prospects for a healthier future are rapidly fading: Four out of ten adults are obese, and seven out of ten are overweight, making them much more likely to suffer from back and joint pain, and, over time, to be stricken by heart disease, stroke, type 2 diabetes, and certain types of cancer. The highest prevalence of mental health problems is among young adults. Our failing health jeopardizes our national security; as of 2014, the Pentagon estimated that seven out of ten young adults in the United States would not qualify for military service, the most common reason being their weight.

The nation is paying dearly for these failures. Companies that cover employee health insurance have seen rising costs that erode their margins and hobble competitiveness. Much of that ever-rising expense has been passed on to employees, often in hidden ways like flat wages over the past 50 years. Workers are also getting hurt directly, as deductibles and co-payments soar. (There is one more insidious hidden cost: since World War II, employee and employer premiums are exempt from income and payroll tax. They aren't a taxable benefit, the way a bonus is, which means that the government foregoes billions in tax revenue—$275 billion in 2016 alone. Taxpayers, of course, make up the difference.)

Health care is bankrupting the uninsured and the swelling ranks of the underinsured, and it's often disappointing the millions who do have coverage. This ailing, failing system is making our nation sick—financially, emotionally, and physically. But within this seemingly barren health care crisis is not a spring but practically an ocean of opportunity.

We Pay More for Less

With health care spending rapidly approaching $4 trillion per year, the obvious but misguided solution would be to reduce expenses by cutting care, but that's dangerous for patients and for our future. It's not care that needs to be cut, it's the wasteful spending that doesn't contribute to better health. We have to stop paying more to get less. Here are a few of the opportunities most of us in health care agree on:

- **We waste.** The Institute of Medicine (now National Academy of Medicine) estimated in 2012 that we waste 30 cents of every dollar we spend on health care. That's over $1 trillion per year. Some of the waste is fraud and abuse, but most of it comes from failures to care for patients properly.
- **We overtreat.** A substantial part of the waste is driven by overdiagnosis and overtreatment. In a 2016 survey, US physicians thought that about 20% of all medical care was unnecessary.
- **We make deadly mistakes.** Medical errors are the third-leading cause of death in the United States—over 250,000 deaths each year. That's about 9.5% of all deaths, behind only heart disease and cancer.
- **We practice medicine inconsistently.** Clinicians make decisions without being fully informed about the latest science and without information about costs (to the patient, and overall). Physicians follow recommended guidelines only one-half to two-thirds of the time.
- **We are choking on bureaucracy.** In the United States, about 8% of spending on health care is spent on administration. Among ten high-income OECD nations, the figure averaged only 3%.
- **Health care professionals are paid generously but waste a lot of time.** The average US generalist physician makes about $218,000; specialists average $316,000. These expensive professionals waste a large percentage of their time on frustrating administrative tasks like computer data entry and disputing with insurance companies instead of caring for patients.
- **We push expensive new technologies and treatments even if they aren't any better than cheaper (or generic) alternatives.** We spend double to triple what Canada and some European countries do on pharmaceuticals, mostly due to high-cost, branded drugs and the overprescription of antibiotics and other medications.
- **We wait until it's too late.** About 8.5% of the US population is unin-

sured, and more are forgoing preventive and primary care because they are underinsured. By the time the health system sees them, we've missed our chance at prevention.

- **We wish patients would enjoy healthier diets and more exercise, but we can't seem to influence them to change their behaviors.** As a nation, we seem to favor sugar- and high-fructose corn syrup–laden sweets and drinks (spending $4 billion on them annually), deep-fried food ($200 billion for fast food), tobacco ($130 billion), and sedentary lifestyles with plenty of screen time and video gaming ($43 billion) over healthier alternatives. Eight-minute clinic visits aren't long enough for primary care providers to have meaningful conversations to influence these habits.

- **We deny the wishes of the dying.** We put people in hospitals who would be better off at home. In the hospital, we attach them to costly life support systems, even when they have asked to be left alone. While four out of five people would prefer to die at home, only one out of five does. Most people still die in a hospital or nursing home.

We are spending plenty, but not always in the right ways, and without getting what we want or what patients deserve.

The Price of Paying for Action

The root cause of this crisis is the fee-for-service system: we pay for each pill, echocardiogram, laboratory test, or operation regardless of whether it makes people healthier. Our system rewards action, not better health outcomes. It encourages overtreatment and specialty care at the expense of prevention and primary care. For example, every headache or backache warrants an MRI in a fee-for-service world, and every episode of chest pain (even if it's just indigestion) justifies a coronary angiogram. This is *the* fundamental flaw of American health care.

It started harmlessly enough. When Medicare began in 1965, it simply paid all bills that hospitals submitted for procedures, tests, and operations.

The more bills they sent to Medicare, the more money hospitals received. Over time, the industry developed what economists refer to as a "supply-driven demand economy." In other words, to make money, every hospital or clinic filled its beds and loaded its patients up with tests, prescriptions, and consultations. Over the next few decades, the skylines of most urban centers were blotted by construction cranes for new hospital towers, imaging offices, and cancer centers, all of which were quickly filled with patients. Between 1967 and 1983, annual Medicare payments to hospitals shot up from $3 billion to $37 billion. By 2018, the figure was a stunning $308 billion.

In hindsight, the results were predictable. When people are paid for doing *something*, regardless of whether it works, we tend to do more and more of it. As Ceci Connelly, the former *Washington Post* journalist turned president/CEO of the Alliance for Community Health Plans, put it, "If you told me when I was a reporter that I was going to be paid by the word, my stories would have been a lot longer but not necessarily better." The pay-for-action (or "fee-for-service") system motivates hospitals and doctors to do things to people, and not necessarily to make them healthier. That's backward. And dangerous.

Demanding Results not Action

Even those of us succeeding in the current fee-for-service model realize that paying for results—better health outcomes at lower costs—would radically improve our system. If our nation stopped expecting quick fixes—a prescription, a referral to a specialist, an MRI, an operation—and instead put a premium on measurably improving lives for good, then prevention would become paramount. The medical world would focus on diet, sleep, and fitness. We would make restoring mental health as important as restoring physical health. We'd try to prescribe only drugs that work and that do so cost-effectively. We'd recommend imaging studies or operations shown to be beneficial. Back operations, for example, would be reserved for the few who truly needed them, and everyone else would be told to rest or undergo physical therapy. Hospitals and clinics would standardize care, making it safer and better. And those who didn't would go out of business.

Who Cares? I Have Insurance

If the answer is so clear, then why isn't the nation moving faster to paying for results?

For one, many have a vested interest in the status quo. Maybe even more important, most of us don't really buy health care, we buy health insurance. That means we don't pay for health care directly, we pay for it *indirectly*, and even that is often subsidized. For about half of Americans, employers pay for most of their health care. For others, health care is a government benefit paid for by taxes. Only the 8.5% of Americans who remain uninsured pay for their health care bills directly—and mostly they can't afford them.

With this insurance-based model, the dynamic between insurers and doctors can put them at odds with patients' interests.

Consider a hypothetical small company, say, a book publishing house or a tech start-up with 200 employees. The president of the company engages an insurance company to provide health insurance to her employees. Each year that insurance company sets the annual premium rates based on predictions of how much health care her employees will need. The employer pays 70%–80% of the premium; her employees contribute the remaining 20%–30% through deductibles, co-payments, or coinsurance (see Notes for definitions). The insurance company then uses that pool of premiums to pay (or "reimburse") doctors, hospitals, pharmacies, and others for the care that employees and their families receive over the year. (Instead of paying premiums to the insurer, larger employers who are self-insured will set the money in reserve to pay the health bills themselves.)

In this arrangement, better health isn't necessarily everyone's goal: Insurers who pay doctors and hospitals for care *are incentivized to spend as little as possible on a patient's health.* The less they pay out, the more profit they make. Conversely, in a pay-for-action model, most doctors and hospitals *are incentivized to spend as much as possible.* This means patients—or more precisely, their premiums—are the rope in an annual trillion-dollar tug of war. Doctors and hospitals pull by ordering more tests and operations; insurers yank back by denying those services or adding restrictions like "prior authorization" paperwork for expensive medications and tests. When hospitals or doctors charge more than insurers are willing to pay, patients can get caught in the middle and be asked to pay the difference, leading to so-called "surprise bills."

Usually, we expect competition in the market to drive innovation that leads to better services at lower costs. Not so here. Because we have an insurance model of paying for health care, the normal economic rules of the market don't readily apply. For the insurance model to work, many healthy people have to enroll in a plan to offset the costs of unhealthy people. That's a great deal for those who need expensive medications or a knee replacement, but a lousy one for those who don't expect to use a lot of services. When healthy people opt out of such plans, leaving just the sicker (and more expensive) in the pool, premiums go up, and even the moderately healthy people are priced out.

This also means people who are insured have more incentive to get care they think they have already paid for, especially once they've spent their deductible. ("Use it or lose it!") That drives costs up for everyone. Leonard Saltz, a doctor at Memorial Sloan Kettering Cancer Center in New York City, explained it to me this way: "It's like a dozen of us go out to dinner, and we're going to split the check. You cleverly realize you might as well order the surf 'n' turf instead of a cheeseburger, because you're going to pay the same amount, regardless. That works until everybody orders lobster, and all of a sudden the check is much higher. That's where we are in health care."

When you take your child with a sore throat to the emergency room for a strep test that could be done in the clinic, undergo an MRI you probably don't need, or fill unnecessary prescriptions—say, for an opioid pain medication or an antibiotic for a common cold—you (or the doctor who prescribed it) are piling on more and more "surf 'n' turf." And all of us are paying that grossly inflated dinner bill at the end of the night, which, in health care, means higher premiums for everyone next year.

What Are We Paying For?

Progress in fixing US health has been held up by its daunting complexity, polarized politics, and many entrenched interests. Some argue for radical change—that the only solution is for the private insurance companies to be replaced by the federal government. Others believe in a totally free marketplace (including moving government-run programs like the Veterans Health Administration and military medicine to the private sector). Regardless of whether the payer is the government, an employer, or an insurance company, the root cause of our problem still needs addressing:

It's not *who* runs the system that matters, it's *what* they pay for that needs to change radically.

A Tectonic Shift Away from Fee-For-Service

The good news is that things are changing. The Centers for Medicare & Medicaid Services (CMS) are shifting away from fee-for-service to new value-based payments and "alternative payment models." CMS pays for $1.3 trillion (37%) of US health care, so it's like the old E.F. Hutton commercial: when CMS talks, "People listen."

In 2012 in Utah, we listened attentively. First, the state's Medicaid office announced that as of January 2013, it would no longer pay our hospital and clinics on a fee-for-service basis for its beneficiaries. Instead, we would receive a fixed allocation to cover care for each person for the year. (The amount would be adjusted depending on the medical conditions the patient had.) Within that budgeted amount, we had to meet expectations of high-quality care to keep the Medicaid contract going forward. We were going to get paid for results, not action.

Second, Medicare announced it would begin the Bundled Payments for Care Improvement pilot project for total hip and knee replacements (two of the most common procedures in the United States). In this program, Medicare would pay hospitals a fixed (predefined) fee to cover preparation for the operation, the surgery itself, and all the medical care necessary for 90 days after the surgery. If the patient got an infection and had to be readmitted to the hospital after the operation, it would be at the hospital's expense. If the hospital spent less than the allotted dollars, it could share in the savings.

These two announcements were a shock to the system. We realized that our future success depended more on delivering better outcomes at lower costs than on how effectively we could bill for yet another MRI or yet another operation. We felt unprepared.

Leading Innovators

Fortunately, at the University of Utah I led a high-performing organization that could afford to think boldly. Our innovative leaders embraced change, and we were keen to put our collective toes—as a community of clinicians, patients, and their families, and as one of the state's largest employers—into that ocean of opportunity. Like other hospitals across the country, we studied industries outside of health care that had spent decades competing on who could deliver better services at lower prices. We had a lot to learn.

For example, in thinking about customer satisfaction, the Utah team borrowed lessons from other high-consumer-experience companies like Apple and In-N-Out Burger. In 2012, we were the first hospital in the nation to post all our patient satisfaction scores and comments online (more on this in Chapter 7). Medical centers like Geisinger Health in rural Pennsylvania and Virginia Mason Medical Center in Seattle taught us how they'd adopted lessons from Toyota's assembly lines to "manufacture" better health (more in Chapter 4). Inspired by the safety checklists that pilots use before takeoff, surgeons in hospitals across the country started requiring completed checklists before each operation to make sure an important step wasn't skipped—for example, making sure the patient was the right Mr. Jones for brain surgery.

These lessons helped make University of Utah Health consistently one of the safest teaching hospitals in the country. Better care, fewer mistakes, shorter stays, and fewer readmissions to the hospital all lowered the costs of care, too. All this made our business stronger than ever. We showed that in this new environment that was challenging us to change, a major health system could both do good and do well.

Minding the Widening Gap

Our challenges of improving health for Utahns were a lot like those facing the nation. Beyond the debates about Medicaid expansion, rising out-of-pocket costs were placing good health care out of reach of even insured Americans. And for the uninsured, lack of access to health care was reaching a crisis, one that has disproportionately affected the poor. In 2018, those living below 100% of the federal poverty level (income of less than $25,100 for a family of four) were five times as likely to be uninsured as those at or above 400% of poverty (16.3% versus 3.4%). Insurance coverage wasn't the only line that divided the haves and have-nots of health care. Rural Americans, like many in Utah, make up 15%–20% of the population and are sicker (more heart disease, more cancers, and more accidents, for example), older, and poorer than their urban counterparts. Race and ethnicity are associated with significant differences in health outcomes. Black Americans are more likely to be afflicted with diseases like heart attacks, stroke, and breast cancer, and more likely to die from them. More education also predicts better health. Any action plan for improving the health of Americans has to recognize these disparities in outcomes and bridge the gaps.

From Utah to Verily

After six years at Utah, I took a one-year sabbatical to do more research to study how other exemplar organizations were improving care in their communities. Besides these visits I interviewed about one hundred patients, clinicians, insurance executives, policy experts, community leaders, employers, journalists, and more. I was also introduced to a wide range of inspirational people and ideas by attending conferences at the National Academy of Medicine and the Institute for Healthcare Improvement, and others, as well as by serving on a number of expert panels and boards such as the Defense Health Board of the Department of Defense (advising on matters of the Military Health System) and the Commonwealth Fund Board of Directors. Across the nation, I discovered more real and practical solutions for how we all, working together, can build a safer, better, and cheaper health care system.

During this sabbatical year, I became convinced that accelerators of change are needed from outside the traditional system, and include technology and Big Data. That's what drew me to a new role: I became the president of Health Platforms, at Verily, the health care company of Alphabet and Google. Verily is using the data, new sensors, and machine-learning capabilities of one of the largest global technology companies to improve health. (In this connection, let me just say unless I specifically mention it, I do not have a financial interest in any product that I discuss in this book.)

A Revolution of Common Sense

This book tells the stories of some of the committed individuals on the front lines who have experimented with new ways of practicing, built pilot programs, tested new technologies, and forged new partnerships to lay the groundwork for better care and a more workable system. In this book, I synthesize and distill our collective ideas for this revolution of common sense into five main imperatives:

1. **Pay for results instead of action** (Chapter 1). The best investments in health engage people and keep them healthy at home and independent and recognize the vital roles families and communities play (Chapter 2). Within hospitals and clinics, paying for health instead of paying for action creates the opportunity for health insurers and physicians to work together (instead of at odds with each other) to keep people healthier (Chapter 3).

2. **Run health care delivery systems like businesses competing to deliver better health at lower costs**. Start with the highest priority of all: Make health care safer. Reduce medical mistakes by adapting better management models from other industries like manufacturing and aviation (Chapter 4). Improve the quality of care by making it easier to learn from experience, and tap into people's intrinsic

motivation to continuously improve (Chapter 5). Build tools that measure the costs of care as the first step to contain rising costs (Chapter 6). Treat patients like customers in the center of the health care universe and engage them as the most important coproducers of health (Chapter 7).

3. **Demand that other health industries also compete on making people healthier at lower costs.** Pharmaceutical and device manufacturers should compete on the cost-effectiveness of their treatments. Entities like Medicare, which represents millions of patients, should be able to negotiate drug prices, armed with data about their effectiveness (Chapter 8). Patients' electronic medical records should be used for the benefit of their health and to help doctors and hospitals improve the delivery of care (Chapter 9).

4. **Learn from the successes of employer-driven** (Chapter 10) **and government-run health systems** (Chapter 11). Invaluable lessons from both models help us imagine a better health care system for America.

5. **Implement an action plan for the Long Fix** that builds on the vital roles that everyone needs to play (Chapter 12).

The journey to better health won't happen with a quick fix. As my old mentor Dr. B used to say, it may take a little more time than we expect, but it'll be worth the ride.

CHAPTER 2

AN APPLE A DAY KEEPS
THE PATIENT AWAY

*How do you give the best care possible to people who
are becoming more frail and more fragile ... so they
get to achieve what they really want, which is to
be home?*

—Nancy Guinn, medical director,
Presbyterian Healthcare at Home

"**G**o see that crazy Chinese doctor who takes care of all the poor
Cubans!"

Chris Chen grins as he tells me how people used to rave about his
father's clinic in Miami. His father had started as a typical primary care
doctor in private practice. He was paid "fee-for-service," which meant the
more patients he saw, the more he earned. Then in south Florida in the early
1990s, a few insurance companies started experimenting with new ways to
pay doctors. Instead of fee-for-service, they gave them a fixed amount per
patient each year. If a patient needed expensive imaging, costly drugs, or

long hospitalizations that added up to more than that amount, it was the doctor's problem.

Chris's dad (the doctor) and mom (the office manager) experimented in this new model. They welcomed referrals, but other doctors sent them only their frailest and poorest patients, the ones they knew would be grossly unprofitable under this new way of paying. That's how Chris's parents began with 250 of the sickest people in Miami—people who would have been almost impossible to keep well at any facility, at any price. It looked as if the Chens had signed up for a financial suicide mission.

Because resources were scarce and their patients' needs were many, the Chens decided to focus on primary care and prevention. Their fragile, elderly patients had to be seen frequently by doctors—once they got sick, it would be too late—so they set up monthly visits, even if there was nothing wrong. Getting to the clinic would be tough for many of them, so the Chens provided free door-to-doctor transportation. (They worked out that averting the cost of just one ambulance ride and hospital stay could pay for a year of shuttle service.) They opened a pharmacy in the clinic so their patients could conveniently, cheaply, and reliably fill prescriptions. And since their patients often had complex needs, physicians in the clinics conferred several times a week about how best to treat those who weren't doing well.

Somehow, that "crazy Chinese doctor" and his wife not only provided outstanding care for their patients—including many who often didn't have enough to cover co-pays or deductibles—but they also managed to make them *healthier*: they reduced hospitalizations, and even more amazingly, they broke even financially. Out of desperation, the Chens invented a better way to do health care.

The Chens' model of care was particularly well suited to the Medicare Advantage programs that were rolled out starting in 2005. In the new model, Medicare allows insurance companies like Humana or Blue Cross Blue Shield to make special arrangements with physician practices. From Medicare's payment for health care for a group of seniors, the insurers can take their share up front for administrative costs plus profits—15%, say— and give the remaining 85% to groups like the Chens to run their clinics,

cover prescriptions, pay doctors, run shuttles, and even pay for hospitalizations or nursing home stays. If, at the end of the year, the Chens and their
colleagues spend less than the 85% they received from the insurers, they
pocket the difference. By 2020, Chris Chen, a doctor and the CEO of his
family's company ChenMed, introduced this model to more than 50 primary care practices for seniors in states like Florida, Illinois, Louisiana, and
Pennsylvania.

The catch is that in order to get paid, these groups must meet stringent
goals for keeping patients healthy and satisfied. People in these Medicare
Advantage plans can change doctors at least once a year, so quality and
patient satisfaction are high priorities for medical groups like the Chens.
(Their free shuttle service and onsite pharmacy are not only good for
health, but they also keep their patients happy.)

The ChenMed model is also surprisingly attractive to physicians, who
enjoy having the time and the tools to take better care of these seniors.
Instead of signing up as many patients as possible, which is the only way
to make money in the traditional pay-for-action model, physicians in these
Medicare Advantage programs have fewer patients and spend more time
with each of them. Primary care doctors in the United States typically
manage over 2,000 patients each; a ChenMed physician has between 350
and 600. Sofia Recabarren, a primary care physician who sees patients at
a ChenMed clinic in Miami, treasures the 40 minutes allotted for each
new-patient visit and the 20 minutes for follow-up appointments—twice
the time she had in her old job in New York City. "You actually know their
meds," she says. "You know what's going on in their lives."

That extra time matters. Chris Chen told me about a 400-lb. woman
who, whenever she was asked what she had for breakfast, lunch, and dinner, always gave answers that suggested she was eating sensibly. Chen was
baffled over why she couldn't lose weight. One day, the woman's daughter
came with her mother for a follow-up visit. She thanked Chen for continu-
ing to try to help her mom and then asked, "Can you get her to stop eating
that bucket of Kentucky Fried Chicken at midnight?"

ChenMed makes money by keeping patients out of the hospital. To reduce the risk of falls and broken hips, Recabarren created a class for her patients in which she tests how well they can see, checks their balance, makes sure their shoes fit well, and even gives tips for staying hydrated. She also encourages them to sign up for the clinic's free Tai Chi or yoga courses.

ChenMed clinics also understand that a person's health is inextricably tied to their happiness. That's why they host monthly birthday bashes for patients. Their vans will bring patients to these popular events and take them home after they've had their fill of cake, dancing, and gossip. The ChenMed doctors aren't the only ones who understand that loneliness is a killer. All over the world, physicians are starting to treat social isolation as a disease. In 2018, the British government appointed its first "minister for loneliness."

The profound lesson learned by Chris Chen and his parents is that it's far more effective to care for people *before* they get sick, and it's also cheaper. In Miami, ChenMed lowered the number of days spent in the hospital by 38% for their patients compared to the regional average. Because their clinics can usually find a way to see patients immediately, they also have fewer expensive emergency department visits. Chen says clinics that adopt the ChenMed model see at least a 25% increase in profitability. Applying similar models, California's CareMore Health, Chicago's Oak Street Health, Providence, Rhode Island's Coastal Medical, and Boston's Iora Health also have had impressive results.

Rushika Fernandopulle, a Harvard-educated physician born in Sri Lanka, founded Iora Health in 2011. He has given a lot of thought to the challenges of scaling this kind of medical care across the nation for seniors, and more broadly, for all Americans. He shared with me the key challenges:

First, when people move to clinics like Iora Health or ChenMed, they often have not been getting all the recommended screenings, filled all their prescriptions, or gotten all their vaccinations because their rushed clinicians haven't had the time. Iora Health makes sure they do when they sign on. That's good for the patient, but it can be a costly onboarding for the medical practice. Preventive medicine take time to prove its worth. It's not a quick fix.

The second challenge is that it's more costly to run these primary care clinics than the usual 30-patient-per-day fee-for-service office. Fernando-pulle estimates that an Iora clinic costs twice as much per patient for a regular clinic visit. Clinics also employ health coaches—three per doctor—who come from the community, speak the language of the people they serve, and help them learn how to eat healthier foods, reduce stress, understand their illnesses, and navigate the health system. And yes, they offer Zumba and yoga classes. To Fernandopulle, just like to Chen, it's worth it. Spending more on primary care reduces hospitalizations, emergency room visits, and specialty care visits by as much as 30% or more.

Finally, for businesses like Iora Health, the capital investment is considerable, especially the need to build homegrown information technology tools like Iora's "collaborative care platform" to coordinate and communicate seamlessly about all dimensions of a patient's care—laboratory testing, follow-up visits, and check-ins—on a single system. (ChenMed also uses their own homemade system.)

On top of all these costs, Chris Chen adds that it isn't easy to recruit and retain the right kinds of doctors, like Sofia Recabarren, who are skilled in practicing medicine the way Dr. Belknap used to in the 1970s. Fernando-pulle agrees.

Despite these challenges, Medicare Advantage is popular and growing. By 2025, about 38 million seniors—half of all eligible—are projected to sign up for the program. Not all of them can get care in practices with shuttles and yoga classes, but if groups like ChenMed and Iora Health have their way, they will soon.

Family Docs

Most doctors aren't accustomed to thinking about prevention. They're taught in medical school to diagnose what's broken and fix it. There are, however, a few notable exceptions who practice holistically. Consider, for example, those who care for our children and seniors.

Christine Stern is a pediatrician at NYU Langone Medical Center in New York City. She's warm, energetic, and endlessly curious, and she always enters her exam room with a smile. Only the stethoscope around her neck marks her as the doctor. She sits at a desk computer but faces her patients as she talks. *How's school? Made any new friends? What time do you go to bed? What time do you wake up? Do you eat school lunch, home lunch, or out lunch? Do you like vegetables? Do you play sports?* Despite her casual tone, she is intensely focused on the overall health of her kids, which means looking at all aspects of their well-being: physical, mental, emotional, and social.

Primary care physicians—pediatricians, family medicine doctors, and geriatricians, for example—tend to think less is more. Prescribing fewer medications for the elderly can lower the risks of side effects. Avoiding unnecessary antibiotics for coughs and colds reduces antibiotic resistance in kids. Canceling annual electrocardiograms for patients who have no symptoms and are at low risk of heart disease simply makes sense. These clinicians also know it's important to be aware of troublesome social dynamics, whether it's isolation for the recently widowed or bullying in middle school. Their aim is to prevent the preventable, whether it's the flu (Get vaccinated!), falls (Stay hydrated! Avoid trampolines!) or hospitalizations (Take your meds!).

Prevention isn't always attractive for patients, especially when they're feeling fine. No one looks forward to getting jabbed with a needle for a vaccination or probed with a colonoscope. Mammograms are uncomfortable and stressful. Skipping desserts is a downer. Quitting smoking is hard. Even brushing and flossing your teeth can be a drag.

The solution may be to make prevention more fun, or at least more engaging.

A Spoonful of Tech Helps the Medicine Go Down

The first video game designer I ever met was Roger Altizer, a ginger-haired and ginger-bearded fellow who, despite living in Salt Lake City at the base of the Wasatch Mountains, wears Hawaiian shirts year-round. When asked about his favorite innovation of all time, he doesn't pause before replying, "The long-sleeved Hawaiian shirt."

Altizer is a games journalist turned video-game professor at the University of Utah. About two-thirds of all Americans play video games, and they spend over $43 billion a year on this pastime. Altizer and his students invent and design games for them.

When I was CEO at University of Utah Health, I invited him to spend some time with my hospital colleagues. His takeaway: doctors don't understand regular folks all that well. For example, they are always showing people numbers on pieces of paper. He furrows his eyebrows, and asks, "But what do these numbers even mean?" If, say, we are worried about a patient with prediabetes whose blood sugar (glucose) level is 350 mg/dL, we can tell the number is abnormal because it is above the normal limit of 140 mg/dL. But then Altizer wonders: *Is that a little bad, sorta bad or really, really bad? Like do some people have numbers around 2,000?*

A few weeks later, Altizer shows me what he was thinking. He hands me a pair of virtual-reality goggles, and with them I see a plot of hypothetical blood sugar levels over time. I have to look up to see mini-peaks that correspond to numbers that are a bit high, 160 mg/dL or 200 mg/dL. But for a number like 350 mg/dL, I have to tilt my head *way* back just to see the top of that peak. "Now you know—your body knows—that number is way too high," Altizer says. A number on a piece of paper now feels real.

With a little help from people like Altizer, we can be a lot more imaginative about improving health, not just understanding these numbers but also doing something about them.

The Virtues of Virtual Health

Stephen King (not *that* Stephen King—he's quick to point out that he is, unfortunately, not the writer of any best-selling horror novels) hails from Marietta, Georgia. A few years back, he was diagnosed with prediabetes. Then one day, he felt nauseated and dizzy. He went to the emergency room, where his blood sugar (glucose) tested high—440 mg/dL—Mount Everest level high in Roger Altizer's virtual world. King was diagnosed with type 2 diabetes, meaning his body can't transfer glucose from his bloodstream into his cells because they've become resistant to insulin. Unmanaged, high levels of glucose in the blood slowly damage the kidneys, the eyes, and blood vessels of the heart and legs.

If diabetic patients like King can keep their blood sugar levels in the normal range—through diet, oral medications, or, when necessary, insulin injections—they can stay healthy and live as long as people who don't have diabetes. But keeping blood sugar levels in the right range isn't easy. To avoid excessive swings in either direction, people with diabetes must check their glucose levels multiple times a day. To do that, they prick their finger and place a drop of blood on a test strip that is analyzed in a glucometer machine.

Despite trying hard for a year, King couldn't keep his glucose levels in the safe range. Then his health insurance company offered him the chance to try a new program called Onduo, a "virtual diabetes clinic." (Onduo is a joint venture between Sanofi and Verily. I am an employee and shareholder of Verily.) King got a kit in the mail that had a new kind of technology, a continuous glucose monitor (made by Dexcom and Verily). It's a quarter-sized device that automatically inserts, almost imperceptibly, a tiny wire under his skin. It stays pasted to his arm (or abdomen) for about ten days. (It is fine in the shower and even in a pool.) And it contains a tiny Bluetooth chip that transmits blood sugar values to a smartphone app, 24 hours a day.

For the first time, King can see directly what happens to his blood glucose levels when he eats a burger or drinks a soda. He can see the difference between a diet soda and a regular soda. Instead of the dreary food journal (a typical part of a diabetic patient's regimen), King takes photos of what he's eating. Computer vision technology recognizes over a million meals and snacks and counting. Some diabetics get a big kick out of having their phone recognize new foods, like the Ma Po Tofu from the neighborhood Chinese restaurant. It's preventive medicine, but it's also fun.

Patients can then visually associate what they eat and how their bodies respond to those foods. They can also collect other information, like exercise data from their fitness tracker. Through texting or video chats, they connect with a health coach who offers tips, like pointing out that the high-fructose corn syrup in King's beloved soda was wreaking havoc on his blood sugars. That one change—eliminating sugary sodas—was key to keeping his blood sugars in range. Just as pleasing, in his first six months in the program, he lost over 20 pounds.

Several doctors I've spoken with believe that all adults should hook up to one of these continuous glucose monitor devices for at least a couple of weeks, even if they are not diabetic. A tech company CEO did just that and told me the experience changed his life. Seeing how a handful of M&Ms from the office candy jar caused his blood glucose levels to spike, and also realizing how closely glucose numbers correlated with his overall sense of well-being, changed his outlook, and his habits.

Mentally Fit

Just as important as physical fitness is mental well-being. In 2017, nearly one in five Americans had some form of mental illness, and one in twenty-five experienced serious mental illness that substantially interfered with life activities. Keeping people mentally well is key to keeping them in good physical health, too, because mental health and physical health are inextricably linked. One study showed that people with mental health or substance abuse problems ended up using 2.5 to 3.5 times as much health care as those who were otherwise the same but who didn't have mental health problems. Most of the extra spending was for medical services.

Smartphone-based digital health solutions, like Onduo for diabetes, can give people access to mental health support any time, any place, and potentially at considerably lower costs. The most popular apps are designed to help manage stress, anxiety, and depression. Some even give you access to a live (streaming) therapist—a doc-in-a-pocket of sorts.

This portable version of videoconferencing between a patient and clinician, referred to as telehealth or telemedicine, can get health care, mental or physical, to people living in remote areas and regions with shortages of specialists.

Tell It to the Telehealth

At the University of Utah, we had plenty of reasons to use telehealth. As a major referral center for Utah, Idaho, Wyoming, Montana, and parts of Nevada and western Colorado, the university cares for patients from a region spanning 10%–15% of the geographic landmass of the United States. When patients go home 600 or 700 miles away from their doctor, they can check in via video. At a session I observed, a young woman from Wyoming recovering from a burn on her right wrist and arm waved hello to us in Salt Lake City via videoconference. She repeatedly bent her wrist forward and backward while the physical therapist measured the angles of her wrist on the screen as she encouraged the patient through her exercises.

Beyond patient-clinician interactions, physician-to-physician video-conferencing can help specialists coach primary care doctors practicing in remote areas as they care for patients with complicated conditions. In this tech-enabled "teach-a-man-to-fish" approach, the computer screen becomes a grid, one box for each doctor calling in from around the region. It's reminiscent of a school show-and-tell; each participant shares the medical circumstances of their patient and asks the convening expert for advice. Terry Box, a hepatologist who himself is a liver transplant recipient, directs the University of Utah's Project ECHO program. I observed a session on hepatitis that had a dozen physicians calling in from across the region. With each case, the bow-tied Box elaborated in his Texan drawl on the underlying principles of his recommendations—how to test for acute versus chronic hepatitis B infection, for example. Sixty minutes later, with all their questions answered, the doctors online had received the equivalent of a short course in acute and chronic hepatitis.

Project ECHO has expanded in Utah to cover a number of other kinds of care, including child and adolescent psychiatry. Primary care doctors and pediatricians call in for advice about teens with eating disorders, depression, anxiety, and other mental health disorders. Board-certified child psychiatrists teach them how to manage some of the most common conditions.

After a while, the doctors learn enough that they can stop calling in as regularly. That's a big win for the doctors and their patients.

Telehealth may prove just as useful in urban and suburban settings, saving patients the need to travel or miss work for care. But it has been slow to achieve national adoption because Medicare and most private insurers have been reluctant to pay for it as they do in-person visits. In the Kaiser Permanente health system based in California, which includes a major insurance plan, hospitals, and a large group of physicians, telehealth has been routine for all physicians since 2014. Doctors can respond to questions quickly, and patients don't have to leave their homes or offices to be seen. Children with rashes or suspiciously red eyes can quickly get a once-over from a pediatrician. The Kaiser health insurance plan encourages doctors to practice telehealth because it is more cost-effective. The same is true for the Veterans Health Administration system. These are the exceptions. If commercial insurers and Medicare were paying for results instead of action, they'd recognize the value of telehealth.

From Farm to Farmacy

Health systems like ChenMed that are paid to keep patients healthy recognize that what happens to patients in their clinics is often less important to their health than their circumstances at home: whether they are financially secure, have access to fresh food, live and work in a safe environment, and have adequate access to transportation and housing. It makes sense for them to care about these matters, to visit patients at home to see whether carpets are fraying (a tripping hazard), whether the shower needs a support rod (to prevent a fall), and even peek inside the refrigerator to make sure their patients have enough to eat. That is preventive care at its smartest and most caring.

For example, one Kaiser Permanente patient with diabetes was struggling to keep her blood glucose levels under control, and her doctors were worried. When Nirav Shah, a physician who was then the chief operating officer for Kaiser Permanente in Southern California, asked her what the problem was, he discovered that she didn't have a refrigerator for her insulin. Shah said the decision was easy for Kaiser: "Buy her a fridge!"

At Geisinger Health, a health system and insurance company based in Danville, Pennsylvania, a patient can get help stocking that fridge through their Fresh Food Farmacy, a program established by then CEO David Feinberg and his physician wife, Andrea Feinberg. It's hard to worry about eating enough fresh fruits and vegetables when you're uncertain about your next meal (in 2018, 14.3 million American households reported "food insecurity"). Touting the slogan "Food as Medicine," their program signs up diabetic patients who are food insecure and who have difficulty managing their blood sugars. The Farmacy "prescription" entitles them to enough food to prepare two meals a day, five days a week, and includes recipes and hours of online and in-person diabetes education.

Cincinnati Children's Hospital runs a similar program in partnership with Freestore Foodbank to provide shelf-stable food—plus bimonthly offerings of fresh fruits and vegetables—from the pantry in the medical clinic. Cincinnati has one of the highest rates of child poverty in the nation (almost half of all children live at or below the federal poverty level). Besides running the pantry, hospital staff also provide connections to social work, legal assistance, SNAP (Supplemental Nutrition Assistance Program) food stamps, mental health support, and transportation services.

Anita Brentley is the Cincinnati Children's Hospital's community engagement consultant. She talks animatedly about the power of family engagement and activation. At hospital meetings, "I'm a rabble-rouser," she says, "I sound like a broken record. . . . What about the families? Have we asked the families?" She tells me that third-grade reading level is one of the best predictors of long-term health, which is why her community is focused on school readiness for kindergarten.

Brentley introduces me to Mrs. J, the octogenarian who owns her own hair salon and leads the "Granny Group." Her Grannies call families to remind them of their promise to read to their children twice a week. They help collect and distribute over 1,000 books. When the adults don't know how to read, the Granny Group sets up reading lessons for them, too.

Brentley is proud of what the community is accomplishing and hopes others will do the same. "We are not looking carefully enough at the power of our partnerships with our families," Brentley says. Whether it's school readiness, running the food bank, managing domestic violence support groups, or supporting home health visits, she says that families and communities are an untapped resource for improving health.

The medical staff of a children's hospital providing support for non-medical services probably sounds brilliant to Yale researchers Elizabeth Bradley and Lauren Taylor. In their book *The American Health Care Paradox: Why Spending More Is Getting Us Less*, they convincingly demonstrate that Americans spend more to get less health because we spend far too little on social services like housing, nutrition, education, environment, and unemployment support. Those aren't traditional investments for health insurance companies or hospitals, but many are starting to think about it, especially in partnership with community programs. As they do, they begin to learn that, like Mrs. J's Granny Group, communities do more than provide social services—they foster trust.

From Pastors to Beauticians

Gbenga Ogedegbe is equally comfortable in the hospital wards of New York University and the churches and barbershops of Harlem and around New York City. He's traveled the world to get to those two places; from his native Nigeria, he attended Donetsk University in the Ukraine to study medicine, and now he directs NYU's Center for Healthful Behavior Change. Ogedegbe has been a pioneer in engaging community groups to rally around health. For example, his Center's federally funded studies show that pastors, trusted leaders in the community, are effective in persuading African American men in New York City to undergo colon and prostate cancer screening tests and to manage their blood pressure better. Barbershops, senior centers, and beauty salons are also terrific places to educate people about screening tests (talk about a captive audience).

Increasingly, he and others have been exploring how technology can enhance community connectivity, even for those who are housebound.

Housebound but Digitally Connected

An indefatigable woman with a perfectly coiffed puff of silky white hair, Karen Feinstein leads Pittsburgh's Jewish Healthcare Foundation. Among their initiatives for the elderly, the Virtual Senior Academy encourages participants to sign up for a wide range of discussion groups, a culinary tour of Italy, a virtual tour of the latest exhibit at the city's Andy Warhol Museum, a demonstration of how to create a blown-glass vase, and a monthly book club, among other such activities. Peppered throughout those offerings are classes on managing blood pressure and lung disease and other health-related topics. During the sessions, attendees appear on the screen in a modern-day "Hollywood Squares" grid—one square shows a woman at home, another captures a room of eager discussants around a table at a library, a third reveals a man and his dog on a couch. The program is free and easy to use. Anyone in Pittsburgh over 50 can sign up. Chair Yoga is a perennial hit.

Feinstein and Brentley will tell you that people who are connected with their communities are better off at home when they are healthy, and even when they aren't.

Just Say No to Hospitals

Stanley, a 97-year-old former captain in the US Air Force during WWII, had failing kidneys but did not want dialysis. (He did not want the hassle of getting to a clinic three times a week, each time spending four hours tethered to a blood-pumping and filtration machine.) Stanley hadn't been feeling well for a couple of days and came into the Mount Sinai Hospital emergency department in New York City with a fever. According to his chest X-ray, he had pneumonia in both lungs—probably because he had aspirated some food—and very low blood pressure, which meant he was probably dehydrated. In almost any hospital, doctors would have admitted him for intravenous antibiotics and hydration. But Stanley refused to be hospitalized. Each time he had been admitted recently with a bout of heart failure or something else, he had experienced delirium at night and had left a little worse off.

His doctor, Al Siu, was sympathetic. Siu, a geriatrician and former head of the department at Mount Sinai, had secured funding for a Medicare pilot project for patients like Stanley. He made him this offer: Stanley could go home and be cared for by doctors and nurses there. In the Hospital at Home program, Mount Sinai would deliver equipment to his apartment—an intravenous infusion pump for the antibiotics, a pulse oximeter to measure the amount of oxygen reaching his blood, maybe an oxygen tank in case he needed extra oxygen while his lungs were healing. A nurse and sometimes a doctor would visit him every day, in person and also by videoconferencing.

Stanley agreed, and after a few days at home, he started to get better.

Since the mid-1990s, Bruce Leff, a physician at Johns Hopkins Medical Center, has been advocating for the Hospital at Home model. Clinicians send patients home with a range of conditions they ordinarily would be hospitalized for: dehydration, urinary tract infections, and skin infections, for example. Even serious conditions like heart failure, lung disease, or pneumonia can be managed at home. Physicians visit daily; nurses might come for as long as two hours once or twice a day. Home health aides help bathe patients or prepare light meals. The team can help patients manage their medications and maintain a healthy diet. If a patient's condition deteriorates, nurses get to them within 30 minutes.

Hospitals in the UK, Australia, New Zealand, and Japan have been doing this for years. They've shown that caring for patients at home is a sensible strategy. Patients are safer and fare better. In US hospitals, 5% of patients acquire a serious infection. That figure is almost negligible in the home. Most patients sleep much better in their own beds than in the hospital. One in five hospitalized elderly patients suffers from severe confusion or delirium, as Stanley had experienced. Getting out of bed unassisted in the unfamiliar environment leads to falls, broken bones, and often a subsequent loss of independence they never regain. On the other hand, if patients stay in bed too much, they may suffer from blood clots in the legs, bedsores, and often a loss of mobility. Being away from home also spawns other worries, like who is looking after pets or the garden.

Leff has advised hospitals like Mount Sinai and Presbyterian Healthcare Services in Albuquerque, where programs like Siu's are working and cost-effective. Nancy Guinn, the family medicine physician who leads Presbyterian Healthcare's Hospital at Home program, says the majority of patients opt for care at home when offered. Presbyterian's health plan pays the program a fixed rate that is 75% of what the hospital would have recieved had the patient been admitted to the hospital. The actual costs are only 70%–80%. Despite the success of its pilot project at Mount Sinai, Medicare has been slow to pay for Hospital at Home care. Doing it well requires investing in technology, training nurses, therapists, and doctors in new kinds of skills, and fostering a shared sense of responsibility for its success. Under those conditions, it can be a win-win-win for the health plan, the hospital, and most importantly, the patients.

The Action Plan for Proactive Health

A pay-for-results system prioritizes preventive medicine and recognizes that family and community programs can help keep all of us healthier outside the walls of clinics and hospitals. New technologies give people tools to manage their health more effectively, connect them with social support, and provide people in rural and underserved communities access to expert care. Most importantly, addressing poverty, food deserts, inadequate housing and transportation are vital to any health readiness strategy. The stories from the front lines, like Food Farmacy or Hospital at Home, are promising, but progress is slow.

In shifting from a reactive to proactive health care system, we all have a role to play.

As a patient, you should:

- Do what you can to keep yourself and your family healthy, such as making sure you eat, exercise, and sleep as well as possible, and, if applicable, stop smoking.
- See your primary care physician regularly for appropriate preventive care, like vaccinations and cancer and cardiovascular screenings, and both physical and mental health care.
- Take advantage of telehealth, texting, email, and video chat options with physicians and other health care providers. Try mobile health or virtual clinics when offered.
- If you are Medicare eligible, seek out innovative Medicare Advantage clinics or similar accountable care organizations (ACOs) where physicians practice pay-for-results care.

As a physician or other health care professional, you should:

- Work in hospitals and clinics that reward you for better patient outcomes, and emphasize prevention and patient well-being, such as ACOs.

As a payer, such as a self-insured employer, government entity, or health plan, you should:

- Support reimbursement for new models of care such as Hospital at Home, mobile health/virtual clinics, and telehealth, provided that carefully defined quality and safety standards are met.
- If you are in a rural or underserved area, consider taking advantage of and funding physician-to-physician consultation programs like Project ECHO.

If you are a policy maker, you should:

- Invest in social services, like food pantries, housing, transportation, education, and legal aid. Each of these can improve health and are more cost-effective prevention strategies than expensive medical care for the sick.
- Facilitate partnerships between health systems and community organizations to care for patients who require social services.
- Support the training of more primary care physicians and other primary care health care professionals and mental health professionals.
- Develop or expand loan-forgiveness programs that reward physicians and nurses for practicing primary care and serving in rural and underserved regions.

And most important, all of us need to elect leaders who will invest in prevention and social services to achieve better health at lower costs.

CHAPTER 3

AT YOUR HEALTH'S EXPENSE

*There is no turning back to an unsustainable sys-
tem that pays for procedures rather than value. In
fact, the only option is to charge forward—for HHS
[Department of Health and Human Services] to
take bolder action, and for providers and payers to
join with us. . . . We are unafraid of disrupting existing arrangements simply because they're backed by
powerful special interests.*

—Secretary Alex M. Azar II

Libby Rosenthal knows how to start a movement. In 2013, the physician-
turned-journalist started publishing a series of exposés about medical bills,
beginning with colonoscopy, pregnancy and delivery, and total hip replacement. She described everyday Americans struggling with outrageous, inex-
plicable bills, and the stress of negotiating with hospitals and with insurance
companies. *New York Times* readers deluged her with their own accounts of
billing misadventures, so many, in fact, that Rosenthal set up a Facebook

account ("Paying Till It Hurts") and invited readers to post their stories and their bills. It became a self-help network for thousands of fuming, frustrated people seeking solutions to their unintelligible bills.

Dissecting bills line-by-line became a popular exercise in outrage. In his 2013 *Time* magazine cover story, "Bitter Pill: Why Medical Bills Are Killing Us," journalist Steve Brill flagged inflated charges like the $1.50 acetaminophen tablet, the $77 box of sterile gauze pads, and the Accu-Chek diabetes test strips for $18 per strip that he found online for $0.58 a strip. The markups were particularly egregious for some of the most expensive items, like $13,702 for a 660 mg injection of the cancer drug rituximab (brand name Rituxan, manufactured by Genentech, Biogen) for which Brill estimated the hospital—in this case, M.D. Anderson Cancer Center in Houston— would have paid what was still an eye-popping $3,500.

In addition to the staggering costs, people were upset about so many other mysteries surrounding their bills: Why was coverage denied? Why was the hospital allowed to bill the patient when insurance would not cover the service? How could the surgeon be "in network" but the anesthesiologist be "out of network?" People who trusted the medical system to look after them felt betrayed, lied to, and cheated.

The Battle of the Bills

It's easy to despise hospitals and health insurers for treating people so poorly. Understanding the strategies and casualties in the battle of the bills requires a little background, and the recognition that the root cause of this nasty, debilitating conflict is the familiar problem of our fee-for-service, pay-for-action business.

Each year, insurance companies collect premium dollars from individuals and employers ($1.2 trillion in 2017). During the course of the year, hospitals, doctors, nursing homes, and others try to wrest those dollars from the insurers by sending them bills. (They also sent another $1.3 trillion in bills to Medicare and Medicaid in 2017.) How much they collect from the insurers depends on the deals that have been struck: what services the insurance plans promised employees they would cover and how much they agreed to pay doctors and hospitals "in network" (a preferred group) and "out of network" (everyone else).

What's covered by the insurer depends on the health plan employees have chosen. Plans can have many variables: premiums, out-of-pocket expenses (deductibles, co-payments, and coinsurance), covered benefits (eyeglasses? psychotherapist?), and the network of preferred hospitals and doctors. People who don't expect to use much care tend to opt for plans with lower premiums and higher deductibles and co-payments. People willing to stick to a small network of doctors and hospitals (like a health maintenance organization) save more because medical professionals and hospitals give significant discounts off their list prices to gain "in-network" status with insurance companies. The discounts pay off because insurers steer their members to them.

The annual negotiations to determine which hospitals are in network and how much insurers will pay for each service are complicated. Every price for every service is negotiable, and the agreed-upon prices are secret. They can differ markedly for the exact same service. For example, a chief of obstetrics and gynecology recently complained that for a vaginal delivery of a newborn baby, one insurance company paid three hospitals in his city $3,000, $17,000 and $26,000. Why the difference? It all comes down to what kind of a deal each hospital negotiated with that insurer at the beginning of the year.

Carving Out Mental Health

Because of an artifact of insurance coverage and contracting, mental health is cared for almost completely separately from physical health.

In the 1980s, when rising costs led to complaints that people were over-using mental health care, health insurers began to "carve out" the care, splitting it from the rest of medical coverage. They created separate insurance policies and separate networks of mental health clinicians. Through clever pricing and network schemes like those that discouraged patients with substance abuse or those who are more likely to use services from signing up, behavioral health insurers successfully drove the costs of care down, but these lower costs mostly came from reducing care.

In 2008, Congress passed the Mental Health and Addiction Equity Act, which promised to make behavioral health treatment as accessible as other medical care. It hasn't worked that well. One 2017 study showed that mental health care was still almost six times as likely to be considered out-of-network as medical care. Being out of network means significantly higher out-of-pocket costs for patients. As a result, only about two of five adults with a mental health condition received some care for it in a given year, and only about two-thirds of those with serious mental illness got treated.

Whether it's mental health or physical health, the battle between insurers and clinicians for your health care dollar is preventing people from getting proper care.

Mark It Up to Mark It Down

Each year, every hospital in the United States prepares a list of charges for every supply item and every procedure. This is called a charge description master, or "chargemaster." Think of it as the starting point of a Dutch auction, in which the auctioneer starts at a very high price and then lowers it until a bidder accepts. For as long as most hospital CEOs can remember, there's been no downside to pumping up their chargemaster prices, because they can discount them whenever and however they wish, and until recently, the figures have been confidential. In a 2013 interview, Dr. Brent James, then a leader at Utah's Intermountain Healthcare, explained:

> In a chargemaster, what you're seeing is the old phenomenon called "mark it up to mark it down." Hospitals will make an initial estimate of what something costs, and then they'll mark it up—sometimes four-hundred to five-hundred percent. Insurance brokers measure [their] success in the size of the discount they get. That's how you end up with $17 pieces of gauze. It loses all connection to reality.

A 2016 article, "US Hospitals Are Still Using Chargemaster Markups to Maximize Revenues," reported that in 2013, private insurers ended up paying, on average, two-and-a-half times the rate that Medicare paid for inpatient care. For outpatient care, insurers paid three times the Medicare rates. (Note that Medicare prices are closest to the actual costs of care). Markups varied from state to state and also by services. The biggest markups applied to anesthesiology, CT scans, and MRIs: 13–28 times the Medicare prices.

This game of huge markups and big discounts hurts patients. The uninsured and those who are out of network are billed at chargemaster rates. Even with a discount of, say, 30%–50%, the charges are still at least double—if not more—what Medicare pays.

Decoding Medicare

Untangling the fee-for-service system relies on understanding how Medicare, the nation's largest single payer, pays for health care. Consider, for example, how Medicare pays for an inpatient hospital stay based on its "prospective payment system."

What's Wrong: For each hospitalization, every patient is defined by diagnosis and treatment codes, referred to as ICD-10 codes. These codes are crucial; each extra code offers another opportunity to increase the bill to Medicare. It's not a simple job—there are over 70,000 ICD-10 codes for diagnosis.

What Was Done: For inpatient stays, Medicare mostly tries to pay a single, flat rate per type of discharge, using one of a few hundred diagnosis-related groups (DRGs) that best summarizes the main reason for the hospitalization. One of the most commonly used is DRG-470, major joint replacement or reattachment of lower extremity, typically a hip or knee replacement. Not all patients who undergo a hip replacement are alike. When patients have additional medical conditions, called "comorbidities and complications" (CC) or more serious comorbidities (major CC or MCC), they may receive an upgraded code. For example, patients who are also diagnosed with depression or Crohn's disease may qualify for a CC, while those with severe infection or stroke have a major CC. For Medicare, in 2019, there were over 760 of these DRG categories (referred to as Medicare Severity Diagnosis Related Groups or MS-DRGs), including those with and without CCs or MCCs.

Grouping: Sometimes it's clear from the outset what the right DRG will be for an admission. Other times, when patients come into the hospital without a clear diagnosis (is the fever from a urinary tract infection or a blood infection?), it may take a while to figure out the diagnosis, and even then their condition may change over the hospitalization. They accumulate ICD-10 codes during the stay, which are later mapped to (MS)-DRGs using software programs called "groupers." There's a fair amount of discretion and messiness in this process. Figuring out which codes yield the largest payments is a high-stakes game for the people tallying up your bill.

Math Spaghetti

Medicare pays hospitals and doctors after patients are discharged, based on the submitted codes. The reimbursement calculation for a hospital stay starts with a base rate for each admission. In 2019, the Medicare base rate was around $5,600. That number is then multiplied by several factors, including the disease-related group multiplier, a number that reflects how difficult it was for the hospital to take care of that patient. The multiplier can be as high as 26.4106 for a heart transplant in a patient with a major comorbidity or complication (major CC). A hip/knee replacement is, under the system, twice as complicated as an appendectomy: its multiplier is 1.9898, whereas an uncomplicated appendectomy has a multiplier of 1.0853.

Comorbidities or complications substantially boost reimbursements. The difference between a patient who undergoes a below-the-knee amputation without complications versus the same patient who has a comorbidity or complication could mean as much as a $7000–$10,000 difference in the bill. Multiply that amount by tens of thousands of patients per year and you know why armies of individuals have been trained to trawl through electronic medical records looking for any signs of additional conditions that can be added to a patient's list of diagnoses. Twenty-two years after the comorbidity or complication modifier was introduced, it became the new normal; 80% of patients were coded as having one. (Medicare pushed back and in 2007 revised its definitions to reduce the percentage back to 40%). If you wonder why your clinicians sometimes pay more attention to their computer screens than to you, it could be because their paychecks depend on how many diagnoses they type in.

Surprise after Surprise

In addition to the set of bills that hospitals and clinics send (for the "technical" or facilities costs), doctors send a completely different set of bills (for "professional" services). Because doctors contract with insurers and government payers separately, each group of physicians—surgeons, anesthesiologists, pathologists—may have their own billing office. Laboratory tests may be billed separately, too. That's one surprise bill after another.

Zero-Sum Gaming

Doctors and hospitals want to get paid as much as possible; insurers want to pay them as little as possible. Before the Affordable Care Act took effect in 2014, health insurance companies had more powerful weapons to keep expenses down. They could refuse to insure people who were likely to cost more, a practice referred to as "denying coverage to those with preexisting conditions." For sicker patients who might have comorbidities and complications, insurers could raise premiums (called "medical underwriting"). The Affordable Care Act took bold steps to limit these on the individual exchange and for small employer groups.

That left insurers with only a few remaining options. They can exclude from their networks hospitals and doctors prone to overcharging and create "narrow" networks instead. These limit the choices patients have for where they can get their care. Secondly, the insurers can still say "no." If a physician orders an MRI or recommends a procedure, the insurance company can dispute its necessity and refuse to pay. Lastly, short of saying no, they can require "prior authorization" for expensive studies or drugs. It's a hassle factor—mounds of paperwork for doctors to justify what they're prescribing or ordering.

Meanwhile, in a pay-for-action world, doctors remain incentivized to overprescribe and overtreat. One prestigious hospital, for example, will order a PET-CT scan on a patient with lymphoma, even if it was just performed across town a week ago. Medicare has tried to lower its payments in these settings. Still, nurses have been known to show up in patients' homes with the sole purpose of drawing blood to demonstrate a low blood count. Hopefully they aren't making it worse.

The Wrong Temptation

Tired of being at the mercy of overzealous clinicians and hospitals, some insurers have gotten into the health care business. For example, the nation's largest private insurer, United Healthcare, employed over 30,000 physicians by the end of 2018. Highmark Blue Shield of western Pennsylvania paid $500 million for West Penn Allegheny Health System in 2011 and then added three more to those eight hospitals. In 2011, WellPoint, now Anthem Blue Cross of California, acquired CareMore Health Group, a senior-focused medical practice that had 26 clinics, serving about 54,000 predominantly Medicare Advantage members.

Conversely, many large hospital systems have hired their own physician groups and set up their own health insurance businesses. Kaiser Permanente, University of Pittsburgh Medical Center, Intermountain Healthcare, and Geisinger Health are among some of the largest combined insurance and health systems in the nation. University of Utah Health did the same when it created a commercial employee health plan. Ceci Connelly, president/CEO of the Alliance of Community Health Plans, says that when "payers and providers are more aligned, sharing in the winning and losing, they start being motivated to do different things for different reasons." Health systems that have insurance arms can fund new and better care models, like telemedicine, mental health, and home health care.

Whether this consolidation strategy is the best way to improve quality or reduce costs is doubtful. Competition strategy guru Michael Porter, of the Harvard Business School, laments the market trend. After all, consolidation reduces competition, and rarely does that make costs go down.

Who's Winning?

In the battle of bills, neither side is really winning. Operating margins for nonprofit hospitals averaged only about 1.6%–2.5% in 2017. (These slim margins reflect the balance between losses from Medicare and from caring for the uninsured and underinsured against the profits from privately insured patients.) Similarly, the National Association of Insurance Commissioners reported that in 2017, the health insurance industry experienced an average profit margin of 2.4% and blamed rising administrative expenses for lowering profit. No one is winning.

Getting Paper-Worked

The battle of the bills makes the United States a world leader in health care bureaucracy. One study estimated that about 25 cents of every dollar collected by a hospital is spent on administration, which means American hospitals spend more on paperwork than they do on nurses. Using data from the Organization for Economic Co-operation and Development (OECD), researchers found that administration consumed 8% of all health care costs in the United States, compared to 1%–3% in OECD nations.

One team of researchers figured that it cost Duke Medical Center $14.50 to collect $100 of payment for the work of a primary care physician, or over $99,000 in expenses per physician per year just to bill. That number doesn't even include the gargantuan expense of the electronic health record system (more on this in Chapter 9). The bureaucratic complexity creates an ocean of work and a tsunami of mistakes and wastes everyone's time.

Having fewer payers—or even a single payer—and simpler contractual arrangements could lower administrative costs dramatically. Because Medicare's internal costs for administration are a fraction of those commercial payers, Medicare-for-all could reduce administrative costs from around 14% to 6% or less. Another way to simplify administrative billing and coding would rely on a common set of standards across the industry. Either strategy would help patients act more effectively like consumers in the market—whether for their health insurance plan or for their health care.

That's key because the American model of health care is counting on consumers to play their role in the market.

From Inscrutable to Simple

In 2018, a couple of months after he became secretary, US Secretary of Health and Human Services Alex Azar gave a speech to the Federation of American Hospitals in which he described trying to understand the costs of his own care. It all started when a physician recommended that he undergo a routine echocardiogram stress test. Azar agreed, thinking this would be done in the doctor's office. Instead, "I have a plastic wristband slapped on me," he said. For what should have been a simple test in the room next door, he found himself being admitted to the hospital.

Azar's insurance was a high-deductible plan. Since he knew he would be paying for this test, he asked how much the test was going to cost. He was told that information wasn't available. "Fortunately, I didn't just fall off the turnip truck," he said, and eventually the manager of the clinic appeared and told him the list price was $5,500.

That was the "turnip" rate. When Azar asked what his plan's negotiated rate was, he was told $3,500. Then, he looked up online what the test would have cost had it been performed in a doctor's office: $550.

"Now, there I was, the former deputy secretary of Health and Human Services.... What if I'd been a grandmother? Or a twenty-something with a high-deductible plan?

"This is simply wrong," he told the hospital executives in the audience.

The Price-Is-Right Calculator

In 2014, the University of Utah tried to address the problem Secretary Azar would pose years later: How can patients determine their out-of-pocket costs *before* they get the care? We decided to build an online price estimator. Done right, we knew this could be a natural complement to the patient satisfaction ratings and comments we already posted online (more on this in Chapter 7). Patients could use costs to comparison shop.

Despite a lot of well-intentioned effort over the next few years, the website was only partially successful. Here's why:

To Each His Own Bundle of Benefits

First, every insurance company offers many different—sometimes hundreds of different—plans, with different covered benefits, deductibles, co-payments, coinsurance, annual cost-sharing limits, and lifetime limits. It was impossible for us to know what kind of health plan patients had and what its rules were. The best we could do was to ask people to enter what they knew about their deductibles, co-pays, and coinsurance.

Then there was the question of what benefits were covered. Before the Affordable Care Act, there were few rules governing these plans. After the bill was passed, insurers were required to cover ten essential benefits on their individual and small group plans: ambulatory (outpatient) services, emergency services, maternity and newborn, hospitalizations, mental health and substance use disorders, prescription drugs, rehabilitative and habilitative services and devices, laboratory services, preventive and wellness services, chronic disease management, and pediatric services (including oral and vision care).

Even with the new laws, the definition of "cover" leaves a lot to discretion. Insurers vary the co-pays or coinsurance for each benefit and change what and how many services are covered. For example, coinsurance for a very expensive hospitalization or drug can total thousands of dollars. The government sets limits on the total out-of-pocket amounts ($8,150 for an individual and $16,300 for a family in 2020), but given that in June 2018, the median American household had $11,700 in savings, the caps don't provide much security for most families.

Besides thwarting price transparency efforts, this variability in health plans also makes it very hard for people to choose the right plan. Some states are trying to standardize plans on the individual exchanges that they sponsor. These include Massachusetts, California, New York, Connecticut, Oregon, and Vermont as well as the District of Columbia. Many are also gradually limiting the number of choices of health plans, typically to fewer than ten. That's more than enough for most; one study showed that over 60% of consumers selected their health plan online without leaving the initial screen. Picking the right plan also means being able to understand the complex offerings and to anticipate the health care needs for the coming year. Most people, even seasoned health care experts, have difficulty with both.

To Each Her Own Chargemasters

For the price transparency website, the next challenge was how to provide the menu of services that patients might want to check. Unfortunately, like benefits plans, hospital services (and chargemasters) also are not standardized. The Affordable Care Act required that hospitals make the chargemasters public in "machine-readable format" starting in 2019. Unfortunately, machines may be able to read them, but most normal humans can't. That's because there are no rules governing chargemasters. One hospital might list 8,000 items, while another lists 15,000 or 30,000. The terminology varies by hospital and is undecipherable to the layperson. For example, most people would need help understanding "PERC D-E COR REVASC CHRO SING" (translation: unblocking a single coronary artery in a patient with chronic disease, not an acute heart attack) or "SYSTEM MGMT LINX RELUX BEAD LXC1X" (you'd have to intuit that "RELUX" is "REFLUX," and that this is for preventing acid reflux or heartburn).

The University of Utah initially posted the out-of-pocket costs for about 60 of its most commonly performed procedures, like vaginal delivery of a newborn, a head CT (or "CAT") scan, and a mammogram. The website estimated costs for patients who had commercial insurance or Medicare based on the deductibles and co-payment data that they entered. For those who were out of network, uninsured, or seeking care not offered by their health plan (some dermatology procedures or cosmetic plastic surgery, for example), the estimator used chargemaster prices, less a discount of 30%.

To Each His Own Definitions of Disease (Codes)

Sixty procedures was far from complete. Our price calculator fell short because there is no one price for anything beyond the most straightforward of care. Negotiated rates for complex conditions with comorbidities and complications depend on contracts between payers and the hospital and on the ICD-10 codes and the resulting disease-related groups. Any effort to estimate out-of-pocket costs, without knowing the details about a patient's condition (does the patient also have other ailments like depression or Crohn's disease?) even with large-font disclaimers, seemed futile.

Keep It Simple ... and then Make It Simpler

What we learned from our calculator experiment is that every component of the reimbursement and payment system needs simplification and standardization, starting with common definitions of units of "health care service." Imagine organizing charges according to the ways people seek care: *got pregnant and gave birth, had appendix removed, was treated for and recovered from a stroke,* and so on. Whenever possible, a flat rate would include all the care needed through an expected period of recovery, including mental health support, with appropriate adjustments if the person had other serious medical conditions. By identifying clear units of service and making the prices known, patients and payers could comparison shop, factoring in performance in often-neglected dimensions like quality and outcomes, patient satisfaction, convenience, and amenities.

Bundled Payments for Care Improvement

That's what the Centers for Medicare & Medicaid's Bundled Payments for Care Improvement (BPCI) program is designed to do. In BPCI, Medicare pays hospitals a flat fee for patients hospitalized for conditions like joint replacement surgery, pneumonia, inflammatory bowel disease, coronary artery bypass grafting, and stroke. Unlike the DRG-based payments, the fixed fee covers care during the hospital admission *plus* 90 days thereafter. The fee paid to the hospital also covers physicians costs (no separate billing). And if the patient goes to a nursing home or is readmitted within 90 days, the hospital doesn't get paid any more. (Geisinger Health system offered this same deal to employers and marketed the fixed payment as a "money-back guarantee" [more in Chapter 5].) Medicare expanded bundled payments to 31 inpatient diagnoses and four outpatient diagnoses in 2020 and required participating health systems to meet quality measures to receive full payments.

Prepayments

Bundled payments could obviate most of the complex coding and billing rigmarole. Imagine if a patient could be diagnosed and assigned to a particular bundle of care upon admission (or even before admission). After verifying the success of care (quality metrics met, patient satisfied), a single bill could be paid, undisputed. It hasn't happened yet, but the possibility is powerfully alluring.

With both Medicare Advantage and bundled payments, Medicare is giving health care professionals the responsibility for keeping costs down. The momentum toward pay-for-results models is growing in state Medicaid programs as well. Kaiser Family Foundation estimated in 2019 that two-thirds of the nation's Medicaid beneficiaries received care from managed care organizations with a similar approach. In 2013, Utah's Medicaid program switched to such a model, offering a fixed payment (also called a "capitated" payment) per year for each Medicaid beneficiary. For a patient who visited the University of Utah's emergency room more than 50 times in 2012, the hospital was paid for each episode. Recognizing that would no longer be the case for 2013, the hospital responded in a ChenMed-like way—introducing the patient to a primary care clinic, offering transportation there and back, and assigning a care manager just to make sure she made her appointments and filled her prescriptions.

The Action Plan for Paying for Results

By making the American health care system pay for results instead of pay for action, we can slash the Gordian knot of inscrutable, outrageous billing practices that consume gargantuan resources and frustrate everyone involved. Insurers should be working with clinicians instead of against them.

Successes with pay-for-results pilot projects give us a chance to imagine even bolder steps. Medicare-Advantage-like annual payments incentivize primary care providers to keep patients healthy all year. Those payments are adjusted based on the health (and projected needs) of the beneficiaries. When their patients require hospitalization—for acute illnesses, accidents, or other unexpected needs—primary care medical groups (think ChenMed or Iora Health) could pay hospitals using Medicare-like bundled payments that are again adjusted based on the patient's overall health (a comorbidity and complication adjustment). If doctors and hospitals only got paid if patients did at least as well as expected, it could obviate most of the billing and coding requirements, with considerable potential savings. By simplifying and clarifying services that health insurers, hospitals, and medical groups offer, and by making information about their costs available publicly, people could make choices based on quality, accessibility, service, and other amenities, in addition to price.

To move to new pay-for-results models of care, we all have a role to play.

As a patient, you should:

- Embrace a patient's health plan bill of rights: demand to know how much you likely will have to spend for every hospitalization and every test or drug you have to have. Ask your employer to obtain this information as part of their insurance negotiations. Expect to understand your health insurance plan: what's covered, how much it will cost you, out-of-pocket expenses, and what happens in the event of an unexpected emergency.

- Use consumer-friendly applications that can guide better decision making and take every opportunity to provide customer feedback on websites that evaluate hospitals, doctors, health plans, and any other services.

As a health insurer, hospital administrator, or health care professional, you should:

- Standardize and simplify the units of health care services in understandable terms and replace existing chargemasters. Map standard services to a single price that includes professional, technical, and rehabilitative services. Encourage integration of physical and mental health.
- Offer standardized benefits plans. Deductibles, co-pays, and coinsurance for each covered benefit should be consistent across a limited number of offerings, and the essential benefits, which include catastrophic care, should be the same. Encourage integration of physical and mental health.

As a policy maker, you should:

- Encourage or mandate standardization and simplification, as described above.
- Seek cooperative markets in which care delivery systems like doctors, hospitals, and rehabilitation facilities work together with insurance companies, using models like the new Medicare Advantage arrangements, bundled payments, prepayments, or other alternative payment models.
- Expect health care businesses to compete on costs as well as health outcomes, convenience, supportive services, accessibility and responsiveness, customer service, and more. Empower consumers through better tools including standardized offerings and open pricing.

And most important, all of us need to elect leaders who will drive insurers and health systems to produce better health outcomes at lower costs, collaboratively.

CHAPTER 4

MANUFACTURING OUT
THE MISHAPS

*I've toured piano factories. I can watch them make a
piano and see the care with which they handle every
part of that piano so it isn't nicked or dinged. And I
think about our patients and say: How do we care for
them every step of the way, so that we're not doing the
equivalent of nicking or dinging them?*

—Sarah Patterson, former COO,
Virginia Mason Medical Center

A father brings his daughter to the emergency room because she's having an asthma flare-up. To help dilate her constricting airways, the doctor prescribes a nebulizer treatment. The nurse sets up the treatment, connecting oxygen tubing from the wall to the nebulizer that attaches to the mask and blows the aerosolized medication into her lungs. Another nurse puts an intravenous catheter in the girl's arm, in case she needs more medications. A short while later, one of the medical residents comes to check on her. She's feeling better. He sees that the treatment is finished, and he disconnects the tubing to the nebulizer and removes the mask. Aiming to restore the right connections, he attaches the tubing to a different connector. A few moments later, a giant bolus of air enters the girl's bloodstream and moves from her veins into her heart. She dies almost immediately, in her father's arms.

The resident had connected the oxygen to her intravenous catheter. It was the wrong connector—they all looked the same. His simple mistake caused a tragic death.

The Errors Epidemic

In 1999, the esteemed Institute of Medicine (now the National Academy of Medicine) issued a report, *To Err Is Human: Building a Safer Health System*, which concluded that hospitals and clinics were dangerous places. The experts estimated that up to 98,000 people died per year in US hospitals due to medical mistakes. Subsequent revised estimates placed the number of people killed annually by medical errors much higher, between 250,000 and 440,000.

These figures make medical mistakes the third-leading cause of death in the United States, behind heart disease and cancer. The statistic is shocking, almost unbelievable to most. Twice as many people die from medical mistakes as die from suicides, firearms, and motor vehicle accidents *combined*. Another well-kept secret is that "mistake" is not used on death certificates or in hospital records, so these errors are not tracked in any systematic way. The true number of deaths could be even higher than those alarming estimates. When you consider the number of victims who don't die but are seriously harmed is probably ten times as large, you realize health care in the United States is dangerous.

It's not really possible to quantify the impact of medical mistakes in financial terms, but some economists have tried. In terms of additional health care, lost income and household productivity, and disability, these errors could add up to as much as $100 billion in the United States each year. That doesn't include medical liability. In 2010, researchers estimated that lawsuits and the practice of defensive medicine racked up over $55 billion. The pain and suffering of the victims and those close to them aren't part of those calculations.

First, Do Less Harm

Any plan for better health care must start here: Stop violating the fundamental principle of medicine—*Primum non nocere*, or First, do no harm.

To start, we need to stop making avoidable mistakes that involve physical acts leading to harm, like hooking up the wrong catheter. Ken Kizer, former CEO of the National Quality Forum, coined the term surgical "never events," for mistakes that should never happen in the operating room, like leaving a surgical clamp in a patient or doing the wrong operation. Or nicking the intestine during an operation to remove the gallbladder, leading to infection and death, which is what reportedly happened to Pennsylvania congressman John Murtha in 2010.

Like most medical mistakes, surgical "never events" are not reliably reported. Estimates of their frequency come from medical malpractice data. From 1990 to 2010, 9,744 malpractice settlements and judgments were paid for surgical "never events" in the United States (about 500 per year). In about half (4,857) of those cases, surgeons left a piece of gauze or a surgical instrument inside a patient. The other half of the cases were most commonly either the wrong procedure or the wrong site, for example, operating on the wrong knee or at the wrong level of the spine for back pain. And 27 were for operations on the wrong patient! Researchers estimate that for every "never event" that leads to a malpractice suit, there are about seven that don't. That implies there could be 4,000 or more surgical "never events" in the United States each year.

Instead of doing the wrong thing, sometimes the unfortunate mistake is failing to do the right thing, like not prescribing a needed medication or forgetting to recommend a screening test. Sometimes the system tries to do the right thing but poor communication or coordination get in the way. Surgeons or internists may miss reports from radiologists and pathologists and fail to act on their findings. A misfiled report may mean that a patient is never notified of a positive mammogram or malignant cells on a prostate biopsy.

Diagnostic errors are extremely common but very hard to call out as mistakes because getting the right diagnosis sometimes requires trial and error. A 2015 National Academy of Medicine report found that at least 1 in 20 adults who seek care in an outpatient clinic experience an inaccurate or delayed diagnosis, and most people will experience at least one diagnostic error in their lifetime. Autopsy studies show that diagnostic errors contribute to about one in ten deaths. One of the most common causes of diagnostic error happens in my own field, radiology—where studies show that about 30% of abnormal findings on an exam are missed.

A Hard Pill to Swallow: A Case Study

Over half of all Americans regularly take at least one prescription drug. Those who do, on average, take four different medications. That makes them vulnerable to adverse events because mistakes in prescriptions and dispensing are common. Consider, for example, what happened one morning in 2010 in the cardiac intensive care unit at Seattle Children's Hospital. Nurse Kimberly Hiatt was caring for Kaia, an eight-month-old baby girl with a severe congenital heart condition who had been in the unit since birth, awaiting a heart transplant. That morning, Kaia had a low calcium level, so the physician ordered for her to receive 140 mg of calcium chloride intravenously. As Hiatt was preparing the drug, a colleague came by and chatted with her. Doing the kind of quick math she was accustomed to in the ICU, Hiatt drew up calcium chloride and injected the clear liquid into the intravenous catheter. Not long after, the baby's heart rate quickened and became irregular. A quick blood check showed that her calcium level was much too high. When another nurse reviewed her calculation, Kimberly realized her mistake. She had injected 1.4 g of calcium chloride into the baby, ten times the ordered dose. Five days later, Kaia died.

Hiatt was fired, and the state's nursing commission placed her on probation for four years. She was unable to get a job as a nurse. Seven months later, she took her own life.

Every time a patient receives a medication in the hospital, there's a 20%–25% probability that it involves at least one clinical error—the drug may be given at the wrong time or at the wrong injection rate, or maybe it's the wrong formulation. Sometimes it might be the wrong drug. The mistakes don't always lead to harm, but on average, a hospital patient is subject to at least one medication error per day.

There are so many ways to make a mistake. Start with the similar names for very different drugs. Would you blame a physician, pharmacist, or nurse for confusing Celebrex (an arthritis drug), Cerebyx (a seizure medication), and Celexa (an antidepressant)? The Food and Drug Administration (FDA) and the Institute for Safe Medication Practices regularly publish online lists of dozens of look-alike or sound-alike drug names. Instead of prohibiting confusing names, the FDA recommends writing three of the key letters in uppercase—"tall-man letters"—like clonazePAM, cloNIDine, cloZAPine, cloBAZam, LORazepam. Call me a skeptic, but I am not conVINced this will work.

Even if you get the name right, it can be easy to get dose wrong. A misplaced decimal point is the difference between 12.5 mg and 125 mg, both plausible doses for cloZAPine in patients with schizophrenia. How many daily doses a patient should get can be confusing, too; clonazePAM is often given three times a day for seizures but only twice a day for panic or anxiety disorder.

Digital prescribing is reducing some of these errors, including those resulting from poor penmanship. (One study showed that about one in five handwritten prescriptions by medical residents had an error.) The process still relies on humans to do math. Working out the right concentrations and infusion rates for certain intravenous drugs can make calculating your taxes seem like a breeze. Consider this example with dopamine, a medication used for very sick patients in an intensive care unit. One milliliter (mL, just under a quarter of a teaspoon) drawn from an 80 mg/mL dopamine vial and injected and mixed into a 500 mL (about a pint) bag of saline makes a dopamine solution of 0.16 mg/mL. A 100 kg (220 lb.) patient who should receive a steady dose of intravenous dopamine at 2–5 micrograms/kg/min, where "kg" refers to the weight of the patient, would need about a 1.25–3.125 ml/min infusion from that bag. Easy, right?

Multiply these steps by the hundreds (or thousands) of medications administered each day to the hundreds (or thousands) of patients in any given hospital or clinic, and you'll have an idea of the staggering challenges—and the monumental risk for errors.

Distractions multiply that risk, and they happen all the time in health care. Studies show that nurses are interrupted during medication rounds—by patients, family members, other nurses, physicians, therapists—about once every two to five minutes. It's not just nurses; most clinicians experience frequent distractions. For example, one study reported that emergency department physicians are interrupted once every six minutes, on average, or about ten times per hour. These lead to slips and lapses. It's a system-wide problem that needs solving, and it's taking a toll on everyone.

Welcome to the Stress, Burnout, and Blame Ward

For every mistake in health care, there are the obvious victims—the patient as well as the patient's family and loved ones. And then there is, in the words of public health expert Albert Wu, "the second victim," the health care provider who harmed—or even killed—a patient by accident. In medical environments, conditions are deteriorating. Information is poorly communicated. Electronic medical records, intended to improve that flow, can be burdensome and make information feel less accessible. The frantic urgency to complete each clinic visit in under ten minutes stresses clinicians and patients alike and isn't conducive to good care. And on top of all that, alerts, beepers, and calls distract and produce more anxiety, more mistakes.

More than half of US physicians are experiencing substantial burnout, and the numbers are on the rise. The suicide rate for physicians is more than twice as high as for other professionals. Younger physicians are affected the most—suicide is the most common cause of death among males in their training (residents) and the second leading cause of death among all residents. One survey of US surgeons found 15% suffered from alcoholism, and those who reported burnout were at 25% higher risk of developing alcohol abuse or dependence compared to those who did not have burnout.

The mental health of professionals greatly affects hospital safety. Higher burnout levels among hospital nurses correlate with more health care–associated infections in their patients. Soaring job dissatisfaction also causes doctors and nurses to reduce their work hours or quit, exacerbating the already serious shortages in the United States. That medical resident who attached oxygen tubing to the girl's intravenous catheter dropped out of medicine, throwing away over ten years of post-high school education and training. Shortages of physicians and nurses in the United States worsen the workload for the rest, which in turn exacerbates burnout and increases the risk of mistakes. The vicious cycle needs to stop. And to start, the system needs to own up to the problem.

Hiding Mistakes Is a Mistake

Historically, legal teams have instructed physicians to avoid taking responsibility when things went wrong. Mistakes were shrouded in secrecy, so much so that many patients were never even told when mistakes happened. In the late 1990s, things began to change. Leading medical associations declared that physicians had an ethical obligation to disclose errors to their patients. A few years later, when studies showed that families were less likely to sue if doctors owned up and apologized, admitting a mistake began to gain acceptance. Hospital lawyers changed their exhortations from "Don't ever say you're sorry" to "Say you're sorry!" States began mandating disclosure of "unanticipated outcomes" and passed laws to prevent apologies from being used in litigation as evidence of fault.

Fear of litigation isn't only used to justify being tight-lipped about mistakes. It's also the excuse for overordering laboratory and imaging tests. Even if the risk of a teenager's headache being due to a brain tumor is less than 1%, two factors are enough to make that physician "err" on the side of ordering the unnecessary CT (or "CAT") or MRI scan: first, the fear of a multimillion-dollar lawsuit, and second, a lifetime of having to report that lawsuit (regardless of outcome) on every application form for state medical licensure or hospital privileges for the rest of his or her professional life. Weigh that against the impression that the test costs you nothing to order, might reassure a worried patient, and could increase profitability, and the tendency to overorder makes sense. This happens so often that as many as 30% of laboratory tests and 20%–50% of advanced radiologic imaging may be unnecessary, and as much as 2%–3% of health spending in the United States (over $50 billion) is considered defensive spending.

Many malpractice lawyers argue our health system would be even more dangerous without the fear of lawsuits. This may have been true in ancient Babylonia, where the Code of Hammurabi declared that any physician who caused a death would have his fingers cut off. These days, there's little evidence that the threat of being sued (or having your fingers amputated) improves the quality of our care. Malpractice cases in the United States frequently make headlines with huge payouts ($5.72 billion per year), and yet we still have one of the worst safety records in the developed world.

Nations like New Zealand (starting in 1974), Sweden, Finland, and Denmark have a completely different system of compensating patients when things go wrong, called a medical malpractice "no-fault" system. Akin to workers' compensation or automobile insurance in some states, patients who are harmed file claims with the government. In Denmark, about one in three are compensated, with an average payout of $30,000, one-seventh the average in the United States. Importantly, patients can qualify for compensation even if their injuries were not caused by negligence.

No-fault doesn't mean no accountability. The Danes hold physicians accountable and start disciplinary proceedings when poor outcomes are due to wrongdoing. Nevertheless, their process seems to encourage doctors to be more open—about 10% of the claims are filed by a physician on behalf of a patient. With that openness, mistakes are more commonly reported, and systems are set up to prevent them from happening. From one cluster of claims, the Danes identified an error in the computerized pharmacy ordering system that was delivering doses of the drug methotrexate daily instead of weekly. Another study showed that doctors and midwives were misreading fetal monitoring strips of women in labor. That led to a nationwide training and a new recertification program. These examples may explain why nations with no-fault systems are among the highest performing in the world.

In the United States, experience with no-fault is limited. Virginia and Florida enacted similar no-fault programs that cover the lifetime costs of infants who suffer neurological injuries during birth. The larger of the two programs was initiated in Florida in 1988, when skyrocketing malpractice premiums made it hard to find an obstetrician. Here's how it works.

In Florida, families with newborn infants who sustained neurological injuries at birth file a $15 claim petition with documentation, and a hearing officer decides the case within 45 days. Most awards are for the actual expenses for medical and custodial care. Pain and suffering awards are capped at $100,000; most parents receive the full amount (in Virginia, this benefit is not available). The no-fault pool is funded by a one-time $40 million allocation from the state, participating obstetricians (who pay $5,000 per year), other Florida physicians (who are required to pay $250 per year), and most private hospitals. If the fund runs out of money, a provision of the statute says that insurance companies may be taxed.

An analysis in 1994 showed that the compensation of injuries was comparable, and administrative costs were substantially lower for no-fault than tort law. In 2019, the program was still solvent. While there haven't been any studies to examine the impact of no-fault compensation on safety in Florida, other data show that states that eased medical tort laws didn't make medicine less safe.

If It Flies in Aviation, Why Not Here?

Aside from making it easier to make mistakes apparent, the question is why can't we make medicine safer? Other industries offer invaluable lessons.

Consider, for example, the aviation business. Distractions in the cockpit can be just as deadly as distractions in the intensive care unit. In 1981, after distractions caused a series of crashes, the Federal Aviation Administration required pilots to refrain from nonessential activities during critical phases of flight, typically below 10,000 feet. Hospitals have tried adopting guidelines similar to this "sterile cockpit" approach, including draping nurses with "Do Not Interrupt" sashes or vests while they dispense medications and cordoning off silent zones around medication dispensing stations.

Checklists are also moving from cockpits to intensive care units and operating rooms. They cut down on distractions and make sure minimum safety and operational standards are met. For example, central venous catheters, often called "central lines," are common in hospitals. Used for patients who need intravenous antibiotics, chemotherapy, or supplemental nutrition by vein over weeks or months, the slender tubes that deliver medications directly into the bloodstream require careful management. The skin around the catheter as it enters the body needs to be clean and sterile because bacteria that enter the bloodstream via the catheter can cause fatal infections. About 250,000 patients in the United States get catheter-related bloodstream infections each year but, as anesthesiologist Peter Pronovost showed, these infections can be prevented with a simple five-step checklist. The commonsense actions include washing hands before the insertion process and cleaning the insertion site with sterilizing solution.

When implemented at 100 Michigan intensive care units, the central line infection rate declined by two-thirds. If used across the United States, Pronovost's checklist could save many of the 28,000 lives lost each year to these infections. Using a similar approach in operating rooms, surgeon-writer Atul Gawande led a worldwide study in which eight hospitals implemented the World Health Organization's Surgical Safety Checklist. Infections dropped from 11% to 7%, and death rates were cut in half.

If health care were like any other industry, a "never event" would be grounds for shutting down a hospital. That's what happens with airplanes. On October 29, 2018, one of Boeing's new 737 Max jets crashed in Indonesia, killing all 189 people aboard. On March 10, 2019, another 737 Max jet went down in Addis Ababa, killing all 157 passengers. Three days later, regulatory authorities around the world grounded all 737s.

The number of deaths due to medical mistakes in the United States equates to somewhere between two and six 737s crashing every day, depending on which estimate you believe. Despite this, it's almost unheard of to "ground" a hospital. In 2014, the *Wall Street Journal* found that 350 hospitals had violations issued by the Centers for Medicare and Medicaid Services that ranged from failing to provide lists of home health agencies to surgical "never" events to fraud. Twenty hospitals had violations considered likely to cause "serious injury or death." Sixty percent of those hospitals also had violations in the previous three years. Despite these violations, almost all remained accredited.

Similarly, few physicians are grounded for their serious mistakes. In 2017, out of almost a million licensed doctors in the United States, 711 were put on probation, 656 had their license suspended, and 248 had it revoked. About one-third to one-half of the time it was because of negligence, incompetence, or inappropriate prescribing. The rest were because of issues like fraud, alcohol or substance abuse, or inappropriate/sexual contact. In 2018, *USA Today* reported that about 500 physicians disciplined in one state just moved to another state and kept working. (Medical licenses are issued by states.) The congressionally mandated National Practitioner Data Bank was supposed to prevent this, but few state medical boards check it, and it's not open for public searches.

Stop Paying for Mistakes

Instead of getting penalized for mistakes, most health systems get paid for them. Until 2008, Medicare covered the treatment of infections acquired in a hospital and the care of patients who received the wrong blood type in a transfusion. They even paid hospitals for surgery to remove objects accidentally left inside a patient. If additional nights in the hospital were needed because of a medical mistake, the hospital might make money off of that, too. For mistakes that Medicare or insurance audits don't detect, this continues to happen today.

Expectations are so low that in the early 1990s, instead of grounding hospitals, the federal government rewarded them simply for not making serious mistakes. Here are a few of the main things it rewarded hospitals for NOT doing: accidentally cutting into intestines, liver, or other organ in an abdominal operation; causing an infection; allowing patients to fall and break a hip after surgery; inadvertently allowing patients to develop a new bedsore while in the hospital, and . . . killing a patient.

Champions of this approach point out that it worked. Between 1999 and 2013, far fewer patients suffered from adverse reactions to medications, got new infections, or developed bedsores. "Hospital-acquired conditions" decreased from about 14% in 2010 to just under 9% in 2017. That's over three million fewer hospital-acquired conditions, and over 125,000 lives saved per year. The financial impact has also been substantial. Between 2010 and 2017, reductions in hospital-acquired conditions created over $27.5 billion in savings.

Skeptics believe these improvements in safety reflect administrators gaming the system—teaching to the test rather than developing a culture of safety. For example, to lower their reported rates of hospital-acquired bedsores, some hospitals assigned a physician the task of thoroughly examining every newly admitted patient from head to toe for a preexisting bedsore—because documenting its existence meant it wouldn't count as a new bedsore that would be the hospital's fault. Plus, it defined the patient as sicker to start (more codes!).

Hospitals and doctors that care for sicker patients are expected to have worse outcomes than those that care for healthier patients. To convince payers like Medicare that their patients are *really* sick, some might recommend ordering tests such as an echocardiogram just to prove that a patient has mild heart failure so that they can add this condition to their list. This "upcoding" or "coding inflation" helps hospitals justify poorer outcomes and gets them paid more, too.

Progress toward safer health care is slow. In 2017, there were still 2,550,000 hospital-acquired conditions in the United States. Rather than tackling the problem case by case, it pays to consider how hospitals and clinicians can change altogether how they approach care.

Factoring In the Human Factor

Designing products and processes for the harried users in the complex, distraction-filled hospital environment can go a long way to making them less harried and less vulnerable to distraction. Pronovost showed his checklist could improve the catheter insertion process. What about keeping the catheters clean over the subsequent days thereafter? Carrie Charlesworth, the nursing leader in the burn unit at the University of Utah, enlisted the help of a human factors expert, psychologist Frank Drews, to see if together they could prevent central line infections by making the process mistake-proof.

Drews and team designed user-friendly dressing change kits that hold all the supplies needed for one dressing change. The nurse doesn't have to hunt down all the supplies or worry about forgetting something. As the pouch unfolds, each of the necessary supplies for the next step is revealed. It's practically fool-proof. With this and other initiatives, the infection rate in the burn unit declined dramatically. After four years, the ward celebrated *zero* central line infections. Now that's "never."

Hospital as Factory

It's not much of a stretch to think of hospitals as manufacturing plants— sick patients are the "input" and healthy patients are the "output." Doctors, nurses, and therapists, among others, are the line workers. Unlike today's slick, robotically-driven manufacturing plants, hospitals are strikingly inefficient and frequently chaotic. Every shift has its own way of running the line. Every person on the line has a phone that receives calls or texts 10–25 times an hour. Safety gear is optional. Maybe half of the assembly-line safety alarms work. Most workers don't feel empowered to stop the line even when they suspect something bad is happening. In light of all that, it's no surprise the "products" are "faulty" one-third of the time and that the workers have crushing levels of stress. What could go wrong?

Right after World War II, Japanese auto manufacturers might have felt as disconsolate as Americans do about health care today. Their reputation was so poor that some companies set up plants in the Japanese village of "Usa," just so that they could say their products were "Made in USA." Asked to help rebuild these devastated industries, American management scientist W. Edwards Deming traveled to Japan and devoted the next two decades to that job. He championed a new kind of industrial engineering— Total Quality Management—that gave rise to a new culture of management in manufacturing, later labeled Lean manufacturing and six sigma. Deming showed that engaging and empowering frontline workers to eliminate waste and defects, reduce variations in practice, and improve quality continuously could transform industries and revitalize an entire nation.

His lessons inspired Toyota, and in the mid-1990s, when Toyota signed a big contract with the airbag manufacturing giant Autoliv, his teachings spread to Utah. To make sure the airbags would be worthy of its brand, Toyota sent Lean manufacturing expert Takashi Harada to the Autoliv plant in Ogden, Utah, for three years. Over the next couple of decades, Autoliv embraced the Toyota way.

When leaders from the University of Utah Health toured the Autoliv plant in 2012, we could see how seriously they took their motto, "Saving More Lives." Their processes were completely standardized. Visible dashboards reminded everyone of the company's performance goals and tracked progress toward them. It was a calm and controlled environment. Distractions were rare. Supplies were organized impeccably. When Autoliv leaders shared data on their error rate, we were put to shame. Their goal wasn't one in a million. It was zero.

A decade earlier, CEO Gary Kaplan had led Seattle-based Virginia Mason Medical Center on a similar tour—he and his leadership team visited a Toyota plant in Japan. Sarah Patterson, the former hospital COO, was on that tour and recalled how these lessons taught them that leaders needed to spend their time on the front lines, with patients.

Patterson pointed out that health care is more than treating patients like widgets on an assembly line. She draws on her observations from a piano factory tour. After the automated steps on the assembly line are done, the piano goes into a soundproof house for tuning. There, the tuner is given as much time as he or she needs to tune the piano. The company does not rush this critical part of the process. Patterson looks for that same balance and judgment in health care. She says, "We must be sure that we create the environment for that craftsman (nurse, doctor, other clinicians) to do their work, so that it can yield the best results." To help others learn to incorporate Lean into their health systems, Sarah Patterson runs a 35-person consulting business at Virginia Mason, teaching others how to find that balance.

In Salt Lake City, former chief quality officer at Intermountain Healthcare Brent James explained how Lean manufacturing worked in his health system. He says it's all about applying the scientific method to medicine. At Intermountain Healthcare, clinicians used data from their homegrown electronic health record system to measure how patients with conditions like pneumonia or diabetes or acute respiratory distress syndrome fare depending on the different treatments they receive. The team takes the protocols that work the best and keeps improving them over many iterations. The best protocols become the default approach—not just for one or two doctors in the hospital, but for all of them.

Raj Sethi, spine surgeon and chair of the Virginia Mason Neuroscience Institute, admits that embracing the Lean way means giving up some autonomy—the right to use whatever implant you want, for example—but in return, you get an "impeccable patient experience." Following evidence-based guidelines also means that surgeons don't always recommend surgery. That's how Virginia Mason attracted employers like WalMart, Lowe's, and JetBlue to fly their employees to see the Seattle doctors for care (More on this in Chapter 10).

Another Deming acolyte, Don Berwick, founded the Institute for Healthcare Improvement in 1991 to teach health systems about the science of quality improvement. A pediatrician and former administrator of the Centers for Medicare and Medicaid Services, Berwick's nonprofit research and education organization offers training programs, case studies, white papers, and a wide range of toolkits. By 2019, about 6,000 people from all over the world attended its National Forum, learning and sharing lessons of Lean.

Many hospitals are just starting to implement Lean management. A 2018 survey found that about 62% of hospitals were doing some Lean work, but only 12% had spread the management style through the entire hospital. In a pay-for-action world, consistently practicing high-quality medicine isn't as important as building more surgicenters and adding more codes. In a pay-for-results world, mistakes and overtreatment are costly, and Lean makes you profitable.

The Action Plan for Eliminating Errors

Setting expectations of zero tolerance for serious medical error, embracing Lean manufacturing, and employing human factors design are key parts of the strategy to break the vicious cycle of distractions, mistakes, and despondency. With these priorities, built-in safety and quality systems should detect problems before anyone is hurt. Drugs should have simple and distinct names. Tubing connectors and other supplies should be designed for safety. Computerized processes should make things flow better, not worse. When clinicians make a mistake, they should admit it—supported by a combination of no-fault medical malpractice with more effective oversight of professional competency. Members of the public should be able to trust a hospital as much as they trust the airbags in their cars. A hospital should be at least as safe as an airplane and run at least as well as an airbag manufacturing plant.

To improve safety and reduce medical mistakes, we all have a role to play.

As a patient and consumer of health care, you should:

- Be attentive and engaged in the care you or your family receives, especially medications and their instructions for use.
- Use trusted online web tools like Leapfrog or Medicare's online Hospital Compare tool to look at the safety records of hospitals and physicians.

- Report mistakes. Inform the hospital or practice, the accrediting bodies, state licensing boards, and the state department of health if you believe someone has been harmed by a medical error.

As a physician or other health care professional, you should:

- Work in hospitals and clinics that embrace best practices like Lean manufacturing, safety checklists, and reliable information technology systems.
- Follow evidence-based medicine and best-practice guidelines. Do your part to reduce variations in care.
- Expect your organization to invest in human factors design.
- Support a culture that avoids blame and focuses on improvements, but doesn't shelter physicians or other clinicians who should not be practicing.
- Work closely with your risk management team if you are involved in or make a mistake. Be open with the patient and the patient's family about what happened. Seek assistance from peers and others for support.

As a payer, such as a self-insured employer, government entity, or health plan, you should:

- Set a high bar for safety with aggressive timelines to achieve zero "never" events.
- Regularly review data about your employees and members, and seek information about any adverse events (medical mistakes or otherwise). Don't pay for mistakes.
- Expect organizations that care for your employees or beneficiaries to have a continuous quality improvement or Lean manufacturing culture. Ask what quality-improvement initiatives are underway, and request updates.

- If your employees have suffered from poor care (hospital-acquired infections or other conditions, for example), ask for evidence that the hospital is addressing the issue at a system level.

As a policy maker, you should:

- Expect that all entities in health care—health care delivery systems, suppliers, service contractors, and others—track the safety of their products and services and hold them accountable for improving safety in health care.
- Address pharmaceutical naming practices to discourage look-alike and sound-alike drug names.
- Require improved standards across the medical supplies industry to lower rates of medical mistakes, taking into account human factors design.
- Explore no-fault insurance models that compensate patients fairly for injury.
- Encourage health systems and clinicians to report and manage mistakes, manage clinician performance and professionalism, and maintain robust internal quality-improvement programs.

And most important, all of us need to elect leaders who expect health care systems to deliver safe care and who hold everyone accountable including themselves.

CHAPTER 5

LEARNING TO DELIVER
PERFECT CARE

*Every hospital should follow every patient it treats,
long enough to determine whether or not the treatment has been successful, and then to inquire, "If not,
why not?" with a view to preventing similar failures
in the future.*

—Ernest A. Codman

Ernest Codman was born in 1869, during the heyday of surgical innovation. It had been about 20 years since the first public demonstration of
surgical anesthesia at the Massachusetts General Hospital in 1846 marked
the beginning of modern surgery. Until then, operations had been well-
intentioned torture—far surpassing what we now consider the limits of
pain tolerance—and they were only performed when the alternative was
clearly worse. In the 1860s, British surgeon Joseph Lister discovered the
benefits of cleanliness and sterility. He applied carbolic acid, a disinfectant,
directly on wounds and on surgical instruments and showed that not only

were infections prevented, but healing also improved dramatically. (Back then, surgeons were not required to wash their hands or a patient's wounds.)

Around that same time, Florence Nightingale applied statistical data analysis to improve survival of soldiers during the Crimean War (1854–1856). She used data diagrams to show that the unsanitary conditions—overcrowding, "verminous" laundry, and the lack of essential medical and surgical supplies—were contributing to the high incidence of typhus and cholera. The epidemics were so bad that patients arriving at her hospital were more likely to die of these infections than from the injuries sustained on the battlefield. By improving sanitation, chief nurse Nightingale reduced mortality rates from 42.7% to only 2.2%.

With these two breakthroughs—sanitation and anesthesia—hospitals transformed from squalid places where the suffering went to die to clean, controlled environments that offered hope. Just as barbers and quacks in blood-encrusted, thick black coats evolved into surgeon-scientists in clean laboratory whites, Ernest Codman came of age. Ambitious, assertive, and irreverent, Codman was, like Nightingale, naturally inclined to apply data science to medicine. As a student at Harvard Medical School, he and his classmates were responsible for administering anesthesia during surgery. Codman bet his friend and classmate Harvey Cushing (who became a founder of the field of neurosurgery) that he could better manage the anesthesia of his patients. To quantify their success, they plotted patient vital signs like pulse and respiration rate before and after administering anesthetics and other drugs. Their system gave rise to the first anesthesia charts—a universal standard today. After graduating from Harvard Medical School in 1895, the year Wilhelm Roentgen discovered the imaging properties of X-rays, Codman also taught himself radiology and became the first "skiagrapher," or radiologist, at Boston Children's Hospital.

Codman was especially skilled in the operating room. He developed the first techniques for surgical repair of the shoulder and published innovative surgical methods to treat a wide range of conditions, from duodenal ulcers to tumors of the bone. In this era of medical firsts, Codman became obsessed with measuring and recording his surgical results. In his coat pocket, he kept index-card-sized "End Result" cards, one for each patient, on which he recorded a brief description of the patient's symptoms, his diagnosis before and after the operation, the operation performed, and the condition of each patient at one-year follow-up visits.

As exceptional as it was for the time (and even today), Codman thought his End Result approach was obvious and crucial. He was sure surgeons were overconfident and misleading themselves about how much good they were doing for patients. That overconfidence wasn't good for the trainees, either. Codman said, "If some arrangement could be made by which the house officer should see these late results, it would be very instructive for them, for I feel sure that the house officer in graduating from this institution gets a very much more favorable idea of the results of surgical operations than he is really justified in having."

Codman's End Result cards were not popular, nor was he, their unabashedly arrogant advocate. Codman argued that surgeons should be hired and promoted on the basis of their End Results. He advocated that End Results should be made public. Rather than judging surgeons on their "nerve," "steady hand," and "graceful" operating style, patients could judge their abilities by their End Results. Naturally, Codman thought that his colleagues at Harvard and at Massachusetts General Hospital should elect him Surgeon-in-Chief because of his superior End Results. They did not, and he resigned his faculty appointment. Later that year, in 1911, he opened a ten-bed facility called the End Result Hospital. Every surgeon there (including his friend Cushing, who by then was a distinguished neurosurgeon) was required to collect End-Result data, and each year, Codman published them. After five years, *A Study in Hospital Efficiency: As Demonstrated by the Case Report of First Five Years of Private Hospital* detailed the End Results of the 337 patients discharged from his hospital in those five years. Remarkably, the report included every one of the 123 errors identified (not much higher than today's error rate). The most common mistakes were attributed to lack of judgment, lack of equipment, incorrect diagnosis, and cases where the patients refused to accept treatment. Codman described his own mistakes, including a missed gallstone, symptomless hernias (bulges at the surgical scar), and even a missed stomach ulcer.

Don Quixote with a Scalpel

According to his biographer Bill Mallon, Codman "would spend much of his life attempting to convince the medical world of the importance of the End Result Idea—to little avail. It was the windmill at which he tilted but never managed to topple." But his ideas did make their way into broader hospital practice through his lifelong friendship with Edward Martin, a Philadelphia-based gynecologist. Martin built the first program to evaluate hospitals based on outcomes, which later became the leading hospital accrediting body, the Joint Commission on Accreditation of Healthcare Organizations. The Joint Commission, as it later became known, gained authority when a 1965 law required hospitals to meet its standards in order to participate in Medicare and Medicaid programs, partly fulfilling one of Codman's dreams: tying End Results to payment.

Codman was convinced that sharing End Results would not only lead to improvements in care, but it would also give people better information about where to seek care. In 1989, nearly 50 years after his death, the New York State Department of Health decided to test that theory.

Codman and CABGs

The goal was to lower the state's death rate for coronary artery bypass grafting (CABG), one of the most commonly performed operations at New York hospitals. CABGs made up three-quarters of all heart surgery operations, and at the time, one in 25 patients did not survive. To motivate hospitals to improve, the department released data on the percentage of patients in each hospital who died (adjusted for how sick patients were before going to surgery). They also published how many of these operations were performed at each hospital that year—they suspected that those who performed more operations might be better than those who performed fewer. Shortly thereafter, *Newsday* took the public reporting one step further—it sued to get individual surgeon data released and then published the CABG death rates for each cardiac surgeon in the state, *by name*.

Surgeons were furious. (Not much had changed since Codman's day.) Hurt pride aside, they had a few legitimate concerns. For one, they feared that very sick patients would no longer be able to find a surgeon willing to operate on them because if they had a poor outcome, it would hurt the surgeon's statistics. Teaching hospitals were worried because they tended to attract sicker patients and had higher death rates due to the more complex operations their surgeons tended to do. Many feared that the risk adjustment (the statistical correction that factors in the higher likelihood of complications and death for sicker patients) wouldn't adequately reflect these differences. It seemed unfair to be humiliated for taking on the more challenging and often underserved patients.

Despite these concerns, the effect of publishing End-Result data was irrefutable. Over the next four years, the risk of dying from CABG in New York dropped from 4.2% to 2.5% and continued to decline. By 2010, the rate had fallen to 1.6%.

Did the surgeons learn how to operate better? Not necessarily. Death rates improved mostly because the poorer-performing surgeons (for example, those who tended to do fewer than 50 operations per year) stopped doing the operation. Some did so voluntarily; others, because their hospitals forced them to. Some hospitals also assigned especially complicated patients to surgeons who had better outcomes for sicker patients.

Many doctors remained skeptical about public reporting despite the lower death rates. In a nearly identical effort conducted a few years later in Pennsylvania, the majority of surgeons and cardiologists dismissed the effort. Only 10% thought the data were "very important" in assessing performance. They didn't believe the numbers accurately reflected surgical ability largely because they doubted that the statistical risk adjustment was sufficient. Most also said tallying how many patients died was not an adequate measure of the quality of care; it would be better to measure outcomes like physical activity after surgery, for example.

Some of the physicians' fears proved legitimate. After public reporting began in Pennsylvania, 59% of physicians reported they had a harder time finding surgeons willing to operate on their sickest patients, and 63% of surgeons admitted that they were less inclined to do so.

Could there be a better way of measuring and improving performance? Is there a more inspired way to motivate doctors? Yes, but to do so, you must understand first what drives them.

Diagnosing Doctors

In his popular 2009 book *Drive: The Surprising Truth about What Motivates Us*, Daniel Pink talks about how to motivate everyone from truculent teens to highly specialized scientists. Extrinsic motivators, such as money or a promotion, incentivize people whose work involves repetitive, assembly-line-type tasks. For solving complex problems, it's easier and less expensive to tap into intrinsic motivation—the inclination to do something because it is satisfying. That would be how most physicians approach their work.

Pink says if you want to leverage intrinsic motivation, you need to incorporate three elements: purpose, autonomy, and mastery. In other words, align what you want physicians to do with what matters to them, and they will be deeply motivated to advance the cause.

Purpose is the simplest. The health profession is full of people imbued with a strong sense of purpose, eager to do things in the service of a greater good—to help others, to heal the sick, and to comfort patients and their families.

Autonomy is expected. Doctors synthesize evidence and make decisions for their patients. Because no two patients are alike, autonomy to make judgments is integral to the art of medicine. That's why physicians react defensively when administrators try to oversimplify their profession into "cookbook" medicine, where step-by-step care protocols take the "art" and autonomy out of the practice. That's also why efforts to measure a physician's performance by adherence to guidelines frequently fall flat.

Mastery motivates. Physicians are a group of individuals driven to achieve mastery. Most were the hypercompetitive "premeds" of college organic chemistry classes. They often expect to "out-master" others. They want to win and to be the best.

Ernest Codman exemplified these three traits. He didn't define mastery as picking the correct leg to operate on or avoiding bedsores. He wanted to outperform his peers. He aimed to be the best surgeon, and he didn't mind if everyone knew it.

Fee-for-service models of care divert these admirable ambitions with financial incentives to overtreat and overprescribe. The hundreds of hospital quality-reporting requirements crowd out intrinsic motivation. To transform health care, we need to align purpose, autonomy, and mastery with the delivery of better, safer, and more affordable care.

Here's What Perfect Care Looks Like

Programs at three hospitals systems in the United States run by physician leaders show how to leverage intrinsic motivation to improve care: Perfect Care at the University of Utah, ProvenCare at Geisinger Health System, and AskMayoExpert at the Mayo Clinic.

The University of Utah developed a program called Value Driven Outcomes, a modern version of Codman's End Results. Its digital scorecards measure the quality and costs of care (more on costs in Chapter 5) that individual doctors provide their patients. Instead of imposing their definition of high-quality care, hospital leaders invited staff to define it for them. They asked the clinical teams: What should "Perfect Care" look like?

The orthopedic surgeons started with their most common procedures, hip and knee joint replacements. In their definition of Perfect Care, they included some nationally-defined metrics—avoiding infections and bedsores—and grudgingly conceded that satisfying Medicare's expectations and getting paid were important goals. But these weren't sufficient. For example, the surgeons knew that patients who got out of bed and walked on the day of surgery (while the anesthetic is still in effect) had speedier recoveries, they added "ambulate on day of surgery" as a condition of Perfect Care. They also insisted that all their patients be cared for on the orthopedic surgery ward, with its specialized nurses and therapists. With the right home care planning, surgeons even began to send some patients home right after surgery, without a stay in a rehabilitation facility or a nursing home. "Discharge to home" became part of Perfect Care for select patients. In the spirit of W. Edwards Deming and continuous quality improvement, the Perfect Care scorecard evolved over time, setting higher expectations with each iteration.

The orthopedic surgeons did the same for other common conditions, like broken hips and spine operations. They *voluntarily* created a standardized admission order set—the doctor's orders for every patient admitted to the hospital for a given condition—to be sure all steps would be pre-entered into the computer to automate the process. And they *voluntarily* used the same set for all surgeons. Each individual surgeon received his or her own Perfect Care scorecard, and that sparked competition. Each wanted to master, and to out-master the others, and that was good for patients and for business.

Geisinger Health System's ProvenCare similarly created standardized protocols for many common conditions. For example, the cardiac surgery team identified 40 steps for coronary artery bypass grafting, the complex operation to treat patients with blockages in their coronary arteries. These included preadmission documentation of the patient's heart function, orders for the right doses of heart drugs and antibiotics, and counseling for smokers on how to quit, for example. As in Utah, each protocol was programmed into the electronic medical systems so that orders would automatically follow the ProvenCare steps unless the physician chose to override them.

ProvenCare for CABG was a quick success—it led to better outcomes, and patients were less likely to get sick and have to return to the hospital. It was also a financial success. Geisinger estimated that it saved about $1,300 per patient.

Geisinger became so confident in the quality and consistency of its work that it agreed to a fixed price for all the care needed for operations such as CABG and spine surgery. Like the bundled payments Medicare was piloting, Geisinger's fixed price includes the presurgical evaluation, the operation, and even a 90-day "warranty": If a patient had to go back into the hospital for a complication after surgery that could have been prevented,

Geisinger would cover all the costs. Former CEO Glenn Steele said, "We shouldn't get paid if we don't do the right thing."

The doctors and their teams at the Mayo Clinic in Rochester, Minnesota, also created protocols for how to care for patients with specific conditions such as joint replacement surgery, CABG, atrial fibrillation (a heart arrhythmia), lipid management (cholesterol, LDL, HDL), heart failure, and more. To access Mayo's 115 Care Process Models (and counting) and the expertise of the doctors who developed them, dozens of hospitals across the country have joined Mayo's AskMayoExpert program. For the physicians at the Mayo Clinic who serve as Mayo's Expert Advisors, that's a satisfying way to demonstrate mastery.

AskMayoExpert isn't an End Results system yet but, like ProvenCare and Perfect Care, it's a pivotal step in defining high-quality care.

Scorecards for Prevention

For primary care physicians taking care of people in outpatient clinics, ProvenCare- or Perfect Care-type scorecards are already so extensive that following the recommended guidelines is almost impossible. For example, the top priorities on Medicare's primary care scorecard include controlling blood pressure; counseling about smoking cessation; keeping diabetic patients' blood sugars under control and checking their eyes, feet, hearts, and kidneys; counseling about weight loss; performing screening tests for breast, colon, and cervical cancers; carefully checking all medications; treating depression; and clearly communicating these, all in under ten minutes a visit. One study showed that for a typical primary care doctor with 2,500 patients under her care, it would take approximately 21.7 hours a day just to follow all the recommended acute, chronic, and preventive care guidelines, never mind discussing what's on the patients' minds.

Tom Sequist, an internal medicine physician and the chief quality and safety officer at Partners Health Care in Boston, says it could be much simpler. He argues that there are just three areas that need measuring: how good the clinicians are at making the diagnosis (this, he admits, is hard), how effectively preventive services are delivered, and how well chronic diseases are managed. Since our current approaches aren't that effective, Sequist says, maybe we should start from scratch.

He imagines things this way: If the main goals of the hypertension quality measures are to prevent a stroke or heart attack, then why not measure doctors on whether they are lowering those risks? Instead of requiring them to do smoking cessation counseling, weight-loss counseling, and exercise counseling, and to measure lipid levels (what patient can tackle all of these anyway?)—have them apply the American College of Cardiology's online risk prediction calculator, and challenge them to reduce their patient's risk in whatever way works. For example, consider a 56-year-old woman who has high blood pressure and high cholesterol (hyperlipidemia) and smokes. The prediction calculator gives her an 8% risk of heart attack or stroke in the next ten years. Lowering her blood pressure would drop that risk to 5.7%; reducing her cholesterol, 6.4%; doing both would almost halve her risk. Getting her to quit smoking alone would drop her risk to 3.5%. Sequist doesn't care which strategy the doctor and patient decide to take. He says, "However you think you can do it, just knock yourself out!" Both doctors and patients might respond better if they had the autonomy to choose, especially the patient.

The Missing Voice

In the national effort to improve quality, one set of voices has been notably missing: the patients'. Avoiding bedsores and infections might be enough for Medicare to deem a hospitalization a success, but would the patient concur? Charlie Saltzman, department chair of orthopedic surgery at the University of Utah, decided to find out. In 2013, he placed digital tablets in waiting rooms so that patients could complete the standardized surveys about how they were feeling physically, mentally, and socially. The ten-minute adaptive questionnaire asks people to rate statements like the following: "I am satisfied with my ability to do things for fun outside my home" (*Not at all* to *Very much*), "In the past 7 days I felt hopeless" (*Never* to *Always*), and "I am able to run 100 yards" (*Without any difficulty* to *Unable to do*). Every person receives a score of 0–100 for each category, such as physical function, psychological well-being, social activity, and others.

At the end of the first year, over 60,000 surveys were completed, and surgeons could begin to see patterns—a typical 67-year-old, slightly overweight man who'd had a knee replaced might be able to climb a flight of stairs, say, five weeks after the operation and get back to jogging again by twelve weeks. A similar person who had arthroscopy might recover faster, but have to stick with the exercise bike rather than running. (Eventually, this information could guide patients in deciding which treatment might be best for them.) Clinicians were also alerted to early warning signs of social isolation or depression in their patients. At the same time, these patient-reported outcomes gave surgeons another way to define whether they'd truly delivered perfect care—the patient's view.

You Can Lead a Patient to Water . . .

Besides using End Results to learn and improve, Ernest Codman hoped that publicly sharing them would drive patients to better doctors. As hard as it is to sell physicians on quality scorecards, it can be just as difficult to get patients to use them. When the New York State Health Department made End Results for heart surgery available to the public, patients still went to the better-rated and worse-rated hospitals at the same rates. Why? Because most patients followed the recommendations of their cardiologists, and those doctors didn't change their referral patterns. One-third felt the reporting on cardiac surgeons to be "not at all accurate," and only 38% reported that the information affected their selection of surgeons for their patients "very much" or "somewhat."

Patients themselves might be influenced if data were presented in more consumer-friendly ways, more relevant and accessible. For example, Medicare has a website, www.medicare.gov/hospitalcompare, that compares quality measures for most hospitals in the United States. Sure, a five-star hospital is better than a one-star hospital. But beyond that, the data are designed more for policy makers and payers than consumers. For example, if on your 50th birthday you were interested in finding the best hospital to undergo a screening colonoscopy, chances are the two quality measures on that site would not be useful for you. They report the percentage of patients who were appropriately recommended for follow-up colonoscopy three to ten years later, but they do not tell you whether the doctors found polyps or cancers in the colon, or missed them, or even how pleasant (or not unpleasant) the procedure was.

Other hospital quality scorecard programs such as Leapfrog, Vizient, U.S. News & World Report, Healthgrades, and others, provide useful data, but their scorecards all differ, and the inconsistency is confusing. Also, knowing how a hospital performs is useful, but data about each physician or team of clinicians would be more relevant for the patient-consumer.

This vital information does exist. It's buried in hospital electronic medical records and very difficult for people to access, much less interpret, their results. Ateev Mehrota, a physician turned health policy expert at Harvard Medical School, is trying to change that. He's helping to launch a competition to get technology companies to design apps that make the data usable. He reminds me that the US National Weather Service makes its extensive datasets widely available. The information can be shared with people through a wide range of channels, like television, websites, and even combined with location information to produce simple, ubiquitous weather widgets for smartphones.

Making such data accessible and usable would transform the patient experience. Imagine looking for an ob-gyn for your daughter-in-law or a dermatologist for your teenage son. An app could search all publicly available data on quality (and cost and patient satisfaction) and show you the clinics or physicians in your town with the best outcomes and lowest costs. It could even recommend those who specifically care for patients with conditions you are concerned about. It could tell you how much it will cost, depending on your health plan. Even better, maybe the app could schedule your appointment and automatically order a ride-share or taxi to get you there and back or map parking or public transit options for you.

That sounds great, and feasible, except for one hitch: few systems have that data about individual doctors readily available and are willing to share it. But they could, and should, for the sake of patients and for the clinicians. After all, it's their End Results.

Staying Expert

In his article in the *New Yorker* magazine, "Personal Best: Top Athletes and Singers Have Coaches. Should You?" Atul Gawande writes about his feeling of stagnation as a surgeon. He was in his eighth year of practice, and his own End Results data weren't getting better. An impromptu tennis lesson made him wonder why there were tennis coaches but not surgical coaches. To explore the possibility, he invited an esteemed colleague to observe him perform a routine thyroidectomy (removal of the thyroid gland in the neck). He confessed that offering himself up for criticism wasn't easy. He wrote, "I'm ostensibly an expert. I'd finished long ago with the days of being tested and observed ... Why should I expose myself to scrutiny and fault-finding?" One operation later, the answer became clear.

His mentor observed Gawande perform what *he* thought was an error-free, 86-minute operation to remove a cancerous nodule from a patient's neck. He hadn't made any mistakes, but there were opportunities to improve: Be careful that your right elbow is rising to the level of your shoulder, consider repositioning the surgical drapes so that your student and resident can assist you better, be mindful of the operating lights drifting away from the wound, and more.

In one twenty-minute session, that retired surgeon gave Gawande more feedback than he'd received in the previous eight years. He admits it can still feel awkward, but he's continued to invite his surgical coach to observe him and provide more tips. Maybe in the future, coaching and learning don't have to be uncomfortable, and maybe they can be built into everyday work.

R2D2 Meets the OR

With laparoscopic surgery, operations like hernia repairs, appendectomies, and nephrectomies (removal of a kidney) can be done through tiny incisions. Guided by a slender tool with a video camera on its end—called a laparoscope—inserted through a small incision (usually in the belly button), the surgeon can see the inside of the abdomen on a monitor in the operating room. Through another couple of small incisions—each the width of a finger—the surgeon can pass more long instruments into the abdomen with useful tiny tools like staplers or scissors on their tips that can be controlled from outside the patient. In the early 1990s, when I was a surgical intern fresh out of medical school, laparoscopic surgery was just starting to be used to remove inflamed stone-filled gallbladders. Today, increasingly the arms holding the instruments are not human, they're robotic, and the surgeon is sitting away from the patient at a video game-like console wearing goggles and controlling the robot through joystick-like devices.

These modern technologies make video cameras omnipresent in modern operating rooms, and their recordings lend themselves to learning and coaching. Surgeons watch replays of operations like professional athletes breaking down game film. They can dissect their performance, step by step. By feeding thousands of these recordings into computers, artificial intelligence and machine-learning algorithms can glean more insights. Imagine a future in which surgical technologies can provide real-time recommendations during an operation about what to avoid (cutting a nerve, inadvertently clamping the ureter or bile duct) or where to cut. They could give surgeons feedback that feels less judgmental and much more routine, timely, and helpful. They could even incorporate patient outcomes data from the electronic health record to help surgeons learn how some of their decisions in the operating room affected patient recovery later.

A Chance to QURE

Nonsurgical doctors need coaching, too. John Peabody, a physician at the University of California, San Francisco, founded a company called QURE that gives doctors in "cognitive" specialties like internal medicine, oncology, rheumatology, and cardiology a chance to test and improve their skills using patient simulations. A clinician is introduced to a virtual patient on the first screen and prompted to ask about her recent medical history, vital signs, and physical exam findings. As he would in practice he can order any imaging or diagnostic test. Once he has made the diagnosis—for example, acute pyelonephritis (kidney infection)—the doctor is prompted for treatment recommendations like what antibiotic should be prescribed. At the end of the case, the system grades the clinician's performance (on a scale of 100) and also benchmarks his score with his peers. Each case concludes with a review of recommended guidelines.

Peabody and his colleagues at QURE have demonstrated that physicians who go through these case studies perform better in actual practice. They order fewer unnecessary tests and procedures and save money. Imagine if this coaching could take place with real patients in real time within electronic health records (more on this in Chapter 9).

For the visual specialties like radiology, computer vision powered by artificial intelligence can coach doctors in real time. For example, consider the interpretation of chest CT ("CAT") scans. Under current guidelines, about 6.8 million people in the United States are supposed to undergo an annual chest CT scan because they've had a long history of heavy smoking and are at higher risk for developing lung cancer. Cancers look like small white dots on a sea of white crisscrossing lines and dots (the blood vessels and airways in lung tissue). Imagine doing "Where's Waldo" puzzles *all* day (mixed with short intervals of dictating into the computer where you found Waldo) and you've essentially understood the life of a radiologist tasked with reading these scans. (And don't forget to add the pressure that someone's life may depend on your ability to find Waldo.) As primary care doctors start to recommend screening CT scans more consistently (only about 4% of heavy smokers have had the scan so far), the potential workload for interpreting these studies is daunting.

By highlighting suspicious dots automatically, commercial computer-assisted diagnosis programs can support radiologists in their search, and they can probably do it more reliably. It's also likely that they will soon be able to distinguish between cancerous and noncancerous nodules, like scars from prior infections. When it's not provoking fears of future unemployment, the support can be welcomed, especially if it makes them better doctors and relieves them of tedious work.

The Action Plan for Codifying Codman

Ernest Codman's greatest hope was for physicians to get better at their craft by learning from each other *and* their End Results. A hospital that routinely extracts End Results from its electronic health data can help its doctors, nurses, and their teams learn and improve. Artificial intelligence could accelerate the pace of change. Learning health systems are figuring out that higher quality care is not only better for the patients, it's better for their businesses. Fewer complications, fewer readmissions, and shorter stays in the hospital all cost less. Those savings can, in turn, be invested into more improvement. When End Results are shared publicly, as Codman always hoped, patients can reward high performers with more business. It becomes a virtuous cycle, and we all get better.

To develop a learning health system we all have a role to play:

As a patient and consumer of health care, you should:

- Provide feedback about your health care experiences, especially whether the outcomes of your care or your loved ones' care met your expectations.
- Use trusted online web tools like Leapfrog or Medicare's online Hospital Compare tool to look at the quality and safety records of medical facilities you are considering for care.

As a physician or other health care professional, you should:

- Expect from your hospitals and clinics routine feedback on your individual and team performance.
- Refer patients to physicians and facilities that have high ratings on quality, outcomes, and affordability.

As a payer, such as a self-insured employer, government entity, or health plan, you should:

- Demand that your health care facilities and individual clinicians establish ways to assess quality and outcomes and share them in a timely fashion with clinicians and with you.
- Expect health systems to factor in patient-reported outcomes in their assessments of performance. These should include measures of physical, mental, and social well-being and incorporate the patient's health expectations.

As a policy maker, you should:

- Make sure part of the accrediting and national oversight of hospitals and physicians includes how favorable the environment is to learning and improvement.
- Expect that clinician training and coaching, whether by peers or through electronic teaching or artificial intelligence-assisted methods, are a part of continued licensure for physicians and other health care professionals.

And most important, all of us need to elect leaders who encourage the public sharing of quality and outcomes data about both facilities and individual physicians (and insist on accurate risk adjustment so sicker patients aren't neglected).

CHAPTER 6

THE PRICE ISN'T RIGHT

For a field in which high cost is an overarching problem, the absence of accurate cost information in health care is nothing short of astounding.

—Michael E. Porter and Thomas H. Lee

The day after Labor Day 2015 was a quiet one for news . . . except in my office. Journalist Gina Kolata had written a front-page story in the *New York Times* with the headline: *What Are a Hospital's Costs? Utah System Is Trying to Learn.* The article highlighted our efforts to rein in costs by measuring the costs of care for every patient and every doctor in our hospital. It was the most emailed *New York Times* story of the day, and the university's email inboxes were swamped with requests for more information from other hospitals, insurers, state governments, and more: *Could you explain how you measured costs? Could you meet with our legislature? Could our team visit your hospital to learn more? What state is Utah in?*

Amid the hundreds of inquiries, one stood out. It came from Dr. John Wong, chief executive of National University Health System of Singapore, the top health system in a country that many health policy experts believe has the best health care in the world. An American-trained oncologist, Wong asked if we would welcome him and his team for a visit.

Wong told me that despite their impressive statistics, the Singaporean government was deeply worried. At the time, the average Singaporean lived four years longer than the average American, even though the island nation was spending about one-fourth as much on health care per person. But the Ministry of Health budget was growing at double-digit rates, and with an aging population and a workforce shortage leading to high labor costs, health spending was expected to rise to 6% of their GDP—a 30% increase. We found his concerns almost laughable, since that would still be only one-third of what the United States spends, but there was an urgency in his voice. Before a month had lapsed, he and 23 members of his leadership team arrived in Salt Lake City, tablets and laptops in hand, ready to learn.

The Sick Elephant in the Room

The next time you visit your doctor, ask her how much your care costs. Ask how much the flu vaccine costs or the X-ray or blood test or your last hospital stay. She won't have a good answer. First, she may assume you are asking about the *price*—how much you, your insurance, or Medicare will pay. Most doctors won't know, unless they are in cosmetic dermatology, dentistry, or cosmetic plastic surgery, for example, where patients pay cash. (Those doctors may even post their prices online, just like at the beauty salon or barber.)

Most doctors will explain that they can't really know how much you're going to pay because it's impossible for them to keep track—insurance companies have so many plans with different deductibles and co-pays. Fair enough.

Instead, ask her not the price, but how much it costs her clinic to provide your care. How much does it cost *them* to give you that flu shot or blood test? It's not an unreasonable question. Every business, from Jiffy Lube to the neighborhood deli to GM, knows how much it costs to deliver the products and services on their menus—whether it's an oil change, a pastrami on rye, or a full-loaded Yukon truck. (In accounting terms, that's the costs of goods or services sold).

Does it cost her medical group $5 or $50 or $500 to care for you during a single visit? She won't know. Her boss won't know. Her boss's boss won't know. Even the CFO won't know.

And they're not the only ones stumbling around in the dark. I've asked thousands of physicians and other professionals, "Do you know what it costs to provide health care for each of your patients?" It's rare that a single hand goes up. They don't know how much it costs to run the MRI scanner or the echocardiography machine. They don't know how much every minute a patient stays in the emergency department or intensive care unit costs. They mostly don't know how much the drugs they prescribe cost—what *they* pay or what *you* pay. The prescription pads and medical orders they fill out have no prices on them.

Let this astonishing situation sink in, and consider its implications. The individuals responsible for most of the spending decisions—Generic or branded drug? Imaging study or a blood test? Coronary catheter brand A or brand B?—have no idea what the bill is for any of that. It's as if you are shopping in a grocery store where nothing has a price tag on it. And you won't get your final bill until six months after you've eaten what you bought that day.

Maybe you don't want doctors to know all those costs because you want the very best care, regardless of price. Maybe you think the "at any cost" approach is great because you are covered by insurance. You're wrong. Eventually, you pay that bill. We all do. (Remember the surf 'n' turf trap in Chapter 1?) In fact, you may pay two or three times: employer-based insurance comes out of your paycheck (and is subsidized by your taxes), your co-payments and deductibles come out of your wallet, and government-based care comes directly out of your taxes.

That's why it's important for you, me, and all of us to get costs down. And to do that, we all—patients, doctors, hospitals, and insurers—must know what everything truly costs, because we can't manage what we can't measure.

Sticker-Shock Therapy

Harvard Business School professors Michael Porter and Bob Kaplan marveled at how obvious the problem was to them in an article titled "The Big Idea: How to Solve the Cost Crisis in Health Care," where they wrote, "Accurately measuring costs and outcomes is the single most powerful lever we have today for transforming the economics of health care."

In Salt Lake City, we set out to build that lever (and later got Porter and Kaplan to help).

We had a rudimentary understanding of our costs at the University of Utah. The hospital knew overall how much it spent on labor (over half of all costs), supplies (like catheters and oxygen monitors), and contracts with service providers (like laboratory testing companies). It knew how much it cost to build a wing or a clinic and how much it cost to run the cafeterias. One huge problem: All that information was calculated at the department level—nursing, obstetrics, intensive care units—and averaged across all patients and doctors. That averaging made the numbers meaningless because it hid differences and erased the power to motivate individuals to change how they did things. Charlton Park, then the leader of the team of hospital analysts, summarized the data challenges for me: "It was just useless. It never left the finance department ... it wasn't actionable." His colleague Cheri Hunter, who oversaw the data warehouse, agreed. "People didn't see data in a way that was clinically relevant," she said.

That realization motivated one analyst, Cary Martin, to think about how to calculate the costs of care for *each* patient. It was a bold idea, and fortunately, he had a head start on the problem. About 20 years earlier, Jim Livingston, chief technology officer, had started designing one of the nation's first data warehouses for the hospitals and clinics. It automatically captured, organized, and stored detailed data about how the University of Utah was caring for every one of its patients: how many minutes people were spending in the emergency room, operating room, or intensive care unit; what laboratory tests were ordered or drugs prescribed; which therapists, doctors, and nurses were caring for each of them. If he could assign a cost to each of those components (How much was a minute in the operating room? How much did the surgeon's time cost?), he would be able to total up the costs of care for each patient's visit or stay.

Martin started with an estimate Medicare used, called a cost-to-charge ratio. This rough calculation starts with the amount the hospital bills Medicare and then applies a fixed fraction, say 0.8, to estimate what it actually cost to produce the service. It wasn't anywhere close to perfect. Martin knew he could make it better. He just needed some coconspirators.

Fortunately, Ken Kawamoto, a brilliant informatician (and doctor) was eager to join Martin's crusade. He and the chief medical quality officer, Bob Pendleton, had told physicians that they were ordering too many unnecessary lab tests and echocardiograms and overprescribing antibiotics. The doctors ignored them. Kawamoto thought he could get their attention by accurately measuring costs for each doctor and showing them how much their overordering was wasting. He also knew that getting doctors to adopt more consistent protocols would cut costs, reduce mistakes, and improve patient outcomes.

What's a Gauze Pad Worth?

To do what Martin, Pendleton, and Kawamoto wanted, the system needed to itemize the cost of every step of care for every consultation, procedure, and operation. It was a monumental undertaking that would require talented people from across the organization: biomedical informatics, information technology, decision support, finance, quality and safety, and clinicians. Toward the end of a six-month blitz fueled by late-night pizza and Diet Coke, the team produced version 1.0 of a program they called "Value Driven Outcomes," consisting of 135 million rows of data accounting for every element of clinical care necessary for any kind of patient visit. A knee replacement wasn't just one line on that costing table; it aggregated 1,300 costs in 20 categories, from surgical supplies (gauze pads) to facilities costs (operating room time) to labor expenses (physical therapists, nurses, and physicians, including the surgeon, anesthesiologist, and hospitalists).

With this tool, the system could calculate the costs of care for every one of the 1.7 million patient visits to the University of Utah hospitals and clinics each year.

Looking at the itemized costs in the Value Driven Outcomes tool reminded me of when we discovered as children that snowflakes are six-sided crystals or that butterfly wings are scaly. It was so unexpected, so granular, and so beautiful. We learned that each minute in the emergency department cost us 82 cents. Each minute in the surgical intensive care unit was $1.43. Each minute in each operating room for an orthopedic operation cost a whopping $12. And these were just the costs to run them; they didn't cover the opportunity costs—the revenue that could have been collected had the operating room been busy, which can be multiples more. For the operating rooms that tended to start 15–20 minutes late each morning, putting a price on that tardiness was a powerful motivator to be more efficient. Martin and Kawamoto were right. Capturing specific cost dollars did grab everyone's attention. After all, who wanted to start each morning having already wasted thousands of dollars?

Taking a Scalpel to Costs

The Value Driven Outcomes tool arrived just in time. Medicare was launching the Bundled Payments for Care Improvement pilot project that would pay hospitals and doctors a flat fee for each patient who underwent either a hip or knee replacement. If surgeons and hospitals could keep costs below the bundled payment price and meet quality standards, they could pocket the difference. If not, they were on the hook for the overages.

Utah's orthopedic surgeons realized they could use the Value Driven Outcomes tools to handicap those bundled payments. And what they uncovered shocked them. Like an archaeological dig, every layer of costs in the joint replacement "excavation" revealed more differences and more opportunity. For the eight surgeons who performed routine hip and knee replacements, the overall costs of care—what it cost the hospital to care for patients—could differ by thousands of dollars for each patient, and the procedures varied in every possible way: type of artificial joint used, time in the operating room, pain medications prescribed, laboratory tests ordered, number of days in the hospital, and more. Each surgeon had his or her own way of doing what should have been the same operation because they had trained in different hospitals with different mentors. (Medicine still embraces the apprenticeship model.) Their instructors had taught them to replace a hip using a specific brand of artificial joint, using a specific protocol, and that's what they brought with them to Utah.

We knew that if we were going to get better, safer, and cheaper care, we needed to standardize all this. But we also knew that we'd never get our doctors to change how they'd done things their entire career just because we asked them to, even if it would save money. We need to help them see this would make them better doctors and tap into their intrinsic motivation.

Change Is Great, but You Go First . . .

Most physicians hate to talk about the costs of care. The sanctity of the doctor-patient relationship feels violated by such pedestrian money talk. What most of them care about is that their patients get better. Aside from the perverse incentives of fee-for-service medicine, they are taught to order whatever they think the patient *needs* — drugs, laboratory tests, imaging studies, even operations—never mind the price tag. That's why both the Utah and Singaporean teams didn't start their Value Driven Outcomes initiatives by talking with their doctors about money. They started with patient outcomes. They took the hospital-wide quality measures and made personal scorecards so that each physician could see how his or her patients compared with other doctors like them. The differences were revealing.

For example, patients at the University of Utah who had their hips or knees replaced in the late afternoons didn't seem to have as good outcomes as early morning patients. It turns out the afternoon patients were arriving on the hospital floor after the physical therapists had gone home for the day and were not getting the chance to walk on the day of surgery. Consequently, on average, they were healing more slowly and staying in the hospital longer than expected. This was an easy problem to solve. The hospital moved some of the physical therapists to a second, later shift. Within weeks, all patients were getting out of bed on the day of surgery. They did better. And the hospital did better—reducing costs by more than 10%.

Taken together, the outcomes data and the cost data told a compelling story. It was obvious that bad patient outcomes were more expensive. They resulted in longer stays in the hospital, extra tests and procedures, and higher risks of having to come back to the hospital after discharge. *Higher* quality led to *lower* costs. The lowest-cost physicians were among the best, unlike cars, and unlike theater tickets.

It was also obvious that there were needless and wasteful variations in how care was provided. For example, Utah's orthopedic surgeons were struck by the differences in the prices of commonly used artificial hips— the most expensive was three times the cost of the least expensive, yet patients did not do better with the pricier implants. Armed with data, the surgeons complained to the manufacturers and in some cases secured lower prices. In other cases, they asked colleagues to teach them how to operate using a less-expensive artificial joint. It was collegial and voluntary.

Many decisions in the hospital were made easier with the outcomes and costing data. When the analytics team showed that a $15 asthma inhaler worked as well for most patients as a more popular new one that cost $200, it was easy to persuade the doctors to change. "We can . . . have a 15-minute conversation between physicians, and within two days we can change care delivery to save several hundred thousand dollars a year," said Chief Medical Quality Officer Bob Pendleton. "We're just talking about one tiny grain of sand in the beach of opportunity."

That Job Is Beneath You

Harvard Business School's Bob Kaplan is one of the fathers of cost-accounting. Having made a career out of helping companies like John Deere and Siemens run more efficiently, and hence, more profitably, he had thought that his cost-accounting work was mostly done. Then his colleague

Michael Porter persuaded him to look at health care. He did and was flummoxed by what he saw.

When I first met Kaplan in 2014, he was lecturing at a course with Porter on "Value-Based Care" at Harvard Business School. He told the classroom full of eager hospital CEOs that the opportunities for them to reduce costs and increase profits in a pay-for-results environment ("value-based care") were bountiful. In every hospital he visited, he saw surgeons hunting around for medical charts or calling up pharmacies to clarify prescriptions. These highly trained professionals were doing the work of a medical assistant or an aide. He also saw huge variation in the range of costs—more than two-fold—that even the busiest of hospitals incurred to perform a standard operation, such as a total joint replacement. In describing this, his voice rose. He seemed disbelieving that such simple problems could be so easily identified and fixed.

Kaplan lasered in on personnel costs because that was where the opportunities were the greatest. Labor consumes over half of all health care costs, and Kaplan knew that assigning the right jobs to the right employees, and eliminating tasks that did not lead to better patient outcomes, could save most hospitals millions of dollars. He explained the calculations in simple terms: To approximate the cost of an employee's time, first calculate all the expenses associated with that person: his or her compensation and benefits, a pro rata share of costs related to supervising the individual, the costs of equipment and information technology, space, and others. Then estimate the total amount of time the employee has to do his or her work: starting with 365 days a year and deducting weekends, vacations, sick days, and so on, and multiplying the number of days by the number of hours available for work each day. Divide the total expenses by the total amount of time, and Kaplan says, you have a "capacity cost rate" for that individual, in dollars per minute, for example.

As a rough estimate, Kaplan suggests this quick shortcut: start by estimating the person's annual salary plus benefits and then divide that number by 100,000 to arrive at an approximate cost per minute. A typical nurse, paid $82,000 in salary and benefits, costs about $0.82 per minute to do his or her job; a cardiac surgeon, $8.80 per minute; a medical assistant, $0.37 per minute.

Any job done by a nurse that can be shifted to a medical assistant—tracking down supplies, double-checking computer documentation, or bathing a patient—could save $0.45 per minute (or $27 per hour) and reduce labor costs by more than half. Any task performed by a cardiac surgeon that could be managed by a nurse—changing a wound dressing or removing stitches—could save around $8 per minute (or $480 per hour). Having a medical assistant help a surgeon track down old X-rays or type laboratory test results in the electronic medical record could save even more. Best of all, having each person doing what they're trained to do —nurses with patients, surgeons in the operating room—makes them happier and more satisfied.

This exercise inevitably leads to an obvious observation: there wouldn't be so much to save if there weren't such large salary differences. Kaplan, an expert in labor costs, says the gap between the highest- and lowest-paid working professionals in health care is the largest he's seen in any industry, except maybe professional sports teams.

Improving Your Image

When it comes to highly compensated physicians driving up the costs of care, radiologists have long borne the brunt of this criticism. (One friend used to call my profession "Radi-holiday.") Radiologists are a little defensive and quick to point out that imaging science has radically transformed medicine. Guided by MRIs or CT ("CAT") scans, people who suffer strokes can now be treated with clot-dissolving medicine and recover completely. Whole body PET scans can spot and track metastases from head to toe in a single scan. Despite the gibes, general internist physicians rated CT and MRI as the most important medical inventions of the prior century, above coronary artery bypass surgery and hip replacements.

The widespread reliance on expensive imaging technologies has, however, come at a high cost. At their peak, in 2006, imaging costs consumed 13% of all Medicare expenses. Most people think imaging is expensive because of the technology. After all, when was the last time you saw a CT scanner or MRI machine at a garage sale? But that's not the real reason. The truth is that the prices of scans are set at whatever hospitals have been able to negotiate for them (rather like some drug pricing, as we'll see in Chapter 8). When Medicare and insurance companies pushed back, reimbursement rates tumbled. By 2012, imaging costs fell to only 2.1% of Medicare expenses, mostly through reduced payments.

To maintain their businesses, radiologists had two choices: either perform and interpret more scans (the default option in a pay-for-action world) or match declining revenues with lower expenses. University of Utah's department of radiology decided to study the latter, starting with one of the most popular studies, CT scan of the abdomen and pelvis.

The abdominopelvic CT scan is like the Swiss Army knife of radiology. It helps doctors find kidney stones, characterize abdominal cancers and their spread, and spot the telltale swollen worm-like appendage that marks the diagnosis of appendicitis, to name a few examples. Looking at how much it cost to perform an abdominopelvic scan, University of Utah radiologist Yoshimi Anzai and colleagues discovered that the CT scanner costs made up only 6% of the total costs. Another 14% went for the supplies (the contrast material or "dye," intravenous catheter, and syringe, among others). Surprisingly, the overwhelming portion—80% of costs—were to cover personnel: the radiologist who interpreted the images (40%) and the technologist and nurse (another 40%) who operated the scanner and looked after the patient.

In theory, the radiologist should have taken about 10–15 minutes per scan, reviewing the images and dictating the findings into the electronic medical record. However, like the surgeons tracking down old X-rays, the radiologist was spending time calling up the doctor who ordered the study to ask questions that should have been answered in advance, like: Why was the study ordered? Or she was searching for previous scans to determine whether the cancer had grown. Or hunting down a relevant laboratory test result. With radiologists costing about $5.80 per minute, these amounted to the biggest unnecessary costs.

More effective and interoperable electronic health records should obviate some of this drudgery (more in Chapter 9). Until then, it's worth noting that while physician assistants and medical assistants are common in surgery and cardiology, they have yet to make an appearance in radiology. Maybe now is the time.

It's a Wonderful Paycheck

Many health care professionals are highly paid (especially doctors, dentists, and administrators). Analysis of 2016 data showed that the average generalist physician in the United States made $218,173 a year, double the average of generalists in ten other high-income countries (including the Netherlands, UK, Canada, Australia, and Germany). Specialists averaged $316,000, also higher than in any of those nations. US nurses also make more than their international peers, averaging more than $74,000 per year compared to $42,000–$65,000.

Across the board, wages for physicians, dentists, and nurses in the United States have risen over the past 50 years, in parallel with soaring health care costs. While high salaries undoubtedly worsen the US health care crisis, the impact on the economics is not that big. Health care economist Uwe Reinhardt showed in 2007 that higher salaries added about 2% to total national health care spending. Nevertheless, drivers of higher wages are important to understand.

One built-in expense for physicians is the high cost of medical litigation in the United States. Malpractice insurance varies significantly by specialty and by geography. Obstetricians typically pay between $100,000 and $200,000 per year for professional liability insurance. In Nassau County, New York, obstetricians paid on average $214,999 in 2017, while those in Illinois paid $177,441. Surgeons have lower malpractice premiums than the obstetricians. Internists pay the least—their annual premiums averaged $20,000 to $40,000, depending on the state.

Malpractice premiums in California are the lowest in the nation across all specialties. That's partly because the Medical Injury Compensation

Reform Act of 1975 limits noneconomic damages awarded by juries in California to $250,000, and it also caps plaintiff attorney's fees.

Medical school (and undergraduate) debt is another factor driving expectations of higher compensation. The Association of American Medical Colleges reports that about three-quarters of all medical students graduate with debt, and the median amount of debt was $200,000 in 2018. Medical school is expensive—the average cost for public schools for four years of training is $243,902; for private schools, it's $322,767. There is another pernicious factor here: graduating with significant debt motivates some students to pursue more lucrative specialties and shun areas of greatest need like pediatrics, family medicine, geriatrics, and internal medicine, professions that are most needed in a pay-for-results world.

Another factor is the shortage of doctors in the United States, which is expected to worsen as the population ages and physicians retire early. The shortages may be partially mitigated as pay-for-results systems evolve into team-based care models and employ more nurses, pharmacists, medical assistants, health coaches, and social workers. As in many other industries, the artificial intelligence revolution will gradually redistribute the work among health care professionals. My specialty, radiology, might be one of the first to experience this radical change.

Doing Good *and* Doing Well

Over the period from 2013 to 2015, fueled in part by Value Driven Outcomes initiatives, the University of Utah health system reduced expenses and doubled its operating margin to 10%, considerably better than the national average of 2%–3%. It shared some of the savings with the teams who'd made it happen, like the orthopedic surgeons and hospitalists. As a nod to physician autonomy, administrators let the physicians choose how to spend their share, provided they didn't use the funds for their own compensation.

How did the doctors elect to spend the savings? They hired more medical assistants to help them type notes in the electronic medical records.

They hired research assistants to do more quality-improvement work (like the project to ensure that all patients walked right after surgery). They traveled to national conferences to share their results with others. In short, they used the savings to make their lives more manageable, to generate more savings, and to provide better care.

Feeling more confident about managing costs and quality, Utah doctors also began to view Medicare's bundled payment pilot projects more positively. Getting paid for results instead of for action was starting to look like a survivable path forward for both the hospital and for our doctors, and maybe one that might even help them succeed and provide better care.

The National University Health System of Singapore saw similarly impressive results. After their Utah visit, they developed their own version of Value Driven Outcomes and used the tool to standardize care. After three years of working on areas like better care for patients with heart attacks, pneumonia, hip fractures, gout, and cataracts, among more than 40 others, their efforts have proven successful. Between 2016 and 2019 they saved about 7% in costs. That was lower than the rate of savings we got in Utah, but they were still celebrating. And to be fair, they were already one of the lowest-cost systems in the developed world; they didn't have as much fat to trim. Buoyed by their success, the Singapore Ministry of Health announced one year into this effort that the measurement of costs and quality would be required across all hospitals in the country.

The Action Plan for Collaring Costs

In a new pay-for-results world, it's vital to engage physicians and hospitals in improving outcomes and costs in ways that are intrinsically motivating. Better care results in shorter stays, fewer mistakes and complications, and fewer readmissions. Higher quality often means lower costs. How we engage the most important people of all—the patients—presents the ultimate challenge and opportunity in the journey from paying for action to paying for results.

To reduce the costs of care, we all have a role to play.

As a patient and consumer of health care, you should:

- Ask your physician if she knows what it costs to care for you—what you will be charged, and what it actually costs her system to provide that care.

As a hospital leader, physician, or other health care professional, you should:

- Measure costs and outcomes for each patient, and make that information available to all your clinicians. Consider making it available to the patient and the public.
- Evaluate variations in patient outcomes and in costs of care across physicians, benchmarked where possible. Challenge each other to reduce unwarranted variation.
- Evaluate your labor force and consider whether additional medical assistants or other types of health care professionals should join the care team.

As a payer, such as a self-insured employer, government entity, or health plan, or as a policy maker, you should:

- Demand that all health care businesses quantify both patient outcomes and the costs of care at the individual clinician level, and at the clinic or hospital level.
- Develop incentives to reduce variation in how care is provided, and encourage clinicians to practice according to recommended guidelines.
- Consider loan-forgiveness models to alleviate the debt of students who choose to become primary care practitioners and mental health clinicians and serve in underserved geographies.

And most important, all of us need to elect leaders who are committed to improving quality and lowering the costs of care.

CHAPTER 7

FROM CARING TO COPRODUCING

We need to embrace the reality that doctors and clinics don't provide care. The parents, family members, caregivers, and patients themselves provide care.

—Justin Masterson

It was 2008, and poor patient ratings placed the University of Utah hospitals and clinics in the bottom quartile nationally in patient satisfaction. Seething letters of complaint were stacked on CEO Lorris Betz's desk, and neighbors accosted him in the grocery store to rage about a five-hour wait in the emergency department or a battle with a grumpy receptionist at the clinic. Betz's wife had suffered a kidney stone, which had launched a series of encounters with the medical system that had infuriated them both: an hourlong wait for the radiologist to confirm the kidney stone on her CT ("CAT") scan that the radiology resident had seen immediately; the three-hour wait for her lithotripsy procedure to shatter the recalcitrant stone; the urologist who performed the procedure and yet never introduced himself (much less apologized for the delay); and the calls to the clinic that went unanswered.

His wife's kidney stone debacle was the last straw. The CEO had finally had enough.

The Exceptional Patient Experience

Betz invited his system's leaders to his home for a retreat. He challenged them to rethink their roles: No matter how great doctors thought they were, he said, "Medical care can only be truly great if the *patient* thinks it is." He articulated a new expectation for his team: everyone who received care from the University of Utah would leave feeling that they had received extraordinary care. Everyone would have an "Exceptional Patient Experience."

Betz set the university hospital on a completely new course that required reimagining every element of the patient experience, every step of care. Examples of exceptional customer service in health care were so rare that his team turned to exemplars in other industries, like the Apple store and In-N-Out Burger. They noted how those businesses collected meticulous measures of customer engagement and satisfaction and used them to power continuous improvement.

The Utah team designed a questionnaire to do the same. They asked patients: Did the physicians communicate clearly? Did you feel a part of the decision-making process? Did you feel respected? Did you wait longer than expected? Would you recommend your physician to a friend? They carefully avoided topics that physicians had little control over, like food and parking. (Separately, the hospital invested in free valet parking and a la carte room service.)

The hospital mailed (or emailed) surveys to patients right after each clinic visit or hospital stay. To encourage candor, they promised that the feedback would remain anonymous. By using questions from a commercial question bank, responses for Utah doctors could be compared to those for 100,000 other doctors in the national database. In addition to receiving raw scores (on a scale of 1 to 5), doctors also were told what percentile their patient satisfaction scores placed them when compared to peers nationally. That stoked a competitive drive that was powerfully motivating for Betz's doctors.

Where Everyone Is Well above Average

Once the surveys were collected, the team knew the feedback could have the power to motivate change. At the same time, they realized they were sitting on a potential powder keg. Physicians genuinely believe they are well above average and don't always take criticism well. Negative feedback could backfire—it could make them more defensive, more hostile, less inclined to change. (Plus, with the national shortage of physicians, any disgruntled doctor could easily find a new job if he or she was irked by patient surveys.) The team had to manage these results very carefully.

In the beginning, the Exceptional Patient Experience team distributed patient satisfaction scores confidentially and individually. Only physicians and their clinic teams could view their patients' scores and comments. Jim Ashworth, the new head of child and adolescent psychiatry, appreciated that discretion. In the beginning, his patients scored him poorly—at the *bottom* 1 percentile in patient satisfaction, compared to other doctors like him in the United States. It wasn't that they didn't like him—they just didn't like the way his office ran. Many were frustrated at the long waits in the waiting room, the lack of communication from the staff, and the lack of coordination among staff members.

Instead of dismissing that carping, Ashworth saw it as invaluable feedback. "We really only have one chance with some of these patients," he said. The surveys gave him and his team a way to get feedback quickly about their efforts to make the clinic a happier place for his adolescent patients, like a new training program for receptionists or a new template for scheduling clinic appointments. Within six months, Ashworth's scores were better than 90% of his peers nationally. The staff in his division vied for the top ratings. "Everyone wants to be *the* star employee," said Ashworth's chief administrator, Ross VanVranken. Within a year, the entire psychiatric hospital was in the top 5% of all psychiatric hospitals in the United States. VanVranken said, "It's like a love fest around here. It's really a team deal."

Stories of exceptional performance spread, and teams sought to replicate the successes of superstars such as Ashworth and Norm Zabriskie, the university's glaucoma expert. Zabriskie could see up to 80 patients a day in his ophthalmology clinic and still average a score of 4.8 out of 5 on patient satisfaction. A self-described "efficiency freak," Zabriskie worked with five ophthalmic technicians who took the time to talk with each patient, not just about their eyesight, but about new grandbabies and other important matters. His waiting room was almost always empty because patients were seen as soon as they arrived. They didn't feel like they were on a conveyor belt because they got personalized care.

Across the hospitals and clinics, satisfaction scores improved for almost all clinicians, and it began to feel safer to share the ratings more publicly. Satisfaction score charts appeared on a hallway bulletin board, anonymized—"Dr. A, Dr. B, Dr. C, Dr. D . . ."—so a cardiologist, for instance, would know where he or she ranked within the department. A few months later, real names started to show up on those charts, and before long, the dermatologists could compare themselves to the orthopedic surgeons and cardiologists. And they did.

Within a year, about one-quarter of all physicians at the University of Utah were in the top 10 percentile nationally, and over 10% were in the top 1 percentile in patient satisfaction. By the time I joined the University of Utah in 2011, glowing reviews from patients had become the norm. Then one of our pancreatic surgeons had a conversation with her friend that set us on a new path.

Think YELP with a Stethoscope

Courtney Scaife spends her time in the operating room removing deadly tumors embedded in the pancreas, a gland that, other than producing hormones like insulin, is primarily a factory and storage space for enzymes. As the chemicals that help digest food, enzymes are not finicky—they digest anything they touch. Any damage to the pancreas—from a car accident or an operation—that inadvertently spills those enzymes out of their safe pancreatic stores can wreak havoc in the body. It's tough to be a great pancreatic surgeon.

When, at her friend's suggestion, Scaife searched online for information about her performance as a surgeon, she was shocked: A commercial physician rating site had three anonymous, nasty comments about her. "My vet has more compassion," wrote one.

Thanks to the university's survey system, Scaife had received hundreds of anonymized patient survey responses and was accustomed to being praised for being a thoughtful and considerate cancer doctor who was "very thorough in answering my questions ... alleviated many of the fears I had." Criticisms mostly arose when that thoroughness took longer for some patients than their scheduled time, making the clinic run behind; one patient cautioned, "Be prepared to have a long wait." In terms of compassion, patients were consistently positive, writing that Scaife had "put me at ease," and was "very kind and informative." Some patients were effusive in their praise: "Dr. Scaife was awesome."

Although the commercial online comments didn't necessarily come from real patients—anyone could post a comment or rate her on that site—Scaife knew that potential patients, trainees, or recruits who searched her online might take them seriously. With the determination of a cancer surgeon, Scaife asked hospital leaders to post all her patient scores and feedback online. She was willing to post every comment—positive or negative—as long as it was from a verified patient.

Her request prompted heated discussions in my office and across the hospital. Many of Scaife's colleagues were not as eager to share this information. Not everyone felt comfortable with the world reading unfiltered critical feedback about them. On the other hand, many of us knew the information would be valuable to our patients and would show our community how seriously we took their feedback. After nearly six months of discussions and a few lively townhalls, I approved her request. In December 2012, the University of Utah became the first hospital in the nation to post patient satisfaction scores and feedback on the web. We never imagined its impact.

Unexpected Perks Percolating

After the scores were posted, web traffic for the University of Utah Health nearly doubled. Community leaders put pressure on the other hospitals in town to collect and post their results. Health systems from across the country consulted and visited us—Cleveland Clinic, Stanford, Geisinger Health, Wake Forest Baptist Health and Piedmont Health in North Carolina, and Northshore LIJ Health (renamed Northwell Health) in New York, for example—and after a couple of years, they and others began to share their patient feedback online, too.

Online search tools like Google prioritize websites that have real consumer feedback in large numbers. Our patient satisfaction scores were just that. When people searched online for an obstetrician, internist, or cancer surgeon, University of Utah physicians consistently appeared at the top of search results. More patients than ever sought care at our facilities.

Besides driving more business to the university, improved patient satisfaction also meant fewer malpractice suits. Malpractice premiums declined during the first five years of the Exceptional Patient Experience, despite having more doctors and more business. Patients also got better care—improved communication and decision making probably helped. From 2011 on, the hospital consistently ranked each year in the top ten in quality and safety of all teaching hospitals in the country.

Five years after the start of the Exceptional Patient Experience journey (and one year after we began posting patient comments), physician satisfaction scores reached new highs—half of our clinicians were in the top 10 percentile nationally (ordinarily, you would expect only one in ten to have that ranking). One-quarter of all our clinicians were in the top 1 percentile (99th percentile or above). In some of our clinics, every doctor was in the top 1 percentile in patient satisfaction.

Best of all, these results sustained themselves—without much tending. The university achieved significantly improved patient satisfaction without offering any financial incentives to the doctors. Their reward was all that positive feedback, more patients coming to them for care, and a strong sense of personal satisfaction in knowing that they were, indeed, well above average.

The Anti-Ratings Leaders

Nationally, the patient satisfaction movement has made uneven progress. While the University of Utah was rolling out its Exceptional Patient Experience initiative for outpatient clinic visits, the national inpatient satisfaction movement took a different turn.

In 2008, Medicare threatened hospitals with a 2% cut in payments if they did not start collecting patient satisfaction surveys (Hospital Consumer Assessment of Healthcare Providers and Systems, HCAHPS or "H-caps"). Within one year, over 90% were participating. The inpatient questions cover important topics, such as communication with nurses and doctors, pain management, responsiveness of hospital staff, cleanliness and quietness of the hospital environment, communication about medications, discharge information, and willingness to recommend the hospital. These patient ratings influence the amount hospitals are paid and also their public scorecards (whether they are a one- to five-star facility, according to Medicare, for example).

Many physicians are still skeptical about the effects of these mandatory surveys on patient care. They point to medical literature suggesting that emphasizing patient satisfaction can worsen overtreatment and overprescribing because physicians are placed at the mercy of unreasonable patient demands. Some policy makers blame the emphasis on pain management in HCAHPS surveys (and in hospital accreditation reviews) for the rise of opioid overprescribing and the subsequent addiction crisis. (Those questions about pain were removed from HCAHPS surveys in October 2019.) Other studies, including ours from the University of Utah and a Harvard study, showed that high patient satisfaction correlates with better health outcomes for patients. Why the difference?

A thoughtful analysis by researchers at Duke University explained that patient satisfaction initiatives can lead to better care if they are implemented in the right way. They say surveys need to be specific and ask about a particular visit to the clinic or hospitalization. They need to be timely (within days of the experience) and focus on the patient-doctor relationship (not on food, parking, or amenities). The feedback is especially valuable when questions focus on things that seem to influence the quality of patient care, such as communication and shared decision making.

HCAHPS questions fall short of these expectations. Instead of every doctor getting direct and timely feedback about their performance, the surveys sample a random set of patients in each hospital, and only the hospital gets an overall rating, not each clinician. The surveys aren't timely: sometimes they are completed several weeks after a visit. Finally, these and other surveys are often tied to compensation penalties for physicians. Bringing money into the situation can "crowd out" the intrinsic motivation to be a great doctor.

When done right, patient feedback can motivate doctors to deliver better care and sometimes even bring joy and delight back to the practice of medicine. In Utah, we encouraged our teams to take the Exceptional Patient Experience thinking one step further and redesign care for the community.

That Empty-Waiting-Room Feeling

In 2011, in a suburb south of Salt Lake City, the University of Utah built a clinic in what became one of the area's fastest-growing starter-home communities. Every step of planning and design was aimed at delivering the Exceptional Patient Experience.

The clinic is at the terminal stop of one line of the city's light rail system, and there's ample parking. An arriving patient is welcomed by a WalMart-like greeter, who helps him check in at kiosks in the lobby and ensures that the receptionists upstairs are ready for him. The easiest (and most common) way to irritate a patient is to make him wait. Clinics adopted lessons from the Exceptional Patient Experience journey to help the clinics stay on time. As a result, the parking lots were full, and the waiting rooms were empty. Staff members were happier. Patients were pleasantly surprised.

The physical setting was also designed around the patient experience. Architects introduced soothing elements from the hospitality industry. Soft mood lighting in the corridors and exam rooms with silently sliding wood-toned doors remind patients of a boutique hotel. Each exam room has a back door that leads to the "backstage" clinician workspaces where nurses and doctors can confer about patients and make calls without disrupting the tranquil patient experience. Every room is laid out exactly the same for ease of use. Room supplies can even be restocked without interrupting patient care.

The staff knew the neighborhoods around that clinic had a lot of starter families in their starter homes—parents and grandparents often came to appointments with small children in tow. Those patients told us they'd love to have onsite child care. The team partitioned off some of that empty waiting room space to create a room with colorful, spongy floor tiles, crayons, and toys. They staffed the child care center with a professional child care worker and an intern from the university's child education program.

With a high concentration of newborns living a short distance from the clinic, Utah pediatricians offered to make home visits for the new babies, harkening back to the days of house calls and black leather bags. Instead, a doctor and nurse arrived in a university-branded, eco-friendly Prius, armed with a digital scale and lactation tips, ready to check the baby for jaundice (yellowing of the skin and eyes, a common problem for newborns). Home visits make sense because clinicians can get a better sense of how the family is coping. They discuss with the mom any nursing and lactation questions and remind new parents and siblings that they must never shake the baby.

Thinking about health care through the eyes of patients makes it obvious that just asking for feedback after the care isn't as useful as codesigning the care together. Justin Masterson would like us to do just that, routinely.

Care That Cares

After her lively fifth birthday party, Justin Masterson's daughter went to bed feeling exhausted and, in her words, "kinda gross." The next morning, she wasn't feeling much better, so they took her to the pediatrician. Masterson described for me what happened next: "The doctor walked in, and without looking up from the chart said, 'Your daughter has diabetes. You should go to the hospital.'"

After rushing to the emergency room, he felt even more overwhelmed. Instead of talking *with* them, he says the hospital staff talked *at* them. For example, one person handed him a giant binder entitled "The World of Diabetes"—"It sounds like the world's shittiest theme park," he said. Besides the binder, he was handed blue paper logbooks and instructed to "Write down every carb she eats, every [insulin] dose you give her ... do the calculations with her starter ratios and correction factors ... From here on out, for the rest of her life, just write down all this stuff."

Then somebody handed him an insulin pen. On the box, printed on one side were words that he remembers clearly. "It said, 'Take a breath.' And below those words, 'Three things you should know: You didn't cause this and there's nothing you could have done to prevent it. Your child is going to be ok. Your kid can do everything every other kid can do and have a healthy normal life.'"

"In that moment, I started crying..." he tells me. "Where the care system had failed to meet us where we were, the box had met us where we were."

Masterson works for a market research and innovation company. He has spent his career thinking about how to design products and services that meet customer needs. After he asked his brother, a doctor, how he might help improve the care of people with diabetes, he was introduced to a leading diabetologist and, shortly thereafter, invited to run a session in which 80 diabetes specialists, researchers, experts, and patients and family members were gathered to design new ways to improve care. Having the families there changed the tenor of the exercise from the start. "Why are we mad, but they're not?" Masterson recalled thinking. "We're mad because we actually have to live with it every day."

Instead of starting with a design session, the parents proposed an empathy exercise. If the clinicians didn't understand what mattered to their children and to them, they would never be able to design the right kinds of solutions. The parents put together some real-world scenarios from their experiences. (Later, Masterson turned those into a professionally produced deck of cards, called "Walk a Mile.") There's one scenario per card. Here are some examples:

1. *"You are the only one at the senior prom with an insulin pump under your dress. Activity: Tape your phone to your side for the next three hours."*
2. *"You've just learned that your son's new private school won't have a nurse to help manage his diabetes, and classes start in one week."*
3. *"The school called you at work. Your son checked his blood glucose level and accidentally got some blood on a table. Another child freaked out, and the vice principal is now calling you about 'biohazards' in the lunchroom."*

Masterson says these exercises completely changed the dynamic and turned the innovation session "from an academic, theoretical pursuit to a very heart-based pursuit." Engaging patients and their families begins with empathy.

Coproducing Health

In 1968, noted Stanford economist Victor Fuchs recognized that a new service economy of retail, banking, education, and health care was displacing the old industrial economy of manufacturing and agriculture. This shift had profound implications, in his view, in how we should think about producing value. Unlike manufacturing products, delivering services usually requires some coordination with the customer. With services, the customer and the service provider coproduce value. For example, public security is coproduced by people locking their doors and installing security systems. Public education is coproduced through parent-teacher associations and homework help at home. Waste management depends on customers sorting and bagging garbage and dragging bins to their curbs.

The analogies to health care are obvious. For the most part, health care is a service. The patient's role in producing health can outweigh any physician's or nurse's role. Patients produce health through the choices they make about what they eat, what they drink, whether they climb the stairs or take the elevator, whether they take their medications as prescribed. That's why coproduction, like a health system partnering with Masterson and his daughter, is a natural way to think about health care, especially primary care and preventive health. To coproduce, health systems need to shift to thinking about what matters to patients.

What's Wrong with "What's Wrong?"

Susan Edgman-Levitan is a physician assistant and the executive director of an innovation center for primary care at the Massachusetts General Hospital in Boston. In 2012, she and physician Michael Barry wrote an influential article encouraging clinicians to start their conversations by asking, "What matters to you?" instead of "What's the matter?" Their work has gained a strong international following, complete with its own "What Matters to You?" day, June 6th, when millions of people share on social media their stories of care. One woman on chemotherapy shares the compliment she received for her new wig, and another describes a nurse closing off the curtains in the hospital room so that a patient could watch a favorite movie with her daughter.

When I catch up with Masterson, I ask him how his daughter is doing. He tells me what matters to him and to his daughter: "She's healthy. She's mostly feeling very typical, which is great. I think many days she feels almost like a child without diabetes." He pauses and then adds, "For me, that's the most important metric, because she's probably not going to reject her care."

Masterson relishes the chance to share what he's learned. He's discarded those blue paper logbooks for recording every meal, every blood glucose level, every insulin dose, and instead he uses an app he built to track his daughter's blood sugars. Besides the Diabetes Walk a Mile cards, he has designed infographics to educate parents on the pluses and minuses of finger pricks versus continuous glucose monitors—"They aren't for everyone," he counsels. As a designer, he knows that collaborating with the clinical team is key; otherwise, anything he and other patients build—apps, empathy cards, diabetes education kits—will "just be another tool stuck in a corner somewhere." To him, it's a team effort.

Networking It Out

The empathy among families of children with diseases like diabetes draws them together in strong communities, both in person and online. Some hospitals help these informal networks become more formal organizations. For example, the ImproveCareNow Network, founded at Cincinnati Children's Hospital, supports over one-third of all kids in the United States with inflammatory bowel disease. The network has used federal grants to build websites, organize conferences, and work with pharmaceutical companies to host clinical trials that get children access to new drugs and treatments.

Pediatrician Peter Margolis leads the network and says the partnership between clinicians and patients and their families helps kids in ways he never imagined. The ImproveCareNow website, for example, hosts videos and other guides produced by kids, for kids. A video created by an engaging nine-year-old demonstrates how to insert a feeding tube (via the nose), and there is a guidebook created by teens to help kids manage and live full lives with their ostomies (surgically made openings from the bowel to the skin of the abdomen that allow waste to bypass parts of the intestines in patients with inflammatory bowel disease). The combination of social support, coproduction, codesign of health care, and access to better drug therapies has helped the over 30,000 children in the network do better than ever. In 2019, more than four out of five were in remission, meaning they were free from active disease (up from three out of five when the network started).

The Action Plan for Coproducing Health

Masterson answers instantly when I ask what he would change about the health care system: "We need to embrace the reality that doctors and clinics don't provide care. The parents, family members, caregivers, and patients themselves provide care. . . . If you embrace this, you start to ask questions like, How do I equip you to take care of your child in a way that you can use? You ask patients way more questions and listen to their answers, and build treatment plans that they own and feel accountable to because they've created them."

The key is listening and being open to solutions. Margolis calls Justin Masterson a "Lead User innovator." He is one of those people who cannot help but innovate, and he is effective because he understands firsthand the conditions he is trying to change. He's like the clinic leaders who design onsite child care, the physician assistant who starts a "What Matters to You" movement, and the orthopedic surgeon who decides patient-reported outcomes should matter. Margolis says, "If you can create a system to harness the lead user innovation that's already taking place in your organization, you have an endless source of innovation."

To coproduce health and codesign health care, we all have a role to play.

As a patient and consumer of health care, you should:

- Take responsibility for your health, engage in your care, and treat your doctor like your partner. Share with your clinicians what matters to you.
- Think of the feedback you give as a chance for the learning health system to learn from you.

As a physician or other health care professional, you should:

- Ask your patients, "What matters to you?"
- Treat each patient as a learning opportunity, and learn from them how you can improve.

- Avoid unintended consequences of patient satisfaction efforts, such as overtreatment and overprescription.
- Build teams of patients, patient representatives, clinicians, and administrators that focus on the codesign of health care. Encourage innovation, from inside and outside the organization.

As a payer, such as a self-insured employer, government entity, or health plan, you should:

- Expect clinics and other providers of care to have fully developed patient engagement and experience systems of feedback and improvement (meeting the expectations outlined above).
- Ask that they share their patient satisfaction results with you.

As a policy maker, you should:

- Embrace policies and practices that lead to the coproduction of health.
- Set expectations that health systems, health plans, and employers engage people in the codesign of their health care experiences.

And most important, all of us need to elect leaders who recognize that health care is a patient-centered business.

CHAPTER 8

PHARMACEUTICALS: A WEB OF VESTED INTERESTS

Insulin belongs to the world, not to me.

—Frederick Banting

In 1923, Canadian surgeon Frederick Banting, his assistant Charles Best, and biochemist James Collip were awarded the patent for isolating insulin-rich pancreatic extracts from animals. They sold the patent to the University of Toronto for $1 each. Banting, who early in his life almost became a Methodist minister, wanted everyone with diabetes to have access to the miracle drug.

In one way, Banting's wish has come true. The life-sustaining medication is used by 7.4 million people in the United States and 150 million to 200 million globally. But it's probably not in the way he hoped, because most of the world's insulin belongs to three major companies. Under pressure from shareholders to deliver ever-higher returns, these three have raised insulin prices about tenfold in the past 20 years. Humalog (Eli Lilly), one of the cheapest and most popular brands, went from $21 per vial in 1996 to $275 in 2017; other commonly prescribed insulins cost more than $400 a vial. (A vial can last no more than 28 days.) With these high prices, prescriptions go unfilled and doses are skipped to save money. About one in four patients have said they underuse insulin because of its high cost. Newspapers tell the tragic stories of people dying because they can't afford their insulin.

I asked a former pharmaceutical executive why the price of insulin seemed to be skyrocketing. He pointed out that newer diabetes drugs coming onto the market were costing patients $11–12 per day. Insulin, at $3 per day, clearly had room to rise to at least $9 a day. He concluded, matter-of-factly, "Because we could."

Breaking the Bank

Pharmaceutical spending is the fastest-growing part of health care. It's not so much because Americans are taking more drugs; it's because their prescriptions are more expensive. A lot more expensive. A 2018 US Senate report looked at the 20 most-prescribed brand-name drugs for seniors. Between 2012 and 2017, the annual number of prescriptions for those 20 drugs declined by 48 million for all Americans, and yet, annual sales revenue to pharmaceutical companies from these drugs increased by almost $8.5 billion. Across those five years, their prices increased 12% per year, *every* year.

In 2018, estimates suggested that one in seven to ten dollars spent on American health care went to pay for prescription drugs. One insurance industry–sponsored study found that in 2018 insurance companies spent more on drugs than on inpatient hospital stays. Prescription drug spending will continue to rise, and the high costs are hurting patients. In a survey by the Kaiser Family Foundation, nearly three in ten Americans said they haven't taken their medications as ordered by a doctor because of high cost.

Some pharmaceutical CEOs may be looking after their shareholders' interests more than their patients' health. In 2015, former hedge fund manager Martin Shkreli, CEO of Turing Pharmaceuticals, raised the price of an antiparasite medication (Daraprim, the branded version of pyrimethamine) from $13.50 to $750 per dose, which placed the full course of therapy at a stratospheric $75,000. Despite the negative publicity, Daraprim's new price stuck, and it remained one of the 20 most expensive drugs in the United States in 2019. Valeant Pharmaceuticals (now Bausch Health Companies) jacked up the price of a common heart medication, Isuprel, more than 50-fold, from $440 to $2,700 per dose, after acquiring it from another pharmaceutical company, Marathon. (Marathon had quadrupled the price when it acquired the drug in 2013.) Another company, Mylan, infuriated the public when it increased the price for a pair of EpiPens (auto-injecting syringes that contain about $1 of the drug epinephrine and are used for severe, life-threatening allergic reactions). In 2007, a pair of the injectors cost $100; by 2016, they cost $600.

Zero-Gravity Economics

The pharmaceutical market in the United States prices drugs at whatever the market will bear. Patent laws and FDA provisions hand pharmaceutical manufacturers near-monopolies that can last decades. Medicare, the nation's largest purchaser of pharmaceuticals, is required to cover all prescription drugs for six major conditions (including cancer), regardless of price. It's not even allowed to negotiate for lower prices. The appetite for profitability among pharmaceutical companies is insatiable, and sometimes relentless. Valeant's former CEO, Michael Pearson, reportedly often said, "All I care about is our shareholders."

In *New York* magazine, science writer Stephen Hall called it "zero-gravity economics."

It is, of course, costly to bring a drug to market. Industry-sponsored estimates place the costs at about $2.7 billion. Independent researchers calculate that it's closer to $648 million. The most expensive and risky part of developing new drugs is typically the earliest phase of drug discovery, and most drugs that look promising in the laboratory still don't make it to the market. Of the registered clinical trials of 21,143 proposed new drugs between 2000 and 2015, only about one in ten made it to the market.

A distinguished cardiologist and President Obama's commissioner for the Food and Drug Administration (FDA), Rob Califf points out that the high failure rate is closely tied to the rigorous standards that the pharmaceutical industry must meet to get products to market. The approval process demands "evidence" (and by that he means research that proves a product is safe and works). Califf has spent much of his professional life working with pharmaceutical companies to generate that evidence. Califf also points out that the high standards of evidence for pharmaceuticals don't apply to most of medicine, "including what doctors do." Physicians don't have to prove that the way they treat patients is better or safer than alternative approaches.

Decades of collaboration have taught him the value of the pharmaceutical industry's commitment to science and research: "The industry is full of highly motivated people who want things to work," he tells me. For him, the heart of innovation is the "uniquely American ingenuity and creativity" of academic medical centers and the National Institutes of Health which funds them. That ingenuity is underpinning most of drug discovery.

Universities, Inc.

In the late 1970s, western European–headquartered companies were introducing about twice as many drugs to the market as American companies. Meanwhile, almost 28,000 patents—full of potential to spur a US competitive comeback—were languishing in the US Patents and Trademark Office. The bipartisan Bayh-Dole Act (or Patent and Trademark Law Amendments Act of 1980) aimed to fix that. It took the rights to those inventions from the government and gave them to universities, small businesses, and nonprofits instead. These entities could, in turn, license the intellectual property to companies, and if lucky, generate stunningly lucrative returns for their organizations and inventors.

When I was the chief scientific officer at NYU Langone Medical Center, we hit the Bayh-Dole jackpot. Years earlier, two of our microbiology professors, Jan Vilcek and Junming Le, had made an antibody that, when infused intravenously, could put rheumatoid arthritis and inflammatory bowel disease into remission. The antibody became the drug Remicade (infliximab, Janssen), which entered the market in 1998. By 2005, Remicade was generating sales of about $2 billion a year.

In 2007, the university sold a portion of its residual rights to Royalty Pharma for $650 million, with additional payments for exceeding sales milestones. The payout made NYU the top-grossing technology transfer office of all universities in the country that year. Vilcek and Le, through NYU's intellectual rights policies, collected handsome payouts. A Holocaust survivor from Czechoslovakia, Jan Vilcek, along with his wife, were generous with those returns. In 2015, they made one of the largest gifts ever to a medical school, committing $105 million to NYU to support biomedical research and education.

Drug discovery has been a boon for many universities. Stanford's recombinant DNA patent licenses generated over $250 million in licensing revenue. Northwestern University sold royalty rights for the pain and fibromyalgia drug Lyrica (pregabalin, Pfizer) for $700 million. Faster than states could create new lotteries, universities have established innovation centers to look for the next Remicade or Lyrica. Seeing scientists like Vilcek in his dark turtleneck and wool trousers strolling the corridors of NYU Langone Medical Center reminded other scientists that they too might be harboring the next big blockbuster drug in their laboratories.

Between 1996 and 2016, academic institutions spun out over 12,000 companies. At the University of Utah, three start-ups grew to earn hundreds of millions of dollars in revenue and employed thousands of Utahns: ARUP Laboratories (Associated Regional and University Pathologists), a national reference laboratory company; BioFire Diagnostics, an infectious disease diagnostics company; and Myriad Genetics, the company that made headlines with its Supreme Court case on whether genes (specifically, breast cancer genes) can be patented. At least 50% of biotech companies began as a result of a university license, and three-quarters of biotechnology companies have at least one license from a university.

The pace of discovery and its impact on human health are breathtaking. Consider the discoveries, for example, made by Carl June, a board-certified oncologist and researcher at the University of Pennsylvania. After decades of research supported largely by taxpayer-funded federal grants, the FDA approved in 2017 the first treatment that genetically alters a patient's immune cells to attack an aggressive type of leukemia, B-cell acute lympho-blastic leukemia. This remarkable gene therapy, based on June's work, and referred to as CAR T-cell therapy, is marketed as Kymriah (tisagenlecleucel, Novartis). One of the earliest patients, Emily Whitehead, was treated at age six for leukemia, and she was reportedly healthy and cancer-free six years later. The University of Pennsylvania has filed 428 patents for 54 separate inventions for this science and stands to profit handsomely. But commercial-ized products that stand on the shoulders of taxpayer-supported research are increasingly out of reach for most taxpayers. In 2019, CAR T-cell treat-ment cost $475,000. Including hospitalizations and additional tests and care before and after treatment, overall costs easily exceed $1 million.

The hope is that market competition eventually drives costs down. Take Sovaldi (sofosbuvir, Gilead Sciences), and its sibling, Harvoni (a combina-tion drug of Sovaldi with another ingredient, ledipasvir, Gilead Sciences), both of which cure hepatitis C, one of the most common causes of liver fail-ure and cancer worldwide. When Sovaldi came on the market at the end of 2013, the excitement over the once-a-day pill was dampened considerably by its price: $1,000 per pill. (Harvoni is more.) But it works—twelve weeks and $84,000 later, most (about 90%) patients can be cured for life.

Within one year of Sovaldi coming onto the market, rival AbbVie launched its own hepatitis drug at a list price of $83,000 for 12 weeks. The competition between Gilead and AbbVie drove discounts (or rebates, to be more precise—more on that shortly) to about 46% in 2014. Nonetheless, Gilead brought in almost $20 billion of revenue for its hepatitis C drugs in 2015. By 2019, AbbVie's new hepatitis C drug Mavyret (glecaprevir/pibrentasvir) came onto the market at a bargain basement $26,400 for the eight-week treatment. Shortly thereafter, Gilead announced it would offer its own generic versions of two of its three hepatitis C drugs, priced at—you guessed it—$24,000 for a course of treatment. By 2018, combined sales of all four of Gilead Sciences' hepatitis C drugs totaled $3.7 billion, one-fifth of its peak three years earlier.

Specialty drugs like Sovaldi and Harvoni represent only 1%–2% of the drugs sold, yet they consume about 40%–50% of drug expenses. In one report, about half of the 150 specialty drugs studied cost more than $100,000 per year. The protective laws and regulations in the US market give many of these new pharmaceuticals almost limitless drug pricing potential to start.

Patently Profitable

US patent laws give all new inventions—drugs and otherwise—20 years of protection. The clock starts on the date the patent is filed, even though it may take years for the FDA to approve it. For drugs that turn out to be blockbusters, every year that patent protection can be extended can be worth billions, and every day can mean millions. Besides patent protection, pharmaceutical companies also have rights to "market exclusivity" that keep generics from competing for their business. At each opportunity to extend the durations of patent protection or market exclusivity, the pharmaceutical industry has persevered and prevailed.

For example, to pass the Hatch-Waxman Act of 1984, a law designed to spark the generic drug industry, Congress made several important concessions to the pharmaceutical industry. For one, it extended the life of a patent by the amount of time it was under review by the FDA, up to five years. It also included a promise that the FDA would not approve any generic version of a drug for the first five years following approval. The Biologics Price Competition and Innovation Act of 2009 granted 12 years of exclusivity for "biologics"—such as Remicade—that are made biologically, not synthesized chemically. Through a series of adjustments between 1980 and 2000, the effective patent life of branded drugs increased on average from 8 years to over 14 years.

For their most precious drugs, pharmaceutical companies can get especially creative: AbbVie has extended its market exclusivity on some uses of the drug Humira (adalimumab, a competitor of Remicade) to 2034— 31 years after its introduction. That prompted Senator Ron Wyden (a

Democrat from Oregon) to observe that "AbbVie protects the exclusivity of Humira like Gollum with his ring," referring to a covetous character in J. R. R. Tolkien's *Lord of the Rings*.

Despite the concessions, the Hatch-Waxman Act boosted the generic market considerably. Prior to the bill's passage, generics made up 20% of the US market; by 2017, they represented nearly 90%. The law made some compromises. For example, generics only need to demonstrate "bioequivalence" to existing drugs. That means that the biochemical analyses have to show that the generic drug's active ingredient is absorbed at the desired location in the body as fast and as much as the branded drug. Companies don't have to show the drugs work in patients as well as the branded versions.

Pharmaceutical companies are right to be concerned about the competition. Generic drugs reduce prices. After a six-month period of exclusivity for the first generic that comes to market, prices typically decline to approximately half the price of the branded product. With multiple competitors, they decline to one-fifth or less of the price. Most states have passed laws that permit and even require pharmacists to substitute generic drugs for branded products.

Generics are so effective at lowering prices that manufacturers have taken creative measures to stall their arrival. Some pay generic drug companies *not* to launch one. Others use citizen petitions to ask the FDA to delay action on pending drug applications. By filing petitions near the end of a drug's patent expiration, "citizens" of those pharmaceutical companies effectively limit competition another five months. Another six months can be gained if the manufacturer sells an "authorized generic"—their branded product sold under a generic name.

Bob Walks into a Pharmacy...

Pharmaceutical companies are not the only ones profiting from high drug prices. Many other players have their hand in the till, often less visibly. Here's an example of how others get their share as a drug makes its way from a manufacturer to a patient:

Consider the hypothetical case of Bob. He has high blood pressure that is resistant to treatment. To fill the prescription for his branded blood pressure-lowering drug, he heads to his neighborhood pharmacy. The drug's list price is $100. Bob's co-payment will be $10. The remaining $90 needs to be covered by his employer (or, after he retires, Medicare).

That $90 from his employer doesn't get paid directly to the pharmacy. It first goes to the commercial health insurance company that manages his employee health benefit. The insurance company then pays $71 to the pharmacy benefit manager (PBM), keeping $19 to manage the benefit (including $3 profit). The PBM pays $66 to the pharmacy to cover the costs of the drug and nets about $5 ($2 of which is profit).

The pharmacy has now collected $76 for that $100 drug—$66 from the PBM, $10 from Bob as co-payment. When the pharmacy bought the drug from a wholesaler, it paid $60. Thus the pharmacy nets $16, and about $3 of that is profit.

The manufacturer spent $17 to make the drug, and it was paid $58 for it from the wholesaler, so it netted $41. Of that, $15 is profit, which means a profit margin of over 25%.

In this hypothetical case, the drug is a branded one, and the manufacturer makes the majority of the profit ($15 of the total of $23 of the total profit in the system). For generic drugs, the distribution of profit is different. Manufacturers make about one-third as much as they do on branded drugs. But the other intermediaries do much better; PBMs are estimated to make four times as much on generics, wholesalers 11 times, and pharmacies almost 12 times as much.

Rebate and Switch

Pharmaceutical companies like to shift blame for escalating prices to pharmacy benefits managers. As the brokers who negotiate with manufacturers about the costs of medications on behalf of employers, PBMs can secure better deals on medications than employers could on their own. But it gets more complicated. PBMs also help manufacturers get their medications prioritized on the health insurer's list of preferred drugs (called the formulary). Manufacturers pay the PBMs a "rebate" for doing so, in a confidential agreement. PBMs don't have to share the rebate savings with employers, or anyone, and they don't have to disclose what they've done with them. Pharmaceutical companies say that the PBMs are using rebates to line their own pockets, while PBMs say they are helping employers wrangle better prices, and pharmaceutical companies could just lower their prices directly if they so chose.

Either way, the rebates are often disadvantaging consumers. Here's why: Pharmaceutical companies who list drugs at high prices can offer fat rebates to PBMs, who in turn can boast to employers that they've secured higher discounts. This model encourages higher list prices (a lot like inflated chargemasters for hospitals and insurance brokers to negotiate discounts). Since the rebates are paid only after the drugs are sold to patients, they don't affect what the patient pays. If the PBM negotiates a $20 rebate off his blood-pressure drug, Bob's co-payment is still $10, pegged to the $100 list price of the drug. And if Bob didn't have insurance and was paying the whole $100 out of pocket, he would still have to pay the full amount.

For patients on Medicare, deductibles, coverage limits, donut holes, and catastrophic thresholds make it even more challenging for patients to understand and manage their out-of-pocket costs. With out-of-pocket costs mostly tied to list prices, patients are disproportionately bearing the impact of rising drug costs. Leonard Saltz, an oncologist at New York's Memorial Sloan Kettering Cancer Center, warns patients that even if they think their share is modest, 5% of a cancer drug that costs $11,000 per month can mean $550 per month out of pocket, just for one drug.

The I.V. League

Many of the headline drugs—cancer chemotherapies and drugs for autoimmune diseases like rheumatoid arthritis or ulcerative colitis—are administered intravenously, under a physician's watchful eye. For that supervision, physicians can also cash in on high drug prices. They're allowed to bill Medicare an additional 4.3% of the price (after rebates) for overseeing these infusions. That can add up to as much as $5,000–$10,000 per year for each patient who sits in a chair with an intravenous catheter in an arm a few hours a week.

Safety-net hospital systems, including most university and rural hospitals, also run their own highly profitable pharmaceutical businesses. In 1992, the Public Health Service Act, specifically Section 340B, allowed qualifying hospitals to purchase most outpatient prescription drugs at a big discount, on average, 34% less than the average price. Over one-third of US hospitals qualify for the 340B program; they include certain children's and cancer hospitals, sole community hospitals, and hospitals that care for a disproportionate share of low-income patients.

Under the 340B program, facilities can turn around and sell those heavily discounted drugs at whatever prices they can negotiate with payers, including Medicare. Again, doctors and hospitals are rewarded for using more expensive drugs. A single cancer physician can generate $1 million in profit for himself and his hospital each year.

The 340B program has become entangled in a web of cross-subsidies. Teaching hospitals (university-affiliated hospitals) and safety-net hospitals (city and county hospitals) have a lot to lose if it goes away. In many hospitals, the tens of millions of dollars generated from the 340B program each year offset the charity care for the poor and uninsured. (While I was its CEO, the University of Utah provided over $100 million in unreimbursed charity care each year.) In university hospitals, 340B funds also subsidize the training of doctors and medical research, both of which are critical to the US health system. Untangling this part of the pharmaceutical web means identifying new sources of support for research and education that don't rely on pharmaceutical profiteering.

Exceedingly Overdone ... and Underdone

Harvard economist David Cutler once said to me, "In many ways, health care is exceedingly rational ... things that we pay extremely well for are overdone, and things we pay extremely poor for are underdone."

Consider the opioid epidemic as a tragic case of the "overdone." In

2001, in response to perceived failings, the Joint Commission—the hospital accrediting agency—pressured hospitals to better manage patients' pain. Physicians prescribed more painkillers, and as a result, the prescription opioid industry grew to an $8 billion a year business. Over 76 billion oxycodone (including the branded drug, Oxycontin, Purdue Pharma) and hydrocodone pills were prescribed between 2006 and 2012, which works out to more than 250 of just those two types of opioid pills per American. Manufacturers and distributors were thrilled to see profits boom, turning a blind eye to good judgment and the evidence that they were feeding new addictions. The damage to the nation has been devastating. By 2017, 1.7 million Americans were addicted to opioids, and more than 130 died of overdoses *every day* in 2019. The economic burden of the opioid crisis is estimated at $78.5 billion per year.

Short-Fall Windfall

While the nation was awash in opioids, hospitals in the United States were facing frequent shortages of vital pharmaceuticals, including 282 drugs and biological products in 2019. The list included basic electrolytes like sodium chloride (saline), emergency syringes, antibiotics, and cardiovascular agents. Pharmacist Erin Fox thinks it's an issue of national security. A senior director at the University of Utah pharmacy, she is a recognized authority on national shortages of important pharmaceuticals. Fox says that whether it's a natural disaster or a human-made one, supplies like antibiotics, intravenous fluids, and inhalers are essential. "We should think about some products as critical infrastructure the same way as power plants," she says. "Having saline as a supply is so critical, yet there is no backup plan or business continuity plan required." The FDA cannot mandate production of pharmaceuticals. The only requirements are that manufacturers notify the FDA when they intend to discontinue manufacturing drugs or biological products that might lead to shortages.

This crisis motivated over 800 hospitals (including the University of Utah) to join Civica Rx, a nonprofit generic pharmaceutical company founded by Intermountain Healthcare. The FDA may not be able to manage it, but Civica Rx's CEO, Martin VanTrieste, is determined to ensure that hospitals don't run out of critical drugs.

The Price Is Life

The excesses of drug pricing, according to former FDA Commissioner Rob Califf, are not much different from the problem with hospital prices. "They both jack up the list price. All kinds of middle people take a profit," he says, and when prices are negotiated, "bills are very difficult to figure out." We need to start paying for value, he says emphatically. In an editorial with Andy Slavitt in 2019, the two wrote that "Instituting value-based payments for drugs is the most promising path toward a fair system that rewards innovation."

Mark McClellan agrees. A physician, economist, and former FDA commissioner under President George W. Bush, he too is a big proponent of moving to value-based payments. The goal is to get more for what we're spending—"Let's pay for treatments when they work, and more when they get better," he tells me.

The British, Canadian, and Australian governments use a standard measurement called the costs per quality-adjusted life year ("QALY"— pronounced "quality" without the "it") to decide whether to include drugs on their formularies. This number estimates how much extra it costs for a drug to give a patient an additional year of high-quality life. (Note that a drug does not have to provide an additional full year of life; if it costs $10,000 to provide one half-year's high-quality life, then the drug would be $20,000 per QALY). Calculating the dollars (or pounds) per QALY allows policy makers to compare new drugs with existing ones and to reject those that cost significantly more per QALY.

In the early 2000s, the UK's National Health Service established that it could afford to pay about £20,000 to £30,000 (or about 25,000 to 38,000 US dollars in 2019) per additional high-quality year of life, a figure it reaffirmed in 2015. In the United States, there is no agreed-upon number. It could be based on median annual household income (about $63,000 in 2019) or the per capita gross domestic product ($60,000 in the United States in 2017). Many US researchers use figures between $50,000 and $150,000 per QALY as the threshold for a worthwhile drug or treatment. One of the largest pharmacy benefit managers announced in 2018 that it would use a QALY threshold of $100,000 per QALY to decide what drugs to include in its formulary.

The idea is simple, but it can lead to complicated and heated debates, because it feels like policymakers are putting a monetary value on a year of life. Advocates for the disabled, for example, have objected because a full QALY, by definition, can only be achieved by able-bodied individuals. That's a misunderstanding of what this tool does. Cost-effectiveness analysis provides a measure of our society's willingness to pay. It's not what a life is worth, but what society can afford, and countries may differ on that number.

The arbitrariness of the figure gives former FDA Commissioner McClellan pause. He thinks we should look at whether medications reduce hospitalizations and improve patient well-being, and he worries about putting restrictions on what people can spend, especially when it comes to their health. But for state and federal officials on limited budgets, these calculations can help them support difficult financial decisions.

The US government has been remarkably resistant to this approach, so much so that it prohibits federal research agencies like the Patient Centered Outcomes Research Institute (PCORI) from funding research that uses cost-per-QALYs to evaluate new treatments and drugs. PCORI's website posts the following explanation: "We don't consider cost effectiveness to be an outcome of direct importance to patients." As a result of its policies, US prices are substantially higher than in the rest of the world. A 2015 Reuters study showed that the world's top 20 medications (that account for 15% of global pharmaceuticals sales) cost three times as much in the United States as in the UK. In the United States, one month of the cholesterol-lowering drug Lipitor costs $100; in New Zealand, it's $6. And to cure hepatitis C in Egypt, a 12-week course of Sovaldi costs $900.

If the US government won't do it, Peter Bach will. A pulmonary and critical care physician at Memorial Sloan Kettering Cancer Institute in New York, Bach has fought hard to make drug pricing more rational. His Drug Pricing Lab has built tools like Drug Abacus, an interactive program that allows the user to compare both actual costs and costs per QALY for 52 cancer drugs. Cost-effectiveness data like these for all pharmaceuticals on the market would help payers and patients compare medications based on their value more than on the quality of their marketing and direct-to-consumer advertisements.

The More You "No"

Bach's work made him an enthusiastic partner to his colleague Leonard Saltz in taking on cancer drug pricing. In 2012, as chair of the hospital's formulary committee, Saltz was getting ready to submit a new cancer drug, Zaltrap (ziv-aflibercept, sold by Regeneron Pharmaceuticals and Sanofi) for inclusion on the list of drugs that the hospital would have available to patients. It was a reflexive action, because the hospital carried almost all cancer drugs. Then a colleague from the pharmacy sent him the price—about $11,000 per month—and it shocked him. Zaltrap was more than double the cost of another similar cancer drug, Avastin (bevacizumab, Genentech), despite working no better.

Saltz decided to consult his colleagues. Of the 16 physicians in his hospital who saw colon cancer patients, not one could see a reason for recommending the new drug to their patients.

Saltz withdrew the application to the formulary committee, and for the first time anyone could remember, one of the country's preeminent cancer hospitals would not offer a drug to its patients because of price. In October 2012, Saltz, Bach, and a third colleague explained their decision in a *New York Times* op-ed. Less than four weeks later, Sanofi announced it was cutting the price of Zaltrap in half.

Actually, that's not exactly right. Sanofi did not reduce the list price of the drug; it agreed to offer 50% rebates to doctors.

Say "No" to (Some) Drugs

Unlike Saltz and Memorial Sloan Kettering Cancer Center, Medicare, the single largest purchaser of pharmaceuticals in the United States, cannot say "no." Its plans must cover at least two drugs in each of 57 classes of drugs, and it must include *all* drugs in six "protected classes": cancer, HIV, depression, schizophrenia, organ transplants, and epilepsy. That means it is required to cover Avastin and Zaltrap. Additionally, Medicare is not allowed to negotiate prices. According to the law, it is prohibited from "interfer[ing]" with price negotiations between health insurance plans and the drug manufacturers.

Other government programs have more flexibility. The Veterans Health Administration and Military Health System are allowed to negotiate drug prices and, if they don't like the deal, they can refuse to carry a medication on their formularies. One congressional report from 2018 estimated that if Medicare were allowed to negotiate drug prices, the program and its beneficiaries could save $2.8 billion per year.

The Right Rx for Doctors

Even if Medicare plans and hospitals can't manage to keep low value drugs off their formularies, it doesn't mean that doctors have to prescribe them. Rushika Fernandopulle, founder of Iora Health, believes that physicians, supported by pharmacists, should take more responsibility for making sure patients are on the right medications and stop prescribing the unnecessary ones.

Iora physicians are particularly skilled at deprescribing—taking no longer needed drugs off a patient's medication list—as an antidote to overprescribing. A 2011 survey found that more than a third of women over 65 take at least five prescription drugs. Fernandopulle told me about patients who come for their first appointment at Iora clutching bags of 20–30 different pill bottles. Many of those medications are not only unnecessary, but dangerous. For example, mental health and physical health drugs prescribed by two different doctors can lead to bad reactions between, say, anticoagulants and antidepressants, immunosuppressants and barbiturates, or HIV medications and antianxiety medications. Reducing unnecessary medications can make care safer, easier to manage, and less expensive.

While they're carefully managing medications, Iora clinicians also look for opportunities to swap out branded drugs for generics or other lower-cost alternatives. They save a lot of money, and they could save more if the process were automated. When Mitesh Patel and colleagues at the University of Pennsylvania hospital programmed the computer entry system to default to the generic form of medications, the use of generics in that unit increased from 75% to 98.4% in one year. Another team in that system set a default limit for prescribing opioid tablets to ten tablets per prescription. The percentage of physicians who used the default doubled, from about one-fifth to two-fifths in just four weeks.

Insulin Matters

Patients and physicians are taking resourceful and creative approaches to getting essential medications affordably. Jennifer Lee is an endocrinologist and precision health researcher at Stanford and the Palo Alto Veterans Affairs Health Care System. She's also my sister. When she's not the research program lead at that VA, she sees diabetic patients in her clinic. In the course of writing this book, I asked her about how the rising prices of insulin and other diabetes drugs are affecting her patients. "No issues really with insulin access or affordability," she told me. "Vets get such meds at lower cost, if not free of charge, and insulin is on formulary." But she knows most patients aren't so lucky. When she surveys other endocrinologists in the area, the stories vary dramatically.

One community medical center sees mostly Medicaid patients. Their main barrier, says one physician, is the formulary—not every drug is available. Also, Medicaid often only allows the pharmacy to dispense one vial of insulin at a time, and for many that vial does not last the full 28 days. A doctor at a university hospital says about 30% of the patients there have trouble getting insulin, often because of high co-pays or because there's a limited formulary (for example, insulin pens are often not covered).

Through their pharmacists, physicians, or directly online, patients can access two forms of financial support from some manufacturers: coupons for a particular drug (not allowed for Medicare and Medicaid patients) and patient assistance programs, where the drug company distributes free medicines or donates to independent foundations who then provide patients with financial assistance. Some physicians send their patients to big-box stores like Costco and WalMart or refer them to online resources like GoodRx. One physician admitted to prescribing double the actual doses, so that patients could get extra insulin for the same cost. Other doctors even suggest their patients get their insulin from overseas.

A 2013 report estimated that five million Americans bought medications internationally, either in person or online, even though officially it is mostly illegal for individuals to import drugs or devices into the United States for personal use. In 2018, Utah's Public Employee Health Plan challenged that law directly. It created a voluntary Pharmacy Tourism Program. For its members who use any one of 13 expensive medications, the insurer will fly the patient and a companion to San Diego and drive them to a hospital in Tijuana, Mexico, to pick up a 90-day supply. For those worried about the quality of medications manufactured abroad in sites that are not under US FDA surveillance, the Canadian International Pharmacy Association shares information about certified online pharmacies. Buying overseas may make more sense for branded drugs than generics. One study showed that while branded drugs may cost less overseas, generic medication prices are frequently lower in the United States than in Canada.

The Action Plan for Sensible Drug Prices

Mark McClellan points out that because drug costs are the highest in the United States, manufacturers bring them to market here first. He tells me that Americans are fortunate to have earlier access to many life-saving drugs, "We may be subsidizing the world's drugs by providing manufacturers their global profit margins, but we also get some perks."

Moving from fee-for-service to pay-for-value payment models with pharmaceuticals makes sense. Armed with data about cost-effectiveness, consumers and payers should negotiate effectively with manufacturers (without obfuscating rebate deals). Physicians, partnered with pharmacists, need to bear more responsibility for prescribing and deprescribing medications.

To ensure we get the most value out of medications (and devices), we all have a role to play.

As a patient and consumer of health care, you should:

- Review the medications you or your family members are prescribed and be sure that you understand what each is for and whether each is needed.
- Use online tools like Medicare's prescription cost tools, Memorial Sloan Kettering's Drug Abacus, and verified online pharmacy sites to learn more about the drugs you are prescribed. You may find lower-cost choices than your pharmacy benefits plan offers.
- Ask your employer whether they are receiving a share of drug rebates and whether those savings are reflected in employee out-of-pocket medication costs.

As a physician or other health care professional:

- Use cost-effectiveness data when available to support decisions about the medications you prescribe.
- Review medications (and engage pharmacists to help you) and deprescribe where possible and safe.
- Take responsibility for the financial toxicity of the medications you prescribe for your patients. When possible, use tools that estimate their out-of-pocket costs.

As a payer, such as a self-insured employer, government entity, or health plan, you should:

- Aggressively manage the costs of care for your employees or members. Make sure measures like dollars per QALY are used to decide what drugs are included on the formulary for your members and employees and to determine the price you will pay.
- Demand that the clinicians who provide care for your employers prescribe responsibly and ask for comparative data on drug prescribing to benchmark their performance.
- Expect your pharmacy benefits manager and health plan to make drug rebate deals transparent.

As a policy maker, you should:

- Demand price transparency. Rebate agreements, including those secured by government hospitals (like Veterans Health Administration and Military Health System) should be public. Allow all payers and purchasers (including Medicare) to negotiate prices on behalf of the members they serve and to use cost-effectiveness measures to select which drugs go on formulary.
- Develop a policy to ensure that a national supply of vital medications is always available.
- End the prohibition against studying cost-effectiveness and instead fund more research.
- Ensure that drugs developed with federally funded research (coming from taxpayer dollars) are available to all Americans who need them, at affordable prices, perhaps through a separate insurance pool.
- Eliminate anticompetitive practices that delay generic drug approvals.
- Convert Medicare Part B physician payments to fixed fees rather than a percentage of costs.
- Incorporate prescribing behaviors into quality and safety perfor-

mance measurements. Ask whether medications being prescribed are having the desired End Results and whether the most cost-effective and safe medications are being used.

- Untangle the cross-subsidies of the 340B program and identify alternative sources of funding for charity care, research, and education.

And most important, all of us need to elect leaders who will encourage the development of new drugs and ensure that they are affordable, accessible, and safe for all.

CHAPTER 9

BIG DATA DREAMS

To lower health care cost, cut medical errors, and improve care, we'll computerize the nation's health record in five years, saving billions of dollars . . . and countless lives.

—President Barack Obama, January 24, 2009

$\mathbf{A}$s health commissioner of Washington, D.C., LaQuandra Nesbitt is responsible for its 700,000 residents, of whom 31% are low-income and one in four are covered by Medicaid (or CHIP, the expanded plan for children from low-income families). She's also a family medicine physician. She tells me about a patient she saw at a University of Maryland walk-in clinic: A grandmother comes to the clinic with two small children in tow (her daughter was in jail, and their father was not in the picture). One of her legs is swollen and painful. The woman has a history of heart failure and high blood pressure, but, "of course her [medical] chart was missing . . . so I'm flying by the seat of my pants," says Nesbitt. She is worried that the woman might have a clot in the veins of her leg (which could dislodge, flow to the heart, and cause a deadly pulmonary embolism). It's a Friday, and Nesbitt "can't let this woman go home to die." She orders an ultrasound of her leg and sends her to an imaging facility down the street.

A couple of hours later, Nesbitt notices that the woman is back in the clinic. She's had the test, but no one from the imaging center has bothered to share the results with Nesbitt, and the radiologists have gone home. She tries paging the doctor on call, but he has no idea and guesses that the test was "probably negative." Nesbitt is mad now, so she calls a friend in a nearby emergency room who agrees to do a quick scan. The grandmother, however, says she can't go to the emergency room because the kids haven't eaten all day, and she needs to go home to feed them. The nearby pizza and deli shops aren't an option because she doesn't have the money. There's food in her refrigerator, and the bus ride is free, so she's going home.

Nesbitt whips out her wallet and hands the woman a few bills. "I have no more patience," she sighs. The medical assistants in the clinic are waiting for her to finish so they can go home. As Nesbitt heads out of the office, she sees the woman walking across the street to the emergency room, holding the hands of the children, each cheerfully clutching a Happy Meal box.

Nesbitt ticks off the many things that were wrong in that scenario: the clinic couldn't find the woman's chart, there was no electronic medical record, Nesbitt couldn't get her colleagues to tell her the results of the test, and there was no handoff to the doctor on call when the imaging center closed. Things would have been different had the health system had a functioning electronic health record: She should have been able to pull up the patient's medical history on her computer, better assess the patient's risk of having a clot (in the end, she did not), share the relevant information with the radiologist in the clinic, and receive the radiologist's report electronically (it should have been in her inbox before the patient even arrived back). The fact that the woman had to choose between her health and feeding her grandchildren added another layer to this all-too-common drama. Nesbitt says, "These are the choices people have to make on a day-to-day basis," because the system doesn't work.

From the outset, investing in better computer systems was a cornerstone of President Barack Obama's health care strategy. On January 24, 2009, in his first weekly address to the nation as president, he set a deadline of five years. That job would fall to one of his top health advisors during his campaign, David Blumenthal, a man who deemed Obama's five-year goal "virtually impossible."

Forty years earlier, Homer Warner had already achieved this goal on a smaller scale in his hospital in Salt Lake City. Born in 1922, Warner trained as a cardiologist just as computers were making their way into government bureaus, large corporations, and even university hospitals. ("We're talking about a machine that costs half a million dollars . . . to fill about half of this room," he recalled.) In 1954, he started a cardiovascular lab at LDS Hospital in Salt Lake City, where computers attached to oscilloscopes traced blood pressure waveforms from the arteries of patients who were about to undergo open heart surgery. That first foray into computers in medicine led Warner to think about how computers could help clinicians practice medicine better.

Built on mainframe computers and programmed with punch cards, Warner wrote a software program called Health Evaluation through Logical Processing—HELP. It was one of the first electronic health record systems in the nation, synthesizing information from the pharmacy, laboratory, cardiology department, and more. Beyond record keeping, he imagined the tool might prompt a doctor with useful suggestions, like, "If you're going to give this man [the heart drug] digitalis, you really ought to measure his potassium level first." This was 1967.

In 2009, when Blumenthal, the new national coordinator for health information technology, was tasked with computerizing the nation's health records, only 12% of US hospitals had even a basic electronic system. One of the best was built in the 1970s for the government-run Veterans Health Administration hospitals. Other than theirs and a few other vanguard systems like Warner's, progress in electronic records had been glacial.

To move things along, Congress passed the $22 billion Health Information Technology for Economic and Clinical Health (HITECH) Act in 2009. The goal wasn't simply to put computers in physicians' offices—it was to make health information technology the circulatory system of modern medicine. Over the next two years, Blumenthal traveled all over the country, proselytizing, arguing, and goading hospitals and doctors to convert. He even had a carrot to offer: by simply adopting a basic electronic health record, each hospital or practice could receive $18,000 per doctor.

Between 2009 and 2011, the percentage of primary care physicians with a basic electronic health record nearly doubled, increasing from 20% to 39%. By 2017, eight years after the HITECH Act was signed into law, 87% of Americans had access to their medical records in electronic form, and 96% of hospitals in the United States had an electronic health record.

The adoption rate has impressed skeptics, and there are some signs of better care resulting from electronic records—there are fewer medication errors, and doctors are doing better at following recommended guidelines like cancer screenings. But have electronic health records lived up to Obama's promise? Not yet.

Coding Blues

Ask physicians how they feel about electronic health records, and you will get mixed reactions. Most would not want to go back to paper records, but many do find the systems cumbersome to use. That's not Blumenthal's fault. The problem is that most hospitals prioritized one main application for this powerful technology: "revenue cycle," also known as billing and coding. Dreams of delivering better care have been curbed in the haste to increase revenue. A Northwestern University study calculated that an electronic health record could increase reimbursement by $1.3 billion annually for inpatient services simply by assigning billing codes to patients that result in higher reimbursements. Setting up those computerized records was much more expensive than originally projected—from $5 million to $20 million for each community hospital and $1 billion to $16 billion for large health systems—and many facilities wanted to earn those dollars back.

Increasing revenue has been good financially for hospitals but not so good for doctors or for patients. To secure higher reimbursements, hospitals (and their electronic records) have turned physicians into overqualified and expensive data entry workers. Each night, physicians log, on average, 86 minutes of "pajama time" to catch up on their electronic health records work: documenting care, checking off tasks, searching for test results, digging through other colleagues' notes. In clinic, instead of spending time with patients, doctors and nurses spend time with their computers. That's largely why almost half (45%) of US physicians reported feeling burned out in 2017, and 73% of general internists would not choose the same specialty if they were to start their careers anew. Demoralized physicians are saying things like: "I am no longer a physician but the data manager, data entry clerk and steno girl... I became a doctor to take care of patients. I have become the typist."

Christine Sinsky, a practicing internist for 32 years and vice president of professional satisfaction at the American Medical Association, feels their pain. In leading medical journals, she's published articles like "Physicians Spend Two Hours on EHRs and Desk Work for Every Hour of Direct Patient Care." She has teamed up with Thomas Bodenheimer, a general internist from the University of California at San Francisco, to add a fourth tenet to the nation's triple aim of health care priorities (improve health, reduce costs, improve the core experience): Improve the work life of clinicians and staff.

Improving Efficiency: Just Say No to Steno

Improving the life of physicians and other clinicians could go hand-in-hand with making health care a more efficient business. Both could start by simply making the electronic records more user-friendly. Imagine, for example, a search engine that helps physicians quickly and easily find information in electronic records. Voice recognition and natural language processing features could generate medical notes automatically—not only transcribing conversations, but using artificial intelligence to organize the notes into structured formats.

The same tools could make hospitals and clinics more productive and efficient. Technology-enabled consultants use artificial intelligence-powered tools to improve the flow of patients through clinics, emergency rooms, operating rooms, and inpatient hospital rooms. Ideally, these tools can achieve both better health and increased profitability, and what they all rely on is data, "Big Data."

FAANG or FOE

When investors hear the words "Big Data," they picture the transformative effects (and zero-gravity valuations) of the FAANG (Facebook, Apple, Amazon, Netflix, and Alphabet's Google) tech companies. Whether it's Amazon's product recommendations leading to its 49% share of the US e-commerce market in 2018 or Facebook's insights into emotional contagion helping them ensnare 2.4 billion monthly active users in 2019, Big Data has disrupted businesses in bold, unimagined ways. By collecting detailed information about customer preferences, Netflix developed a powerful recommendation engine that matches films to customers based on their prior selections. Its analytics tools help select new films and create hit shows with extraordinary accuracy and success.

Investors, data scientists, and clinicians are entranced by the possibilities of the same predictive analytics applied to health care. Blumenthal points out that venture capital investments in digital health have already grown vigorously, with a compound annual growth rate of 30% from 2011 to 2016 that resulted in an $8.1 billion investment in 2018. If the rest of the technology sector is any reference, this is just the beginning.

Blumenthal also knows there are many issues to be resolved, including questions about patients' control over their data, whether health data can truly be anonymized, and the use of data for purposes beyond their original intended use. There's also the issue of trust—mounting public skepticism about Big Data corporations in Europe has led to the adoption of stronger privacy rights laws like the General Data Protection Regulation, which requires online businesses to get permission before using people's data. Finding the right balance between encouraging innovation and protecting against exploitation has even more significance when it comes to data about your HIV status, genetic predisposition to cancer, or mental health. Maintaining public trust will be vital because when machine-learning tools are responsibly applied to health care's Big Data, some of the most challenging issues facing medicine suddenly seem solvable.

Consider, for example, the urgent need to improve outcomes, reduce waste, and address the third-leading cause of death in the United States, medical mistakes.

Automatically Avoiding Mistakes

It is hard to improve safety in health care because most professionals are reluctant to disclose their mistakes. The current system of voluntary reporting means that only 10% of inpatient safety events are detected. If computerized records could automatically detect these events, they might also automatically prevent them. For example, about 1 in 30 (3%) of all hospitalized patients have a health care–associated infection. Detecting infectious outbreaks early could reduce these numbers dramatically.

In 1985, Homer Warner had already demonstrated that by analyzing microbiology test results, pharmacy reports, and radiology studies, his electronic HELP program could identify which patients had acquired infections in the hospital, who was receiving the wrong antibiotic, who could be receiving less-expensive antibiotics, and even who had been on prophylactic antibiotics for too long. Over 30 years later, only about half of all US hospitals had acquired this capability. Where available, electronic surveillance software can detect infectious outbreaks 3–9 days earlier than the old paper-based systems, saving lives and considerable staff time.

This same approach can be used to spot all kinds of other untoward events. One federally certified patient safety organization, Pascal Metrics, converted a paper-based tool for identifying preventable mistakes—the Global Trigger Tool—into an electronic version. The algorithm predicted adverse events for almost 3% of all patients admitted, and most were serious enough that they led to temporary harm or lengthened patient stays in the hospital. This system implemented in hospitals could routinely alert clinicians in time to prevent injury.

Clear and Future Danger

Besides looking for adverse events, these computer algorithms are useful for detecting early signs of a patient's worsening, such as imminent kidney failure. Diabetes and high blood pressure—both growing epidemics—are the leading causes of kidney disease. About one in seven Americans has chronic kidney disease (the vast majority don't know they have it because it doesn't produce symptoms until the late stages). In a hospital setting, where drugs and imaging contrast agents can be toxic to the kidneys, as many as one in five patients experiences acute kidney injury. The standard laboratory test for kidney function, serum creatinine, is a crude test; it only detects a problem when about half of kidney function is lost.

Using data from more than 700,000 adults treated in hospitals and clinics operated by the US Department of Veterans Affairs, my colleagues at Google Health developed a machine-learning algorithm that can detect impending kidney deterioration two days before the usual laboratory values start changing. The results have raised a new research question: What is the best way to prevent kidney failure if you have a clue that it might happen in a few days? It's not something physicians had ever imagined. But now there's a reason to start that research.

In contrast, clinicians should know what to do with early warning signs of another condition called sepsis, where patients with severe infection develop failure of the kidneys, heart, liver, and other organs. The clinical signs and preventive measures are well established, and one study showed that machine-learning algorithms that predict early sepsis could reduce the death rate by half. Machine learning algorithms can predict more than imminent decline, they can help clinicians care better for everyone.

Red Ball, Green Ball

Global scientific knowledge doubles every eight to nine years. That's an exhilarating fact . . . unless you're the expert whose job it is to know it all. All doctors, including me, have stacks of unread journals on our desks or queued in our inboxes. It's impossible to keep up. Physicians are buckling under the pressure to be on top of all the latest discoveries at the same time as our patients show up to clinic armed with questions they got from "Dr. Google." Fortunately, help is on the way.

Computers can help clinicians incorporate lessons from the published medical literature into daily practice, by embedding recent learnings directly in the electronic systems. Doctors' order sets can automatically default to follow Geisinger's ProvenCare or Utah's Perfect Care, for instance. They can help physicians deliver up-to-date, scientifically-established care without having to remember everything they've read (or haven't quite finished reading). Paul Chang, a Korean-American physician who leads Radiology Informatics at the University of Chicago School of Medicine, told me about a visit with his primary care physician for a flare-up of gout. When his doctor started to prescribe him the standard medicine, allopurinol, he promptly corrected him. "You can't give me allopurinol, because people of my ethnicity are at high risk of carrying a gene (HLA-B*5801) that makes me likely to get a severe reaction to that drug!" Eventually, after testing proved he did not carry that genetic variant, Chang was put on the medication. Homer Warner would have expected computers to anticipate these issues automatically by now, and increasingly, they are.

Better decision support tools can also help resolve disputes between insurers and clinicians. In 2004, insurers tried to reduce the number of CT scans and other expensive imaging studies by putting in barriers to ordering: they required physicians to complete piles of paperwork ("prior authorization") before agreeing to pay. David Blumenthal's team built a radiology order entry application that asked the ordering physicians to enter details about the patient and why they needed the imaging study. The computer would signal whether medical research supported the use of that imaging test. A red ball indicated the patient didn't need the study—perhaps they just had it at another hospital or it wouldn't help with the diagnosis. A green ball said it was fine, in which case insurance would cover the study. Blumenthal thought it was "like a bolt of lightning." It kept him from making mistakes. It kept him from wasting money. It made him order the right tests and sometimes spared the patient unnecessary radiation. And best of all, Blumenthal never had to deal with another prior authorization for imaging.

Besides streamlining physician practice, electronic medical records could help doctors and patients coproduce their health.

Accessible Health Care: In Your Pocket

Tom Delbanco thinks you should see the medical notes written about you, and maybe even contribute to them. An energetic Harvard primary care physician, Delbanco is a founder of the "OpenNotes" movement that started in 2010 when three hospitals, Delbanco's Beth Israel Deaconess Medical Center in Boston, Geisinger Health System in rural Pennsylvania, and Seattle's Harborview Medical Center, invited 20,000 patients to read the notes their primary care physicians wrote in their medical charts.

The doctors were amazed by the response. Patients loved the opportunity, and reading notes about their maladies and treatments didn't upset them. Instead, the notes reminded them of important next steps, like scheduling a screening mammography, colonoscopy, or important immunization, and helped them with taking their medications as prescribed. With OpenNotes patients felt more in control, and older, less educated, and Hispanic patients reported the greatest benefit. Patients can identify errors, confirm (or correct) what they want to communicate to their doctor, and understand better how that information is influencing their care. Importantly, one in four patients who contact their doctor after reading their notes report a possible error, in some cases, preventing serious problems.

Delbanco encouraged our team at the University of Utah to join the movement, and we did. So did the Veterans Health Administration and hundreds of other hospitals. By 2019, more than 44 million patients in the United States had access to their notes. In 2015, Delbanco's team expanded OpenNotes to OurNotes, inviting patients not just to read notes but also to write in their own medical record. Delbanco is finding that OurNotes can improve accuracy and safety directly.

The next stage of the HITECH Act—furthered by the 21st Century Cures Act of 2016—required that all electronic health record companies make their data accessible to patients, and, if granted permission by the patients, companies also must allow third-party software companies to access the records through application programming interfaces. Apple announced in 2019 that hospital systems could partner with them so that their patients could download their electronic health records to their smartphones using Apple's health app. The apps that they and others could build might make the data not only more accessible but also more useful. For example, imagine being able to look at your last MRI or CT scan on an app that automatically highlights the abnormalities and shows you what normal should look like.

At the same time, electronic health record vendors are racing to improve their own technology, called patient portals, to give people access to their data directly so that they can check laboratory values, review imaging results, and even correct information. Insurance plans are also trying their hand at this, offering online digital solutions for managing benefits and their health.

There is another "win" lurking in the 21st Century Cures Act, one that might seem small and prosaic amid all this Brave New Tech talk. But if you're a patient, you'll love it, because it eliminates a truly aggravating bug in our system. The law addresses the problem of "interoperability," the need for data from electronic systems operated by different hospitals and clinics to be shareable and accessible. A few years ago, when a patient at Primary Children's Hospital in Salt Lake City turned 18, she was referred to an internal medicine physician at the University of Utah's clinic on the same campus. She had to print out her records from Children's Hospital and carry them across the street. With interoperability, if you change doctors or employers, or experience an unexpected emergency while away from home, all of your electronic records should be available for your care.

Learning Health System

A bigger and bolder vision for digital health records turns the data from millions of patient records across health systems into insight-generating research engines that answer questions like: Which medication works better for high blood pressure? Which patients benefit more from robotic surgery? Which genes make a patient more likely to develop sepsis? That's what the Observational Health Data Sciences and Informatics collaborative is shooting for. It pulls together electronic health data from many hospitals and combines it with large insurance claims datasets to understand how treatments are working in the "real world." Using a totally open-source approach, researchers have studied, for example, the performance of 29 classes of hypertensive medications. This kind of research is not as rigorous as a randomized clinical trial, but when the number of patients is large and the analysis is done carefully, a lot of gold can be mined. Plus it's a lot cheaper than those clinical trials. The FDA has tried a similar approach to monitor pharmaceuticals on the market.

Project Sentinel

In 2004, five years after launch, Merck pulled Vioxx (rofecoxib) from the market. The pain medication which had been used by 20 million Americans had been shown to raise the risk of heart attacks and strokes. A *Lancet* article estimated that 88,000 Americans had suffered heart attacks on Vioxx, and 38,000 had died. Merck paid nearly $5 billion to end thousands of lawsuits related to this, without conceding they were aware of the increase in heart attack and stroke risk during the approval process or that their publications intentionally understated these risks.

Had there been better systems to monitor patients taking Vioxx, the FDA would have detected these adverse effects earlier and saved tens of thousands of lives. With this in mind, Congress passed the FDA Amendment Act of 2007, which mandated that the FDA develop a program to track and analyze the safety of drugs after they've come to the market without having to rely on pharmaceutical companies to report potential problems.

Richard Platt, a bow-tied professor of medicine at Harvard Medical School, is one of the leaders of that Sentinel program. Instead of expecting health plans and hospitals to share confidential health data, his team gives them some computer code that can be used to search within the walls of their own data warehouse. That way, the FDA can query data from over 100 million people and ask: Has there been an increase in small bowel problems after the introduction of a vaccine? Or, are patients receiving hypertension medication suffering from a condition called angioedema? By 2019, Sentinel had addressed 113 safety issues and answered questions that otherwise would have required at least 19 standalone studies involving ten products. Platt and coauthors point out that the usual post-marketing studies to investigate these would have cost millions of dollars each, taken a lot longer, and led to more people getting sicker.

It doesn't require significant imagination to think that these data could also be used to assess how cost-effectively drugs are working across large numbers of patients. Knowing patients' outcomes with medications could help pharmacies, insurers, and hospitals decide whether to prioritize specific drugs on formulary and how much to pay for them. With real-world evidence, the cost-effectiveness of drugs can be compared across broader and larger populations than tested in the original clinical trials. When I suggest this idea to Platt, he's enthusiastic. "Absolutely!"

New Data Frontiers

Most activities related to health happen outside of traditional health clinics and hospitals. Knowing this, the digital health industry is creating an entirely new set of health records. Tens of thousands of apps are measuring and recording data from our day-to-day lives: steps counted, calories burned, calories consumed, hours tossing and turning in bed, and more. Others are collecting family trees or DNA samples. Even credit history, shopping patterns, and travel history are believed to hold important insights into health behaviors and medical risks.

Some of the least traditional data may prove instrumental for solving some of the most intractable problems of health care. Mandy Cohen, secretary of North Carolina's Health and Human Services Department, wants to improve the health of some of the neediest two million people in her state. To understand those needs, her department collected data about social health indicators, such as food deserts (areas where it's difficult to buy affordable fresh food), places with poor access to transportation, and substandard housing, and then created a map that highlights those communities that needed the most help. It may not seem obvious why the health department is producing social services maps, but to Cohen, a primary care physician, the reasons are clear.

She tells the story of a patient she cared for a few years back, a college student who looked unwell. After eight weeks of running expensive tests on her, Cohen was stumped. And then a technician suggested gently, "Ask if she has enough to eat." She discovered that the student was living out of her car because she had just escaped an abusive relationship. Cohen realized she didn't have the tools in her medical toolkit to help. "It still stings," Cohen says. "I spent a lot of money, and I didn't make her one bit better."

With the data her department has collected, Cohen and team have built a digital tool that connects patients with community programs like a food bank, a program for adolescents at risk, and a domestic violence shelter. Cohen understands that the ultimate, alluring power of Big Data is making the unseen seen—whether it's a hidden cluster of dangerous side effects of a drug, or the too-predictable side effects of being hungry and forced to live in your car.

An Action Plan for Realizing Big Data's Potential

How can we make traditional sources, such as electronic health records or insurance claims data, more accessible to patients, and with their permission, also to researchers and policy makers? New kinds of data ranging from personal health sensors to genomics to data about social needs like transportation, food, and housing can help paint a more holistic picture of people's health.

To realize Big Data's full potential, we all have a role to play.

As a patient and consumer of health care, you should:

- Ask your physician for access to your medical notes, and if the medical practice isn't part of the OpenNotes movement, ask them to consider joining.
- Look for opportunities to access your health records.
- Consider judiciously whether you want to share your personal health data with vendors and ask yourself whether the benefit of the services to you (app features, for example) outweigh the risks of those vendors using your data for other purposes.
- Provide feedback on all patient portals (such as from your physician's electronic health record system or your insurance company's benefits tools).

As a physician or other health care professional, you should:

- Challenge your organization and vendors to improve the usability of electronic health records for you and your patients, and encourage patients to use their portals.
- Improve the quality of data entered into the electronic health records where possible—the better the data, the more useful they can be.

As a payer, such as a self-insured employer, government entity, or health plan, or as a policy maker, you should:

- Support the adoption of data standards and expect electronic health records vendors and health insurance companies to cooperate with third-party technologies that can use data to help employers (and other payers), clinicians, and patients to improve care.

- Set timely expectations of broad interoperability of electronic health data.
- Encourage research that leverages Big Data, such as predictive analytics, to reduce medical mistakes. Invest in clinical decision support tools to ensure the best care for complex patients.
- Invest in real-world evidence research that uses Big Data to answer questions about, for example, the effectiveness (including cost-effectiveness) of different therapies.
- Set expectations for government agencies and data and technology industries to establish and adopt high standards and best practices that protect the privacy and security of health data.

And most importantly, all of us need to elect leaders who will safely and responsibly unleash the potential of health-related data to improve the health of the population.

CHAPTER 10

EMPLOYER, HEAL THYSELF

The question is ... who bears the blame for this chaotic, private-sector price system. The only fair answer is: American employers.

—Uwe Reinhardt

As the third son, Carl Kjeldsberg knew he'd never get to run the family business—a 100-year-old Norwegian department store chain—but he had accepted that. In high school, he was a skiing champion and could imagine only one direction for his life: downhill, schussing. His father, however, had other plans. He plucked his son off the ski slopes of Norway and planted him in medical school amid the gardens and spires of Edinburgh. There Kjeldsberg discovered he had both a passion and a talent for medicine. After graduation, he came to the United States to train as a surgeon, but his career again took a sharp turn when he developed an allergy to latex surgical gloves. He transitioned into diagnostic pathology and settled in Salt Lake City, a 30-minute drive from multiple world-class ski resorts. Before long, he pivoted yet again and found himself running a business.

Chances are good that if you ever get your blood drawn to test for an unusual hormonal condition or an autoimmune disease, your tube will be sent to Salt Lake City. Every night, up to 50,000 samples of blood, urine, sputum, and tissue from all over the country arrive at the Salt Lake City Airport in big yellow crates destined for a company at the base of the Wasatch Mountains called ARUP Laboratories. That's the business Kjeldsberg cofounded in 1984 with fellow pathologist John Matsen, who was then chair of Pathology at the University of Utah. By moving the clinical laboratory out of the university's hospital and running it as a separate business, they were able to attract entrepreneurial and innovative pathologists who wanted to invent diagnostic tests and technologies and to see them implemented clinically quickly. Besides its hundreds of newly invented lab tests, the company also invested in highly efficient robotic technologies that kept quality and safety high. Business boomed, and ARUP Laboratories grew exponentially.

As the business got bigger, so did the number of employees, and before long, Kjeldsberg, downhill racer turned pathology CEO, had to pivot into yet another new role: large employer and health insurer for thousands of employees and their families.

Employers as Insurers

The distinctly American practice of employers providing health insurance to their employees grew out of efforts by the government to control wages during World War II. With millions serving in the military, economists feared labor shortages would give rise to inflation and destabilize the economy. Crafty employers got around wage controls by offering "fringe benefits," such as pensions, vacations, and health insurance benefits, to attract and retain skilled labor. In 1943, the Internal Revenue Service introduced a policy (later clarified and codified in 1954) making contributions by employers to group insurance plans not subject to wage controls and not treated as taxable income. From then on, employer-sponsored health insurance became a fixture of the US health system. In those early days, the financial impact was modest. In 1940, only 9% of Americans had access to hospital insurance, and it consumed only 0.4% of disposable income. No one could have anticipated the eventual financial consequences of this wage control workaround.

By 2017, the majority of insured Americans (56%, or 178 million people) were covered by an employer-sponsored plan. Medical benefits were available to over two-thirds of private industry workers and nearly nine out of ten government workers. Employers paid for about one-third of all health care in the United States—$1.2 trillion per year—second only to the federal government. In 2018, they covered 71% of health care costs for employees with families and 82% of the costs for individuals, which amounted to a breathtaking $14,156 per employee. This meant a company like ARUP Laboratories, with nearly 4,000 employees, was effectively managing a $50-million health care insurance business.

Economists argue that rising health care costs have driven up the price of American goods and services, making them less competitive in the global market. The Big Three automotive manufacturers claimed they needed a multibillion dollar bailout in 2008 in part because of massive health expenditures. (General Motors was spending $71 per worker per hour on health care, while Toyota was spending $47.) In 2004, Gary Cowger, GM's president of North American operations at the time, said the carmaker was spending $4.5 billion on health care each year, and added, "That's more than we spend on steel." Warren Buffett is reported to have said more plainly: "GM is a health and benefits company with an auto company attached."

The current system of employer-sponsored health insurance has fallen victim to the fee-for-service zero-gravity economics of American health care. That's profoundly and insidiously undermining the vitality of the US economy. From 1999 to 2015, wage gains for all but the wealthiest workers were wiped out by the contributions that employers made to health care. And that's not just burning up present earnings. Retirement savings also took a massive hit. In 2001, employers allocated over half of benefits (58%) to retirement. In 2015, that figure was about one-third (36%). We're paying for today's health care with tomorrow's retirement money.

Despite all the spending, employees aren't doing so well. In fact, the Robert Wood Johnson Foundation estimates that poor care leads to as many as 45 million avoidable sick days per year, or 180,000 people calling in sick every day. Every employer in the country is fretting and fuming about astronomical health care bills for a workforce that isn't necessarily healthier, yet few know how to manage them. Rick Wagoner, former CEO of General Motors, summed up the frustration of many companies: "When I joined GM 28 years ago, I did it because I love cars and trucks. I had no idea I'd wind up working as a health care administrator."

From Insured to Insurer

In the 1980s, many large employers realized that it was more economical for them to pay for their employees' health care directly ("self-insure") rather than pay an insurance company to bear the risk. They set aside funds to pay the bills as they came in (using brokers and third-party administrators to help contract with doctors and hospitals and also collect and pay bills). They also purchased stop-loss insurance to cover exceptionally high claims, like those over $100,000 or $200,000. By 2018, 61% of all employees covered by their insurer were in completely or partially self-insured plans; for companies with more than 1,000 employees, the figure was over 85%. Despite paying the bills, these employers often contribute little to the design of their plans and have even less insight into how to rein in costs, relying mostly on their brokers and third-party administrators.

When I was CEO at University of Utah Health, I too was responsible for the health care costs for our 15,000 employees and their families. Managing our costs were as challenging as—perhaps even more so than—those of our automotive manufacturing peers. Getting an MRI scan for a headache or an antibiotic for a cough can seem irresistible when you work right next to the radiology department or the pharmacy. Carl Kjeldsberg had the same dilemma at ARUP Laboratories . . . until he hired Peter Weir in 2006.

Weir, a family medicine physician, had been slogging away in a primary care clinic, rushing through ten-minute patient visits and working through piles of paperwork every night. When a colleague suggested he consider running ARUP's employee health clinic, he seized the chance. At ARUP's clinic, doctors and nurses cheerfully handed out bandages and administered flu shots, but there wasn't much evidence of lives being saved or cost curves being flattened. That didn't concern Weir, because in that clinic, he saw a tantalizing opportunity. He had recently attended a lecture by Thomas Bodenheimer, a renowned primary care physician from the University of California at San Francisco, who had described a team-based approach for patients with chronic diseases. His model moved physicians out of the center of the clinical universe and relied on nutritionists, pharmacists, educators, and health coaches instead. It made patients healthier and lowered costs. Weir thought ARUP's clinic was the perfect place to try Bodenheimer's model.

To start, he created a health risk–assessment survey that asked employees to volunteer information about their age, gender, race, total cholesterol, HDL cholesterol, blood pressure, and any history of diabetes or smoking. He then plugged those numbers into (now online) risk calculators to work out each individual's risk of developing heart disease or stroke over the next ten years. For example, a 65-year-old African American man with normal cholesterol and blood pressure, who doesn't smoke and is not diabetic, has a 6.9% risk of a stroke or heart attack in the next ten years, while the same man who smokes has almost double the risk (11.6%). Add high blood pressure, and his risk shoots up to 19.8%.

Weir also wanted to know what people were doing to keep themselves healthy, so he asked how many minutes of exercise they did each week, how many servings of fruits and vegetables they ate each day, how much screen time they logged, how many sugary drinks they chugged, and whether they got cancer screening tests like mammograms and colonoscopies.

When some employees expressed concerns about confidentiality, Weir made sure everyone knew that personal health information—including the answers to surveys—was firewalled from anyone in the company who wasn't on the medical team, even the top bosses. He even asked his medical staff not to eat in the cafeteria to reinforce that total separation between them and other employees.

To encourage employees to complete this form, Weir persuaded management to offer a hefty financial incentive: 25% off their share of health insurance premiums. By 2018, about 98% of ARUP employees and their partners or spouses had completed the survey.

With all these data in hand, Weir and team redesigned the employee health programs. Clinic employees became chronic disease health coaches. They focused on reducing the risks of strokes and heart attacks, cancer, and complications of diabetes. As a self-insured company, any reductions in costs would be savings for ARUP. That's why, when the team proposed that the clinic provide free insulin, free generic oral diabetes medications, and even free diabetic supplies like glucometers and glucose strips, ARUP's CFO agreed. He knew that preventing just one hospitalization a year would more than recoup the investment.

Weir was also particularly committed to helping employees with mental health conditions, like depression and anxiety. He used a physician-to-physician consulting program offered by the University of Utah to supplement his team. Employees completed questions about their mental health, and university psychiatrists reviewed them and made recommendations to the employee's ARUP physician via a brief videoconference. Weir and his colleagues eventually learned to manage common conditions like depression on their own.

Along the way, Weir realized that not everyone in the company understood what it meant to work for a self-insured employer. When he recommended that one of his patients—a high-level manager—take the generic version of a medication, the manager responded, "No, no, I want the branded drug . . . because I want to screw the insurance company!" After that, Weir went on a campaign around the company's nearly 4,000 employees to explain what it meant for the company to be self-insured. Their insurance company *was* ARUP.

Five years in, health costs for ARUP employees leveled off. Health measures improved, from blood pressure readings to the rates at which women underwent cervical cancer screening checks. Patients started bringing spouses and children to get their primary care from Weir's team. He says he was overwhelmed by their enthusiasm about the clinic: "They treated me like royalty."

Pepsi Goes Flat

Not every employer has had the same success as ARUP Laboratories, although many have tried. In 2012, about half of US employers with 50 or more employees and more than 90% of those with over 50,000 employees offered some combination of wellness or health programs. Besides a few anecdotal success stories and some encouraging early publications, collective experiences in the real world were not rosy. Most employers who invested in employee wellness saw little impact on their health care bills, even though their employees really appreciated the yoga and weight-loss classes. A RAND Corporation analysis of PepsiCo's program shed light on why most people weren't getting good results. To get a clear picture of costs and benefits, the researchers separated Pepsi's programs into two flavors—disease management and lifestyle management. Lifestyle management included programs that managed weight, nutrition, fitness, and stress, and encouraged workers to stop smoking. They may have made employees feel valued, but they didn't lead to any savings. For every dollar Pepsi put into lifestyle management, employee health bills were reduced by only 48 cents. It may not have been a total waste of money, but it certainly wasn't paying off.

On the other hand, disease management programs worked. Pepsi offered six- to nine-month programs that helped employees manage and prevent ten conditions: asthma, coronary artery disease, atrial fibrillation, heart failure, stroke, hyperlipidemia, hypertension, diabetes, low back pain, and chronic obstructive pulmonary disease. After seven years, Pepsi's disease management program yielded almost $4 in return for every $1 invested and reduced health care costs by $136 per employee per month, mostly because of a 29% reduction in hospital admissions. From 2004 to 2011, Pepsi's employees in the disease management program saw their costs cut by more than one-half. Results like that will put a little fizz into any soda-maker's financials.

Not all employers have been able to replicate Pepsi's results. An analysis by McKinsey consultants suggested some key features—many of which were shared by ARUP's clinic—that increase the success of a disease management program: the responsibility for care should fall on one general practitioner (like Weir), larger programs do better than small programs (100 patients is too small), data on patient outcomes should guide improvements, and incentives can encourage both patients and clinicians to achieve common goals.

Getting Skinned in the Game

Failing to develop cost-effective health management programs, many employers have turned to "consumer-driven health care," or more accurately, "high-deductible plans" (often with a pretax health savings account), where employees trade lower premiums for higher deductibles, co-payments, and coinsurance. About 30% of adults had a high-deductible plan in 2019. Unfortunately, these plans are less "consumer-driven," and more "consumer-gets-run-over." In 2016, employer-sponsored family health insurance consumed, on average, one-third of the median household income in the United States, compared to less than 15% in 1999. That doesn't leave much for most families to spend on food, housing, and transportation.

Employers claim these plans encourage employees to try to stay healthier because they have more "skin in the game." Behavioral economists—backed up by the health outcomes of consumer-driven plans—beg to disagree. The prevalence of obesity, persistently high rates of smoking (and now vaping), and low rates of cancer screening, among other signs, in people who likely want to be healthy call into question the role of financial inducements in helping people make healthier choices. Consumer-driven health care also assumes employees will reduce care that is wasteful or of marginal value. Instead of a frivolous trip to the emergency room at midnight, skin-in-the-game employees should wait for a primary care clinic to open the next day. They should choose generic drugs over branded options. They should opt for less expensive hospitals and specialists.

That all sounds good, but research shows it's only partially true, if at all. A RAND Corporation study found that a family that switched to a high-deductible plan spent 20% less on health care in the following year than a family on a traditional plan. The authors note, however, that the reductions are partly a statistical fluke, because healthier workers tend to choose high-deductible plans, so of course they tend to spend less (so-called selection bias).

To examine how cost-sharing changed people's behaviors, a landmark experiment in 1973 randomly assigned almost 8,000 people across the nation to health plans that were either free or had different levels of coin-surance and out-of-pocket limits, and then tracked how they used health care. The study concluded that the more individuals had to pay, the fewer services they consumed. Those who had to pay more saw fewer doctors, and they were hospitalized less. But their health was worse: blood pressure was less likely to be controlled, vision was less likely to be corrected, and they were more likely to die earlier. Higher co-payments meant that patients didn't fill their prescriptions, and they didn't take their sick children to get care. With high-deductible health plans, people simply stopped seeking care, even free preventive measures like cancer screening.

If you have a crystal ball that can accurately predict that you won't use much health care in the coming year, a consumer-driven, high-deductible plan is right for you. But most of us don't have that fortune-telling capa-bility, and the ups and downs of unpredictable health are pushing families into bankruptcy and hurting both employees and the employers who rely on their work.

The solution is for employers to start thinking less like insurers and more like businesses.

Let's Poke the Skunk

In December 2004, Bob Mecklenburg received a visit that pretty much ruined his Christmas break. Mecklenburg was chief of medicine at Vir-ginia Mason Medical Center. His hospital was paid to provide health care to employees of four of Seattle's biggest companies and employers: Costco, Starbucks, Nordstrom, and King County. In his office that day was the medical director of Aetna, the third-party administrator for each of the four self-insured employers. He told Mecklenburg that the care provided by his hospital was too expensive and that unless something changed, they would dump Virginia Mason.

Mecklenburg, who is responsible for hundreds of millions of dollars in his department's annual budget, most of which was clinical revenue from caring for patients, had a startling realization: "I had never come face to face with people who paid my salary—I thought Virginia Mason paid, but it was these employers."

He wanted to understand the problem better, so he asked the four HR heads what was driving their climbing health care costs and lost employee productivity. Back pain and headaches seemed common, they said. But beyond that, they weren't sure.

Mecklenburg immediately asked Aetna for the data on what treatments and procedures these employees had received from Virginia Mason over the past year. Then he spent his Christmas holiday poring over pages and pages of spreadsheets. "This was kitchen-table research," he says, adding that the reports were not easy to interpret—all of the redundancies and absurdities of the terminology used by hospitals and insurance companies made simple things hopelessly complex. For example, he expected to find one code for back pain, but there were nearly a dozen—it was called sciatica, backache, radiculopathy, lumbago, back pain, and more. He carefully grouped all those into one bucket to better understand how back pain was being treated, and then repeated the process for other common conditions so he could see which factors were driving up costs.

After days spent analyzing the claims data, he found it wasn't the rare patients with cancer or unusual autoimmune diseases or even devastating accidents who were emptying the till. The culprits were everyday illnesses that afflicted many people and were being treated incorrectly. Coughs and colds, generally caused by viruses, were being dosed with bacteria-killing antibiotics that wouldn't help. (Those prescriptions drive up costs and inadvertently produce more antibiotic-resistant strains of bacteria.) Folks with headaches too often had expensive CT (or "CAT") and MRI scans, when the best treatment would have been a couple of aspirin. Lumps in the breast mostly turned out to be benign, but too many women were put through imaging, biopsies, pathological interpretations (sometimes false-positives), and all the attendant worry.

In the pay-for-action model, the overwhelming tendency is to over-treat, and Mecklenburg quickly realized that's what Virginia Mason was doing. "Yestercare" is what he now calls treatment that produces plenty of tests and bills and fees, but not enough health. It is not only expensive for both employees and their employers, but it is also inefficient for companies because it results in their workers being out longer. And don't forget the additional complications from, say, unnecessary surgery or prescription drugs.

Mecklenburg also found another distressing pattern. Headaches, colds, asthma, and benign breast masses were very common, but the treatments varied widely. For example, for diagnosing the causes of back pain, MRIs are no better than X-rays (which are also mostly useless, but a lot cheaper). The medical literature is filled with research showing this, yet back MRI remains one of the most commonly performed imaging procedures in the United States. Similarly, for the seven million children with asthma and their 700,000 visits to emergency departments each year, guidelines recommend against performing a chest X-ray or prescribing antibiotics for an acute flare-up, and yet about one-third get an X-ray, and one in six are prescribed antibiotics.

When I asked Mecklenburg why insurers, brokers, and hospital administrators didn't seem to have the insights he'd discovered on his kitchen table over that Christmas break, he shook his head. "They like it fine the way it is," he said, "Fee for service—why mess with it? We're making billions of dollars. Why poke the skunk?"

Start Pulling the Supply Chain

Bob Mecklenburg gradually realized he was grappling with a business problem, not a medical one, and that his HR partners were extremely well equipped to help him solve it. He explained to them that they had a "supply-chain issue"—a clinic failing to keep an employee from getting ill and missing work was the equivalent of a chip manufacturer delivering a poor-quality part to Intel. Think of it this way: if employees are home sick, Nordstrom can't sell clothes and Costco can't restock shelves. Using that fundamental insight, the four Seattle companies drew up five key "performance specs" Virginia Mason Medical Center would have to meet:

Spec #1: Give Us What Works and Skip the Rest

The HR directors told Mecklenburg they would no longer pay for procedures, tests, and medications that didn't work. Virginia Mason's doctors and hospitals would now only do things that were proven effective, also known as "evidence-based medicine." Costco wouldn't sell stale bread and expect to be paid. Why should they settle for less from their employee health providers?

Spec #2: 100% Customer Satisfaction

Business students study Nordstrom because it sets the standard for customer satisfaction. Their representatives asked: Why couldn't health care providers deliver a consistently good, customer-centered experience? They expected the health system to demonstrate respect for the patient as a member of the health care team and to include them in decisions about their care. They challenged Virginia Mason to drastically improve customer satisfaction. (They did, and later even added a warranty.)

Spec #3: Same-Day Care

The Starbucks representative pushed Mecklenburg on this point: imagine ordering a skinny tall white latte and being told it would arrive in two to four weeks. Their ailing employees needed to be seen promptly. In what other business do customers *wait* to get their calls returned, *wait* long beyond their scheduled appointment times, and *wait* for hours in the emergency room, without so much as an apology, much less a snack or a beverage?

Spec #4: Rapid Return to Function

Hospitals and doctors assess their performance in terms of quality and safety. They almost never measure how quickly patients recover and never consider how long it takes for patients to return to work. The King County representative challenged Virginia Mason to minimize down time and maximize productive days for their employees. From now on, an employee's time would be as valuable as a clinician's time, or more so.

Spec #5: Predictable and Consistent Prices for Buyer and Seller
As these employers compared notes on what they spent on care for the most common conditions, they found wide variations. From now on, if a patient needed a total hip replacement, the employers expected to pay a fixed amount for the entire procedure, including rehabilitation. The fee would be negotiated up front and be affordable for both the doctor/hospital and the patient/employer.

These performance specs were good not just for the employers but for the employees. They made sense for the health system. Mecklenburg knew that if Virginia Mason could deliver on these specifications for all their patients, it would be the best health care system in the country.

Reinventing Spine Care

To start, Mecklenburg chose one of the most common ailments, uncomplicated back pain, as a test case. About 80% of people with back pain are categorized as "uncomplicated," meaning they do not have warning signs such as weakness or numbness of the legs or arms which could point to a more serious condition. He knew Virginia Mason routinely failed to meet all five of the performance specifications for uncomplicated back pain.

Working with other clinicians, Mecklenburg created a flowchart showing the experience of a typical employee with this complaint, beginning with that first call to the doctor's office. "It's your lucky day!" he says somewhat dryly. "The doctor can see you in two weeks." Moving his finger to the right on his chart, he arrives at his next box: you finally see the doctor, a primary care physician, who, Mecklenburg explains, "doesn't actually do anything!" She might order a few blood tests and perhaps prescribe something for the pain. You're told to come back for a follow-up appointment in a few weeks. When you return to the doctor's office ("Surprise!"), you're not any better. The MRI comes next ("Unnecessary!"), and then you go back to the physician, who might refer you to a neurologist or perhaps a rehabilitation doctor. A couple of months after you first called the doctor, you are sent to a physical therapist ("Finally!") and begin to recover.

Applying the "Virginia Mason Production System" (their version of the Toyota Production System), the spine clinicians discarded Mecklenburg's flowchart and replaced his boxes with just one, labeled *Spine Clinic*. Rather than the two-month ordeal that entails multiple unnecessary visits and imaging studies, patients with uncomplicated back pain can come to the Spine Clinic *that day* (Spec #3). And see a physical therapist *that day* (Spec #1). And start to improve *that day* (Spec #2), because treatment starts immediately. Employees return to work much sooner (Spec #4). Mecklenburg smiles. "It just takes a couple of hours."

The biggest cost savings, outside of eliminating unnecessary imaging and surgery, came from taking spine surgeons out of the picture until and *unless* absolutely necessary. As Harvard business professor Bob Kaplan loves to point out, having a physical therapist rather than a surgeon evaluate a patient with low back pain saves hundreds of dollars per hour. It seems counterintuitive, but the Spine Clinic was a boon for surgeons, because it allowed them to be much more productive. The clinic could now screen four times as many patients, and spine surgeons saw only the patients they should have been seeing—those who were likely to need an operation.

Raj Sethi, the energetic director of neurosciences at Virginia Mason, confirmed Mecklenburg's impressions. Taking referrals from across the country, he and his fellow surgeons built a reputation for wisely deciding who did and did not need an operation. He tells me about a 46-year-old overweight truck driver flown by his employer from Arizona to Virginia Mason in Seattle. An MRI showed some arthritis in the neck, and his local doctor had offered him an operation to fuse three neck vertebrae. He had had no physical therapy or acupuncture and still needed to lose weight. Sethi told him, "If I do a three-level cervical fusion, the likelihood that your neck pain is going to get better is probably 50%, at best. But guess what happens when you do a three-level cervical fusion? You put stress on the disk above and the disk below . . . and you're looking at another surgery three or four years later." Having flown from Arizona to Seattle to get this candid assessment, the patient got back on the plane home and booked an appointment with a physical therapist.

That's a small example of why many of the largest employers in the country have awarded Virginia Mason a "center of excellence" designation, which means they are willing to fly employees in from hundreds of miles away. It is now one of the best hospitals in the United States and consistently wins top-quality awards (it was one of Leapfrog's Top Hospitals of the Decade in 2010). And it's all because Bob Mecklenburg poked the skunk.

Why Won't They Take Their Medicine?

To answer the perplexing question of why all employers aren't following the lead of Starbucks and Nordstrom, I turned to Bob Galvin, a physician who has spent his entire career trying to fix health care. I met him in his New York office at Blackstone Group, one of the world's largest private investment firms, where he is CEO of Equity Healthcare, Blackstone's health care management program. He advises on the employee health programs of companies held in the private equity portfolio, like Hilton Hotels, Sea World Parks, and Vivint, the home security company. Why is an investment company messing with employee health care? Because every dollar of savings from employee health costs generates a huge multiplier when it comes time to sell the company. Blackstone is in this business to make money, and if they can help employees be healthier, all the better.

Galvin advises over 75 CEOs on their health programs. He sounds a little wistful when he talks about how few of them are taking full responsibility for the health of their employees. He referred me to a paper he wrote with Suzanne Delbanco, former CEO of the Leapfrog Group, a modern Codman's End-Results–type company he helped found. He remembered it being called "Employers, What's the Matter with You?" The printed title is slightly less provocative, "Why Employers Need to Rethink How They Buy Health Care." It was written back in 2005, but the grim facts are essentially unchanged.

Galvin and Delbanco pointed out that fewer than half of major US firms conducted financial analyses on health care costs, and fewer than a third used return-on-investment calculations. Information about quality of care was missing in their procurement decisions. Only about a third of employers provided information about the quality of the health systems employees were choosing from, and fewer than a quarter shared information about price.

So why aren't big employers doing this? Why, after all these years, are they still just shifting costs to employees?

Galvin shrugs. Health care, he says, isn't a C-suite priority. It is assigned to human resources benefits managers and is rarely their primary area of interest. Most employers purchase care through brokers and pharmacy benefit managers and frequently rely on insurance companies and benefits consultants to design their offerings, even if they are self-insured. Rarely do employers even get the detailed claims data on their employees to see how their dollars have been spent. Most HR managers have no relationships with the doctors and hospitals their employees use. Their brokers negotiate with insurance companies and health care systems for them. The brokers take a cut. The insurers generate their fees. The status quo gets everybody paid and home by 5 o'clock. That sentiment is starting to change.

If It's Good Enough for Amazon . . .

What Mecklenburg launched in Seattle is starting to spread across the country. In 2018, Amazon, Berkshire Hathaway, and J.P. Morgan Chase announced they would join forces to solve the employee health problem for their 1.2 million employees, and for others. Walmart, Lowe's, GE, Boeing, and several other big companies have all adopted similar measures in selecting health care systems—like Virginia Mason, Geisinger Health System, and Cleveland Clinic—that they believe can deliver on their specs, even if they have to fly their employees to receive care. Like Medicare's Bundled Payments for Care Improvement, employers are negotiating with hospitals to pay their own bundled rate, where all the services during a hospitalization, including the hospital stay, all the doctors' fees, devices like an artificial hip, and other tests and imaging, are included in a set fee. Typically, that price is 10%–15% less than a fee-for-service arrangement. In return, the health system gets new patients and the prestige of a "Center of Excellence" designation. (When the Employers' Center of Excellence Network opened the bidding process for hospitals to contract with them, they found that fewer than 5% of health care systems met all the quality requirements for consideration.)

Statewide programs are also emerging, modeled after the Employers' Centers of Excellence. For example, the Bree Collaborative, in support of the Washington State Health Care Authority that covers 2 million of the state's 7 million residents, gives state employees and Medicaid recipients the opportunity to choose to receive their hip and knee replacements or spine surgery at state Centers of Excellence with no out-of-pocket expenses.

How do employers justify sending an employee and an accompanying family member to another city just for health care? The biggest savings come from finding highly qualified doctors willing to advise against unnecessary surgery, like Raj Sethi. One study found that of 450 patients with back or neck pain who had been recommended for surgery in their hometowns, only 62% of them really needed surgery when evaluated at one of the Centers of Excellence. Instead, activity-based therapies, pain injections, physical therapy, and weight loss were recommended. Of patients expecting to undergo a hip or knee replacement, 16% were advised not to have surgery when seen at a center. Employee satisfaction ratings for these programs exceed 90%—having no co-pays helps—and nearly all patients end up following the advice of their Center of Excellence physicians not to have an operation, even if their home physician recommended it. That saves the company money and keeps more money in the wallets of employees. Lowe's employees who needed a joint replacement saved on average $3,300 in co-payments and fees compared to those who underwent the same procedure in their traditional health plan.

Centers of Excellence bundled payment arrangements make sense for operations like hip replacements and spine surgery, which can be planned and scheduled in advance. Employers' investments in primary care and preventive medicine are more challenging to manage. Karen DeSalvo, a physician and former acting assistant secretary of the US Department of Health and Human Services, calls it the "wrong pocket" problem. The entity that invests in health isn't always the one reaping the reward. Sometimes the problem is a matter of timing.

The Wrong Pocket

Many employers evaluate their health investments annually, and they seek returns on their investments on this time horizon. They may commit to sponsoring disease management programs for their employees for one year at a time, or perhaps as long as three years. This makes sense because most employees don't stay long. In 2018, across all industries, employees stayed with the same employer for an average of 4.2 years. Younger-generation employees or those working in industries like leisure and hospitality stay less than three years. (In contrast, for those 55 to 64, the median tenure is 10.1 years.)

This has important implications for how employers invest in their employees' health. Take the example that Rushika Fernandopulle, CEO of Iora Health (whom we met in Chapter 2), shared with me about an Iora clinic for employees at a college. The rate of female employees receiving recommended Pap smears (a screen for cervical cancer) had been lower than expected. After getting input from a patient advisory group, one physician decided to start a new program. Once a month, from 5–7 p.m., the clinic sponsored a "Pappy Hour"—with wine, snacks, music, and candles. (One doctor called it a "spa-like experience.") The number of screenings shot up. (Upside.) And when they did, Iora doctors found some early cancers in unsuspecting women. (Big upside!) Those patients went for surgery, and some to chemotherapy. For that year, the costs of care were significantly above expected. (Downside.)

And here's the really tantalizing twist: Fernandopulle points out that the cancers found thanks to Pappy Hour might not have been detected for another couple of years. By then, the women would have had Stage 3 cancer and a much poorer prognosis. That means the program saved a lot of money and a lot of lives, as long as the employee stayed with the employer for at least three years. Many government-run programs have the advantage of durable relationships with their members. With Medicare, military medicine, and the VA, members are often in for life. Investments that pay off in three, five, or ten years make sense because the return always comes to the right pocket.

For employee health, timing isn't always so perfect. When employees stay at the same job for only 2–4 years on average in many industries, employers may not see the return on their investment in prevention and cancer screening. We need a new way of ensuring that employers make the best decisions for their employees, like ARUP's free glucometer strips and free insulin and Fernandopulle's Pappy Hour clinics. For more employers to sign on, they need to believe it will be a "right pocket" decision for them.

A Ten-Point Action Plan for Employers

Employers can radically improve health care in the United States by treating it like any other resource they need for their company and expecting costs to be linked to the quality and efficiency of the service provided. Self-funded employers can design their own benefit packages to improve health and lower costs innovatively. Consortia of companies with the greatest purchasing power can open the doors for smaller companies and their employees to benefit as well. It can happen in just ten steps:

1. **Find a smart health plan administrator.**
   For a 5,000-employee business, health care will consume $50 million to $70 million each year, so it's worth the time and trouble to identify the right person—either in-house or externally—to manage employee health benefits.
2. **Analyze employee claims data.**
   If you are self-insured, you have a right to employee claims data (in anonymized form). Have your health plan administrator help ana-

lyze the data or hire an outside firm to do it. Compare your spending with national benchmarks, adjusting for underlying health conditions, age, and other risk factors.

3. **Develop a health risk–assessment questionnaire.**

This can help your health plan administrator and medical team (see below) identify employees who would benefit from disease management programs that may be run in-house or as part of a separate medical clinic. Make sure there's a clear firewall between medical staff who collect and analyze health data and your management team to protect employee confidentiality.

4. **Partner with other local or regional employers.**

Employers can band together to create critical mass for common services. Joining employer networks like the National Business Group on Health, Health Transformation Alliance, or Catalyst for Payment Reform can provide access to national Centers of Excellence contracts or benchmarking data.

5. **Carefully select hospital and physician partners.**

Public nonprofit health care foundations (Leapfrog, for example) routinely collect and report quality metrics for hospitals and physicians. Many performance metrics required by Medicare (Medicare's Hospital Compare website, for example) and accrediting bodies are available online. Combine this information with your employee claims data to understand differences in costs of care across systems and physicians.

6. **Perform your own evaluation of hospitals and physicians' groups, develop relationships with health care professionals, and define your performance specs.**

Supplement published data with your own homework. Look for systems with a culture of safety, Lean manufacturing practices, high employee satisfaction and retention, reliable data, and a willingness to share. Just as the Seattle business partners were with Mecklenburg, be clear about your expectations, like same-day access to care. Be willing to adjust your benefits to encourage employees to use these systems. Expect to receive data on the performance specifications to guide future contracting decisions.

7. **Negotiate bundled payments for specific medical services commonly used by your workforce.**

   Common medical services, like pregnancy and labor and delivery, total hip or knee replacements, back pain, and headache can be negotiated as bundled payments with clinicians and hospitals. The Bree Collaborative shares templates for some of these contractual arrangements. Consider fixed payment models with progressive physicians' groups in the same way that Centers of Excellence do with Virginia Mason Medical Center.

8. **Contribute your business insights to help your health care partners.**

   Your expertise as a business leader may enable you to help your hospital practice safer, more efficient, and technologically sophisticated care. Get involved and consider joining a hospital or medical board or advisory committee.

9. **Work with your insurance company to standardize your plan offerings and present them so that your employees can understand them.**

   For employers and employees to be informed shoppers, they need to compare plans just as they need to compare hospitals and doctors. If every plan has a different set of deductibles, co-payments, and coinsurance arrangements with every hospital and every doctor, it will remain nearly impossible for patients to comparison shop. Work with other employers to drive greater standardization and simplification. Expect price transparency and out-of-pocket price calculators for your employees.

10. **Engage your employees every step of the way.**

    Educate them about what it means to be a self-insured employee and make sure they know you are committed to coproducing their health. Reward employees for staying healthy and for choosing high value health care.

CHAPTER 11

RESTORING READINESS:
BATTLE-TESTED CARE

*He who would become a surgeon should join an army
and follow it.*

—Hippocrates

When Americans mention government-run health care, we usually
think of Medicare or Medicaid, but both are, for the most part, *health benefits* programs. That is, they are more like health insurance companies than
government-run health care. For that, we need to look at the Military Health
System, run by the Department of Defense, and its even-larger sibling, the
Veterans Health Administration. Both operate health benefits plans, and
they also care for patients. They run their own hospitals and clinics and
employ their own physicians, nurses, pharmacists, and other health professionals. They even run their own mail-order pharmacies.

Both systems have valuable lessons to impart: how to lead change, how
to negotiate better deals for health care, how to train a workforce of health
professionals, and how to measure success. They are driven to improve and

to innovate, and they can't afford to get sidetracked by political infighting or sweetheart deals. For them, health care isn't just a job, it's a matter of national security.

Battle-Tested Care

In his retirement, Major General George Anderson served on the Defense Health Board, a federal committee advisory to the secretary of defense in matters of military medicine. As he welcomed me to the board, he explained the mission of military medicine and why care is an entitlement for active-duty personnel and a benefit for dependents. Military leaders and military medicine have enjoyed interdependency since antiquity, he tells me. "Alexander the Great had a surgeon, and he told them where to put their camps." General Anderson speaks with the wisdom of a soldier and the schooling of a doctor. "Military leaders understand the importance of medicine," he says. "They know what it is to face death and to see people saved."

Because his father was a military doctor, Anderson went to kindergarten at Eielson Air Force Base in Fairbanks, Alaska, and high school in Izmir, Turkey. After attending medical school, he joined the US Air Force and pursued a career in preventive medicine. After a long series of air force assignments and promotions, he served as deputy assistant secretary of defense for Health Services Operations and Readiness from 1994 to 1997, which meant he helped to run the same health care system that had vaccinated him as a child.

With an annual budget of about $50 billion a year, the Military Health System has two vital missions: ensure the readiness of US armed forces for military operations and provide health care (including the health benefits programs) for its 9.5 million beneficiaries. About one-third of beneficiaries are active-duty members and their families, and most of the rest are retirees who qualify for medical benefits, having served at least 20 years of service. Military medicine's Quadruple Aim includes the familiar trio of better health, better care, and lower costs, and adds a critical fourth, improved readiness, which refers to two important dimensions:

a military force that is medically ready to deploy AND a medical force ready to support them.

The large, complex Military Health System operates 932 military treatment facilities, including 177 overseas. Most of its 51 hospitals are small; only six of them routinely have more than 100 inpatients. Additionally, the Military Health System runs 424 medical clinics and 248 dental clinics around the world. Active-duty members and their families get care in these facilities for free. Non-active-duty members typically receive "purchased care" from a network of civilian preferred providers. If they are willing to pay more out of pocket, they can also go out of network. Those over 65 years old can get a supplemental plan for Medicare-eligible retirees.

The military's offerings, referred to as TRICARE, are generous compared to civilian employer-based plans. Premiums for non-active-duty members and families are only about $300 per year for individuals and top out at $720 per year for families. For purchased care, out-of-pocket expenses are set low to encourage in-network care (co-pays of $15–25 for visits, for example, or $180 for a hospitalization). In 2018, total out-of-pocket costs for military families under the age of 65 were much lower—at least $5,800 less—than those for their civilian counterparts.

In terms of quality of care, the Military Health System is overall similar to the civilian sector, although outcomes vary significantly by hospital. The biggest concern about the quality of military medicine stems from surgeons and other specialists not getting enough practice when they are deployed or working in small military hospitals back home. Some studies have shown that surgeons who perform a higher volume of a particular operation have better results, although others have challenged the conclusion that only surgeons who perform a minimum number of cases should be allowed to operate. (Similar concerns also apply to the civilian doctors practicing in smaller or rural critical-access hospitals). Military medical leadership has responded by establishing key competency benchmarks for all surgeons to meet and requiring all surgical military facilities to participate in the national quality improvement program.

Whereas the Military Health System's purpose is to support military operations, the mission of the Veterans Health Administration (VHA) is to provide health and medical services for veterans. The VHA is the largest integrated health care system in the country—it cares for about nine million of the 18.2 million veterans in the United States. The VHA network includes 172 medical centers and over 1,000 outpatient sites, and it employs about 300,000 people. The medical part of its budget was about $85 billion for 2020.

To qualify for benefits, veterans need to have served in the military for at least 24 months, unless discharged for disability or hardship. Because the Veterans Health Administration doesn't have enough resources to meet the needs of all veterans, it primarily cares for those with low incomes, the disabled, and those exposed to nuclear or chemical toxins. (If you don't meet these criteria, then you have to get your health care from another source, like an employer, Medicaid, or Medicare, or you buy insurance on the individual exchange).

Even for the nine million who qualify, resources are insufficient. The Veterans Health Administration made headlines in 2014, when a whistle-blower at the Phoenix VA hospital reported that long wait times were keeping veterans from obtaining life-saving care. In Phoenix, besides the 1,400 veterans officially listed as waiting for an appointment, over 3,500 additional veterans were unofficially listed. And though hospital administrators reported that it was taking veterans an average of 24 days to get seen at the clinic, it was really taking 115 days. Because of those lamentable delays in care, at least 40 veterans died. In August 2014, Congress passed the Veterans' Access, Choice, and Accountability Act of 2014, which included a provision to allow veterans who live over 40 miles from a VA facility to seek medical care from a non-VA facility.

Despite that scandalous failure, champions of the Veterans Health Administration point out that the system delivers care that's as good, if not better, than most civilians get, and at a much lower cost. It is also, on average, safer. A comparison of 129 VA hospitals and 4,010 non-VA hospitals between 2012 and 2015 found that of the nine patient safety indicators used by the Agency for Healthcare Research and Quality, the VA had equal outcomes for three and better outcomes for six, including lower hospital-acquired blood infection and death rates.

Saving Lives . . . and Dollars

Both the Military Health System and Veterans Health Administration are unique microcosms worthy of study for anyone serious about fixing our health care system. Each is a single-payer system that routinely deals with millions of patients. Each faces careful congressional scrutiny and has extensive reporting requirements. Each has dodged the fee-for-service system (except when forced to outsource care to the civilian sector) and instead has implemented a pay-for-results model. Care provided by both is paid for under a fixed budget, annually funded by Congress. The Military Health System's budget has been essentially flat at around $50 billion between 2012 and 2020, compared to an increase of over 30% for the rest of the United States.

As a payer that designs its own health benefits, the Military Health System is experimenting with ways to encourage members to favor care that leads to better outcomes and lower costs. For example, in 2018, it reduced or eliminated co-payments for drugs considered especially beneficial, like low-cost, effective blood pressure medications, because it wanted to encourage their use. When the government systems contract with civilian providers, the payment models are increasingly being converted from pay for action to pay for results.

Change from the Top

Some of the most powerful lessons from the Military Health System come from their efforts at change management.

For decades, each of the services—the US Army, Navy, and Air Force—has been accustomed to running its own military treatment facilities. In 2013, Congress established the Defense Health Agency and put it in charge of ten shared services, including pharmacy operations, the TRICARE health plan, and health information technology. Then came the National Defense Authorization Act of 2017—Arizona Senator John McCain's last. In that act, Congress mandated that operational control and budgets of all hospitals and clinics move from the respective surgeons general to central management by the Defense Health Agency to gain efficiencies from shared operations.

With NDAA 2017 targeted for completion by October 2021, the responsibility for carrying it out fell on the shoulders of trauma surgeon Vice Admiral Raquel Cruz Bono.

"Rocky" to her friends, Vice Admiral Bono is an indefatigable woman with a ready smile and the hint of a Texan twang. Born in the Philippines and raised in the United States, she's a trauma surgeon who headed Casualty Receiving for Operations Desert Shield and Desert Storm. She comes from a line of military medical officers, and until her brother retired in 2013 holding the rank of rear admiral, Admiral Bono was half of the Navy's only brother-and-sister admiral pair.

Under Admiral Bono's leadership, the Defense Health Agency began implementing one of the largest organizational changes in military medicine in decades, shifting the focus from non-active-duty military beneficiaries (who rely more on the civilian sector to provide their care) to the readiness of active-duty members. At the same time, it hopes to keep costs down. As acting principal deputy secretary of defense for Health Affairs Terry Adirim points out, two years after the 2017 NDAA, reform initiatives already contributed to $1.027 billion in savings for 2019.

One Formulary for Success

The Military Health System and Veterans Health Administration have managed their budgets effectively in large part by keeping drug costs down. They negotiate with manufacturers to obtain significantly discounted prices for prescription drugs. They also have another weapon especially designed for them: the Veterans Health Care Act of 1992 mandated that drug companies guarantee them both a discount of at least 24% off the average national sales price.

That's not their only tool. The Military Health System and the Veterans Health Administration each has its own national formulary committee to decide what drugs to offer to their members. Unlike other parts of the federal government, they can make their decisions based on cost-effectiveness research, measuring the utility of drugs in terms of cost per quality-adjusted life years (QALYs), if they wish. Unlike Medicare, they don't have to offer a drug to their members if they believe it is not cost-effective. This gives them extra leverage to negotiate deeper discounts with suppliers of comparable drugs. It also helps curb the rising costs of expensive drugs.

The Veterans Health Administration has the lowest per-prescription costs among all federal purchasers, outperforming even the Military Health System, mostly because they've successfully persuaded their physicians to prescribe lower-cost generic alternatives. In an ideal world, others could benefit from the Veterans Health Administration's work. While it makes its national formulary and price list public, posted prices do not include all the discounts, since manufacturer agreements can (and do) require final prices to remain confidential.

The Veterans Health Administration has also shown that more efficient dispensing, especially through their seven automated mail-order pharmacies, can save money. A 2015 study showed that it cost the VA $1.53 to dispense a prescription by mail order, compared to the national average of $10.50 per prescription reported in 2007. Veterans receive 80% of their prescriptions through the mail, which in 2016 amounted to 119.7 million outpatient prescriptions. Approximately one-third or fewer civilians have their prescriptions filled by mail.

While reducing drug costs has been critically important in managing the budgets of both the Veterans Health Administration and Military Health Systems, the main lesson for civilian medicine to learn is how to manage a fixed budget by paying for results.

Boom! Boom! Boom!

Like his colleagues across the Military Health System and Veterans Health Administration, Commander Andrew Lin is paid a fixed salary. As the senior medical officer on the USS *Bataan*—an amphibious assault ship capable of transporting over 3,000 sailors and Marines—he knows he could be making a lot more money as a civilian cardiologist, but he doesn't envy those doctors, nurses, and technologists who start performing coronary angiograms at 6 a.m. and are often still in their scrubs through dinnertime. "It's just boom-boom-boom!" he says, "almost like a factory, just to be able to bill-bill-bill." In contrast, he says, as a patient in the Military Health System, "once you're in, you are going to get great, great care," because there's no incentive for the doctor or nurse or practitioner to do otherwise. No reason to rush. No reason to overtreat, to overprescribe, or to run up a big bill.

Vice Admiral Bono agrees with Commander Lin's sanguine assessment. Unlike most of her civilian surgical colleagues, she gets paid the same as anyone at her rank in the military, and that's nowhere close to her market value as a trauma surgeon. "But," she says with a grin, "I do get the same pay as a three-star general hunting down ISIS."

Doc of the Medical Bay

Physicians aren't the only personnel saving the Military Health System and Veterans Health Administration money.

On a ship the size of the USS *Bataan*, a senior medical officer like Commander Lin oversees several junior physicians called general medical officers who have one year of training after medical school (rather than the usual three-to-five-to-ten years of residency training plus specialization). Smaller ships with 800–900 onboard may have just one of these junior physicians. And smaller ships with just a few hundred sailors, such as cruisers and destroyers, may be supported by one enlisted sailor without a formal medical degree—an independent duty corpsman often affectionately addressed as "Doc."

I met one of those hospital corpsmen aboard the USS *Cole*, a guided missile destroyer moored at Naval Station Norfolk in Virginia. He was the senior (and only) medical person for the entire ship, having undergone 14 weeks of basic training for the job. His office, the medical bay, was about 8 × 8 feet. (Imagine a room-sized first-aid kit, with a small sink.) Cabinets lining the walls were filled with sutures, gauze, bandages, and antiseptic creams. An operating table in the center of the room doubled as a desk for paperwork. A dusty computer off to one side was for telemedicine and electronic medical records (reception was spotty on the high seas). The treadmills and ellipticals outside his door got more use than his medical facility. We asked him about his medical case load: headaches and back pain, achy muscles and joints, depression and other mental health issues, and an unfortunate ship-wide bout of food poisoning. It was manageable, he said.

Commander Lin explains that this staffing model is effective because the population is very healthy. There's a tight screening process for letting sailors onto a ship, matching their health to available medical expertise. Soldiers who have HIV or complex medical conditions can only serve on ships that have a board-certified physician. They wouldn't be allowed on the smaller ships with independent duty corpsmen or junior physicians. Lin says, "It's a very tailored system that allows us to take care of our patients safely." And cheaply.

This idea of matching training with the needs of those you serve is a capability the military has refined at all levels.

America's Medical School

Tall, lanky and irrepressibly cheerful, Art Kellerman always introduces himself as the dean of "America's Medical School." That's how the emergency medicine physician describes the Uniformed Services University— the military's health sciences university that trains doctors and dentists, nurses and nutritionists.

Run by the Department of Defense, USU is not only free, but students also receive the full salary and benefits of a uniformed officer. After completing their internship and residency, graduates have a seven-year active service duty commitment and a six-year inactive ready reserve commitment. Alternatively, for those outside USU, the Health Professions Scholarship Program enables students at other medical schools to graduate debt-free with a service commitment of at least one year for each year of scholarship participation. While the average civilian physician accumulates about $200,000 in debt from medical school, graduates of the military training program, like Admiral Bono, General Anderson, and Commander Lin, come out debt-free. Except, of course, for the service commitments.

In addition to the usual courses in physiology and pharmacology, Kellerman's students train for battlefield care at the 30,000 square-foot Val G. Hemming Simulation Center, where large-scale simulators recreate battlefield and natural disaster scenarios in an immersive virtual reality experience. Realistic images of gray skies filled with helicopters are projected on screens that surround a 1,000-square-foot mass casualty simulator environment—it's enclosed by one-way see-through panels for instructors to observe from outside. Scattered all over the terrain are bloody mannequins, with torn-off limbs and worse. Soundscapes of flying bullets, screams, and explosions make it hard to hear. Smoke and debris generators cloud the air. Virtual-reality technology isn't just for video gaming—it's readying the military.

In his article for Stanford Medicine Magazine, "Is War Good for Medicine?," Christopher Connell writes, "The crucible of conflict whets appetites for more and better medicine." Nowhere has there been more effort to build a learning health system than at the frontlines of the battlefield.

The Tourniquet Twist

Between the American Civil War and the early 1990s, battlefield survival statistics barely changed: about 90% of fatalities happened before the injured could get to a medical facility, and in recent years, about one in four of those deaths were preventable. The most common killer: soldiers bleeding to death from injuries to the arms and legs.

The history of tourniquets had been rocky, mostly because of anecdotal stories of tourniquets causing gangrene and limb loss after being left on too long out of a fear of uncontrolled bleeding. When one study found that 3,400 service members died unnecessarily in Vietnam because of bleeding from wounds to their extremities, military leaders began to reconsider their position on tourniquets. By 2003, special operations medics and researchers from the US Army Institute of Surgical Research had invented a tourniquet that was remarkably simple and effective: a tough nylon band an inch or so wide, a plastic or metal rod with which to twist it tight, and a Velcro loop to keep things secure. Families of medics back at Fort Bragg were enlisted to sew hundreds of these new combat application tourniquets (CATs). Then they just needed to be tested and proven in the field. That's where the Joint Trauma System, the military's learning health system, played a critical role.

Traumatic Improvements

Established in 2004 by the United States and its coalition partner nations, the Joint Trauma System develops standards for battlefield, evacuation, and hospital-based trauma care. It uses electronic health records to collect all the information about each traumatic event: the characteristics of the soldier, injuries, physiologic parameters, care administered, and outcomes. In 2005, US Central Command issued a directive that every soldier deployed to Iraq and Afghanistan should carry a tourniquet and added training on its use to the Basic Combat Training program. Deaths from extremity bleeding as a percentage of overall combat fatalities dropped from 7.8% in the period from 2003 through 2006 to 2.6% by 2010.

The Joint Trauma System has taught military leaders many other lessons, such as how to keep soldiers warm after injury (hypothermia on arrival to a clinic decreased from 7% to 1%) and how to save the lives of those who require massive transfusions (death rates declined from 32% to 20%). They've established about 45 trauma care practice guidelines. In the Vietnam War, 23% of wounded service members could not be saved. By 2015, that figure had been cut to less than half (9.3%) for soldiers in Afghanistan and Iraq.

The military's learning efforts are working, and those learnings are spilling into the civilian sector.

Leading Leaders

The military knows a lot about building leadership into the job, and Vindell Washington is grateful. Having studied under a military scholarship, Washington knew he'd be a soldier someday. He enlisted in the army right after finishing his emergency medicine residency, and straightaway, he wasn't just working in a busy emergency department: he was in charge of it. Within two years, he also was responsible for a busy urgent care facility and an ambulance service. (When asked whether he knew how to run an ambulance service, he replied, "Well, I've ridden in one!"). He had excellent training opportunities along the way, sometimes formal—a Deming-type total quality management training program (closely related to Lean manufacturing)—and sometimes informal—one colleague had 20 years of supply-chain management experience, and another was a pro at professional contracting.

This leadership training served him well. After completing his army service, Major Washington joined a large private practice with 75 emergency medicine physicians and quickly became head of operations and then CEO. After five years in that role, a large hospital system in Louisiana invited him to be its chief medical information officer. After complaining to his Senator about the new HITECH law's Meaningful Use definitions, Washington was appointed by US Secretary of Health and Human Services Sylvia Burwell in 2016 to be the national coordinator for health information technology to fix them.

The military develops leadership as a core competency, including among its physicians. Nancy Dickey, a family medicine doctor from Texas, who served in several national leadership roles, including chairing the

Defense Health Board, says the leadership training distinguishes military medicine. "They teach leadership all the way down the ranks, because you can't effectively respond to and appreciate leadership if you don't understand leadership, whether you're a private, a corporal, a sergeant, or a general," she observes. The military expects everyone to be a leader.

The Action Plan: Learning from Our Military and Veterans Health Administration Systems

Civilian leaders should take these seven lessons from the Military Health System and Veterans Health Administration:

1. Reevaluate the role of government health: Make the Department of Health and Human Services more like a Health and Readiness Department than a health insurance company. Set expectations for improving the health of the country as national goals.

2. Invest in training: Scholarship or loan-forgiveness models that expect payback through service in underserved communities and underrepresented health professions can help break the cycle of high tuition driving expectations of high remuneration.

3. Allow major payers, like Medicare, to negotiate on drug pricing, use a single formulary, and exclude drugs that do not meet thresholds for cost-effectiveness.

4. Broaden the roles of health professionals to meet the population's needs (for example, formalize the medical assistant role).

5. Consider fixed budgets for hospitals and pay health professionals based not on the volume of services performed but on better outcomes.

6. Expect physicians and other health professionals to maintain their skills through active learning. Use simulation centers for practical training in realistic settings.

7. Create a learning health system. Invest in data and registries and the means to learn from them to test new treatments.

CHAPTER 12

THE LONG FIX

We should be targeting the readiness of all of our citizens . . . to do what they're supposed to do in support of our society.

—Vice Admiral Raquel Bono

When I met with Mike Leavitt in his Salt Lake City home to talk about fixing health care, he had been engrossed in Walter Isaacson's book *The Innovators*, a history of computers, starting with the computing machine that Charles Babbage and Ada Lovelace imagined in the 1830s. According to Isaacson, the move from analog to digital circuitry enabled the first commercially-available computers to emerge by the 1950s. Then, thanks to two key innovations—microchips and packet-switched networks—and the work of key creative visionaries and their teams, these devices evolved into the ubiquitous personal computers and internet nodes of the 1990s. In parallel, Isaacson points out that the field of artificial intelligence was launched in 1956, and four decades later, IBM's Deep Blue chess-playing machine beat Garry Kasparov. Leavitt concluded that the 40-year epochs of computing innovations just might have lessons for how we think about the arc of history in health care.

The current development cycle of health care began in the 1990s. The rise of health maintenance organizations and managed care coincided with Leavitt's election to the first of three terms as governor of Utah in 1993. In 2005, President George W. Bush appointed Leavitt as secretary of the US Department of Health and Human Services, where among many other initiatives, he oversaw the implementation of Medicare Part D (the pharmaceutical benefit). Now back in Utah, he leads Leavitt Partners, a national health care consulting firm whose focus is on changing the payment model to encourage high-quality, low-cost care. By his count, the United States is just over halfway through a 40-year health care spurt.

The defining challenge of this transformative cycle, he says, is the need to align two powerful human drives seemingly at odds: the desire to be compassionate and the desire to be financially successful. A compassionate society wants to alleviate suffering. To many, that means making health care available to all. In 2018, the United States was about 27.5 million people short of that goal—8.5% of Americans had no health insurance. That's significantly less than the 49.9 million (16.3%) in 2010, the year the Affordable Care Act was passed. At the same time, even those with some kind of coverage are increasingly underinsured—in 2018 as many as 45% of adults could not afford their out-of-pocket costs even if they had health insurance.

Providing coverage for the 27.5 million who are uninsured and offering fuller coverage for those who are underinsured seem like quixotic goals when health care is already consuming 18% of the US economy. We might as well declare defeat. And yet, there's that tantalizingly enormous waste in the US health system, estimated to make up at least one-third of all spending. If recovered, those savings could fund the compassionate way forward.

A glance beyond our borders may justify a sense of optimism. Other high-income nations, like Germany, the UK, France, Canada, Australia, Switzerland, and Japan, have managed to contain health care spending to less than 10%–12% of their economies, which is the equivalent of the US rate minus the waste (one-third off of 18%), and they are keeping their people healthier. They show us that it can be done. Better health can cost less.

If the goal is achievable, how do we get there? I've distilled the lessons of this book into three guiding principles for the Long Fix:

Principle #1: Health Care Is a Problem with Bipartisan Solutions

Much of the political rhetoric about health care gets tangled in two contentious points. First, should everyone in the United States be entitled to health care? Some interpret this as asking a different question: Should everyone in the United States be entitled to *free* health care?

Second, what is the government's role versus the private sector's role? In other words, what's the right balance between government regulation and market competition? Finding common ground on these issues could accelerate progress.

IS HEALTH CARE A UNIVERSAL RIGHT?

This question has long divided Americans. We just can't seem to agree. Surveys in 2018 by Gallup and by the Pew Research Center found that about six in ten Americans believed it is the responsibility of the federal government to make sure all Americans have health care. That's a swing of the pendulum from 2014, when about four to five in ten thought so. The Affordable Care Act of 2010 tried to mandate that all Americans have health insurance—creating the individual insurance exchanges and expanding Medicaid as a means of providing more coverage to the uninsured—but this goal of universal coverage was thwarted in 2012 when the Supreme Court ruled that the federal government could not penalize states that chose not to expand Medicaid. As of early 2020, 37 states and the District of Columbia had expanded Medicaid, and 14 states had not. Among all high-income nations the United States remains the only country where coverage is not universal and not compulsory.

As Atul Gawande has pointed out in his *New Yorker* story, "Is Health Care a Right?," there is probably more common ground than the political rhetoric suggests. The debate is less about whether people should have access to care than about whether they should have access to *free* care. State-level opponents of Medicaid expansion often cite fears of rising costs. Even though the federal government (not states) has paid for 90%–100% of the states' expansion costs, they are worried that the burden will fall on them eventually. And they are also nervous about "freeloaders." Over a dozen states want to link expanding Medicaid to new requirements for beneficiaries to seek employment or engage in community work. In his hometown of Athens, Ohio, Gawande interviewed a local librarian who was proud of maintaining her job even though she knew quitting it would entitle her to free health care through Medicaid. He wrote, "The notion of health care as a right struck her as another way of undermining work and responsibility." She told him, " 'I'm old school, and I'm not really good at accepting anything I don't work for.' "

Whether an entitlement or not, health insurance coverage improves health, even if it costs more. In 2000, New York, Maine, and Arizona expanded their Medicaid programs (predating the Affordable Care Act by a decade). A study published 12 years later found that the three expansion states had significantly lower death rates (19.6 fewer deaths per 100,000 adults per year) than their neighboring states, and people reported their own health to be significantly better. Since the Affordable Care Act, several hundred published research studies have shown that Medicaid expansion has consistently improved access to basic health care, and that people have gotten healthier because of that access—their blood pressure and diabetes are better, mental health has improved, and more have been screened for diseases like cervical and prostate cancer.

Universal coverage would improve the health of Americans. At the same time, expecting Americans to take responsibility—both financially (in some way reflecting their means) and in terms of healthful behaviors—is likely necessary for broad acceptance.

WHAT'S THE RIGHT PUBLIC-PRIVATE BALANCE OF RESPONSIBILITY?

The other fundamental question encumbering health care's future is just how much of a role the government should play. Should the government manage all benefits and heavily regulate the delivery system? Should the "free market" and competition drive better care? Or somewhere in between?

Again, we can't agree. But we can learn from the three different models operating in the United States:

First, there's the Veterans Health Administration and the Military Health System, both federal entities that manage the health benefits for their beneficiaries and deliver care (Chapter 11). Second, Medicare and Medicaid are health entitlement programs run by federal and state governments that use mostly private-sector care (Chapters 2 and 3). Third, we have employer-sponsored private insurance with mostly private-sector health care (Chapters 3 and 10). Our three models share similarities with the health systems of other high-income nations who are grappling with challenges similar to our own: the rise of chronic diseases, increasing treatment costs, an aging population, and workforce shortages.

Like the Military Health System and Veterans Health Administration: In the British model (also the Swedish and Danish systems, among others), the government not only covers the health benefits of all its residents, but it also provides care through the hospitals and clinics of the National Health Service (NHS). Some NHS physicians also generate extra income by practicing in private clinics and hospitals just steps away from their NHS hospitals, where privately insured clientele can avoid waiting for care and also receive better amenities. (The NHS suffers from long wait times just as some Veterans Health Administration facilities do—the NHS has a rule that the maximum wait time for nonurgent clinic visits is 18 weeks.) Like the Veterans Health Administration and Military Health System, the UK also expects the pharmaceutical industry to prove a drug is more cost-effective than others on the market before agreeing to pay for it. Individuals have few out-of-pocket costs in the UK (NHS is paid for out of a national tax system), and hospitals receive a fixed budget each year to care for their patients.

Like Medicare and Medicaid: In some countries, the government manages health benefits, while health care is delivered by a mix of public and private hospitals and clinics. For example, in Canada (and Australia), the federal and provincial governments finance health care. While basic coverage is mandatory, supplemental private insurance (mostly for-profit) is also offered by employers to help cover prescription drugs, vision and dental care, rehabilitation services, and private rooms in hospitals. Unlike the US system, the government budgets and pays hospitals a fixed total amount each year (similar to the Veterans Health Administration and Military Health System). Doctors are paid fee-for-service, but they are not allowed to charge more than what is listed on a set fee schedule.

Like the private-sector employer-sponsored insurance model: Other countries have universal health care that is managed and provided almost completely by the private sector and regulated by the government. Take Switzerland, a system with one of the best outcomes in the world, which costs about one-third less than the United States. All Swiss must buy health insurance from private insurance companies that compete for their business. Policies are standardized across the country, and nearly two-thirds of the country opt for the basic level of benefits. Premiums are set for each region by a federal office, and the system expects everyone who can afford it to pay. Unlike in the United States, insurance companies cannot make a profit from basic policies, but they can make money on supplemental policies that offer extra benefits like more doctors to choose from or a higher level of hospital accommodation. In Switzerland, payments from insurers to the health care system are not negotiated. They are standardized. Outpatient care is mostly paid using a national fee schedule, and hospitals are all paid using the same national disease-related group payment system (like the Medicare disease-related group payment system described in Chapter 3).

Although these nations all have universal health coverage, health care is not free in many of them. For example, the Swiss, French, Germans, and Dutch have co-pays or coinsurance (or both) built into their models and subsidies for those who cannot afford them. The Singaporeans do it a little differently: they have mandatory health savings accounts (approximately 10% of annual income is withheld). These funds can be used to cover co-pays and other costs of care as well as to pay for private insurance.

In summary, the health systems of high-income peer nations have a lot in common: (1) health benefits are universal or insurance is mandatory—and most essential care is either free or with standard, affordable out-of-pocket expenses; (2) people have a choice of primary care physicians and outpatient specialists; (3) regardless of whether medical services are delivered by public or private hospitals, the government sets the prices for what it (or private insurers) will pay for basic services, including physician payments; (4) simpler payment models mean lower administrative costs, drug prices, and out-of-pocket spending than in the United States; and (5) health outcomes are better than in the United States.

Mirror, Mirror
What do we conclude from this analysis? There's no one right answer, but there are a few guideposts:

1. Should health insurance be mandatory for all? If the goal is a healthier nation, then universal coverage makes sense, although it will be more expensive in the short term, and, in a pay-for-action world, unaffordable. However, in a pay-for-results world, universal coverage can be the right decision both in financial and health terms.
2. Will there still be special groups who receive government-run health benefits and get care in government-run medical facilities? Most likely yes. Americans do not want to give up Medicare or Medicaid. (In a 2018 Pew Center survey, the vast majority of adults polled believed that it is the federal government's responsibility to make sure all have health insurance; only 4% of Americans said the government should

not be involved in health insurance at all.) Veterans favor keeping the Veterans Health Administration system. The military is proud of their health system. Other programs like the Indian Health Service are unlikely to go away. If anything, they need more funding.

3. Outside of these special populations, how should health insurance be administered? Whether employer-run or government-run, one approach may be to take a lesson from the Swiss: create a distinction between a basic health plan and supplemental insurance. The basic health plan could be universal, like in Switzerland. Everyone would get the same benefits and have the same out-of-pocket costs (with subsidies for the poor and disabled). This could be a basic version of "Medicaid-for-all" except that it doesn't have to be run by Medicaid; it could be offered by employers, too. Either way, the simpler the system—with set benefits and fixed fees—the lower the administrative costs.

Private, for-profit insurance businesses could compete in the supplemental insurance business. A functioning "market" for health insurance plans would need consumers (individuals or employers) to be able to comparison shop—based on services, out-of-pocket payments, the network of available doctors and hospitals, and so on, provided there was enough competition in the market for everyone to have choice.

4. Finally, how should health care itself be paid for and delivered? Under a Swiss-like universal basic health plan, most if not all doctors and hospitals would accept this insurance and get paid according to a fixed fee schedule. For care covered by supplemental insurance and for other elective care, a market-based approach would work best if: (a) people have access to information about products and services and their costs (remember Utah's price transparency exercise in Chapter 3); (b) the market has enough different hospitals, medical groups, and insurers to choose from (mergers and consolidation can put a damper on the market, Chapter 3); (c) the insured are discouraged from overutilizing care; (d) pharmaceutical compa-

nies and other suppliers also compete on value—improving health at the lowest costs (Chapter 8); and (e) people are incentivized for healthy behaviors, but if they do get sick, they receive appropriate care (and aren't refused treatment).

The most important factor in how health care is paid for is not whether employers pay directly, or whether the government pays (funded by taxes on employers): it's what they're paying for. And that brings us to the second principle.

Principle #2: Pay for Results, Not Action

Pivoting a $3.6 trillion business to a pay-for-results model requires Herculean effort. The good news is that the journey has already begun. Clif Gaus founded and leads the National Association of Accountable Care Organizations, which represents groups of physicians and hospitals committed to new value-based care. He believes we are well on our way. It may take another ten years, but, when I mention to him the title of this book, he sighs, "If I say one thing about ACOs, it's a long fix."

There are five key steps in this shift to paying for value: (a) set clear national goals and a timeline; (b) create the right incentives for hospitals, doctors, and insurers to change; (c) reintegrate mental and physical health; (d) change the practice of medicine to reward patients and clinicians for successfully coproducing health; and (e) standardize and simplify billing and payment.

First, No More Stalling

In early 2015, US Secretary of Health and Human Services Sylvia Burwell boldly announced that the days of fee-for-service health care were numbered. By 2016, 85% of Medicare fee-for-service payments would become payments that would be adjusted up or down depending on the quality of care. And, by 2018, half of all payments made by Medicare would be in "alternative payment models," a term referring to arrangements like ChenMed's Medicare Advantage model (Chapter 2) or bundled payments (Chapters

2 and 3). To the industry, Burwell's declaration felt like the moment in the ALS Association's Ice Bucket Challenge just after the bucket tipped: that mixture of fear, shock, and—few of us admitted—also relief. Burwell's ultimatum gave leaders a new urgency in preparing our hospitals and clinics for this new future. Her announcement also inspired private insurers who were eager to rein in spending. Shortly after Burwell's declaration, Aetna's chief executive announced his company would move the percentage of payments in new types of value-based models from 30% in 2015 to 75% by 2020.

Secretary of Health and Human Services Alex Azar and his Centers for Medicare and Medicaid Services Administrator Seema Verma have continued the march toward paying for results. Medicare Advantage is projected to enroll 50% of all seniors by 2025, maybe more. In 2019, Verma announced a five-year Primary Care First initiative to encourage more doctors' groups to directly contract with the government in Medicare Advantage plans. They also hinted that bundled payments might move from voluntary to mandatory. What's needed is a definitive deadline for Medicare to flip the switch to paying for better health at lower costs 100% of the time.

A deadline is critical because hospitals and medical groups can't run their businesses in a split model—where some payers reward for action and others reward for results, especially when the fee-for-service, pay-for-action contracts are irresistibly more lucrative and the status quo is easier to maintain. Hospitals are incentivized to milk as much profit out of the fee-for-service model while they can. They're not focused on the hard work of improving safety, reducing waste, and making the system more Lean. Why bother with all that when you can still charge $25,000 for an MRI?

Paying for results isn't something that can be left to the next administration, the next CEO, the next 40-year cycle. It needs to happen now.

Second, Incentivize Effective Change

To succeed in a pay-for-results system, every hospital and physician practice must be able to do at least the three things: track patient outcomes, measure costs of care, and change the behaviors of clinicians and patients to focus on results, not action. Electronic health records systems should help them and so should health insurers. For example, using information from their pharmacy claims reports, a health plan can alert physicians if a patient fails to fill a prescription and therefore probably isn't taking medications as prescribed.

For systems that aren't delivering the results they expect, training and educational programs offered by organizations like Boston's Institute for Healthcare Improvement can teach quality improvement and Lean manufacturing methodology. The move to pay-for-results care should create demand for programs that bring payers and providers of care together to invent better ways of driving value.

Third, Reunite Mind and Body

Pediatrician and Dartmouth professor Paul Batalden once observed, "Every system is perfectly designed to get the results it gets." A pay-for-results system will restore the connections between primary care and behavioral health. For example, Medicare Advantage practices like Iora Health are teaching primary care clinicians how to manage some of the most common behavioral health conditions, like depression and anxiety, and partnering them with behavioral health specialists and licensed social workers in clinic (like Peter Weir at ARUP managing teens with depression in Chapter 10). It pays off. Patients in better mental health also manage their blood pressure, diabetes, and depression better. A University of Washington study showed that integrating primary and mental health care for depressed, older adults returns more than $6 for every dollar spent.

Fourth, Coproduce Health and Share in the Rewards

When Medicare implements "shared savings" plans, they split the savings from lower costs of care with doctors or hospitals. Patients are left out of the picture. Employer-sponsored health plans have tried to use financial inducements with their employees to incentivize and reward better health but without much success.

Champions of coproduction like Susan Edgman-Levitan and Justin Masterson (Chapter 7) might suggest that these programs are missing the boat by failing to engage employees adequately in their design. If employees could choose, would they want their employers to invest in a weight-loss or smoking cessation program for them? If you asked them for input, their answers might surprise you.

University of Pittsburgh Medical Center's Health Plan and the nonprofit Robert Wood Johnson Foundation worked with a group of stakeholders to build a program to improve outcomes and reduce the costs of care for children with complex medical problems in Allegheny County, Pennsylvania. As part of the program, the families of 262 children living in one of Pennsylvania Medicaid program's costliest counties each got a $500 prepaid debit card to spend however they chose. "It took nothing short of an act of Congress to do that, because you had to be careful you didn't make them ineligible for Medicaid," said Pamela Peele, chief analytics officer at the health plan. I asked her if they knew what the families did with the money.

"Well . . . one family spent their money on a big pizza party," she says. She shrugs and then continues, "One family spent their money on a seamstress." Their daughter was small for her age and going into middle school. Having clothes that fit were important. A two-household family needed a car seat because "Dad couldn't pick up the kid after school because the car seat's in mom's car," and Medicaid only covers one car seat. One family bought a washer and dryer—"If you have an incontinent child, you need a washer and dryer," she noted. Many of the families' choices surprised them, but in the end, the cards were worth it; the program saved $1.8 million.

High-deductible health plans could benefit from redesign, too. Up to the point of the deductible, people are incentivized to avoid using any care—even when it's sensible and necessary. If they do end up reaching the deductible, they are then incentivized to use as much care as possible because it's "free." Korb Matosich, cofounder and president of Asserta Health, pointed out that there could be more effective ways of motivating people to make good choices about their care. Employers could share some of the money they save when employees choose lower-cost, but comparable quality, options. For example, if a knee replacement costs $40,000 at one facility, and the employer has negotiated the rate to $20,000 at a comparable quality facility, then, Matosich said, the employee might be entitled to some portion of the savings for choosing the lower-cost center. For this to work, people have to appreciate that higher costs don't mean better quality, and lower costs don't mean lower quality!

Fifth, Standardize and Simplify: The Holy Grail of Paying for Value

The top reason that the majority of US physicians favor a single-payer system may have less to do with ideology and more to do with the chance to escape burdensome and time-consuming billing, coding, and documentation (Chapter 3). New value-based payments have the potential to simplify bureaucracy but have yet to realize that potential.

With Medicare Advantage-type contracts and bundled payments, doctors shouldn't have to code and bill for every lab test or X-ray. They just need to get the diagnosis right. If their patients' outcomes are as good as expected, they get paid. Physicians could decide on their own whether they really needed to order that extra MRI. After all, it is coming out of their budget.

Medicare's bundled payment program forces hospitals to define standard services—curing a urinary tract infection, repairing a cardiac valve, or fixing a broken hip—and the prices to go with them. Imagine being able to compare three hospitals and knowing the prices up front. With available reviews of quality measures, convenience, and patient satisfaction, you could choose the best facility for you or your loved ones.

Ideally, that flexibility of choice wouldn't be thwarted by the electronic health records. New application program interfaces could allow patients to download their data and bring their records wherever they go. Once empowered to be more effective customers, patients might finally be able to push for better care at lower prices.

Principle #3: Make Health a Strategic Imperative for the Nation

In the military, the Defense Health Agency's goal is "to provide a medically ready force and a ready medical force" to all personnel.

A Medically Ready America

Think about what it would mean if all US medical personnel had a similar mandate: to provide a medically ready America. Imagine if instead of being tasked with lowering the costs of care, our government had a Department of Health and Readiness that focused on health, wellness, and prevention. Its goals would be long term: make people healthier through cost-effective investments.

This wouldn't be easy. Let's face it, we have a lot to work on to have a "ready" population. We could improve smoking cessation (one-fifth of American adults smoke or use electronic cigarettes). We need to tackle diet and weight management—almost 40% of adults are obese, two out of three are overweight, and one-fifth of all children are obese. Three out of four don't do enough aerobic and muscle-strengthening exercise. Nearly one in five Americans live with a mental illness. About one-half have hypertension, and one in three adults don't get enough sleep. The Department of Health and Readiness would want to partner with other departments such as Agriculture, Housing and Urban Development, Transportation, Veterans Administration, Department of Defense, and others because readiness is not just a health problem.

The Department of Defense would share in this readiness mission. The unreadiness of the American population destabilizes our military readiness. In 2014, the Pentagon estimated that 71% of 17–24-year-olds in the United States would not qualify for military service because of issues partly related to health and education. About 27% of the potential candidates for military service do not qualify because of excessive weight, and those ranks are swelling.

Vice Admiral Raquel Bono put it best: "We should be targeting the readiness of all of our citizens." Whether it's policemen, firefighters, or teachers, the nation needs to make sure that "all of our citizens are ready to do what they're supposed to do in support of our society."

To do so, we also need a ready medical force.

A Ready Medical Force

New systems need leaders with new skills. Clay Johnston and Mark Schuster, deans of two of the newest medical schools in the country, are dedicated to producing some of them. Johnston, a neurologist and researcher, became the founding dean of Dell Medical School in Austin in 2014. He embraces eminent physician William Osler's comment that "The good physician treats the disease; the great physician treats the patient with the disease."

At Dell Medical School, medical students learn about value-based care from the beginning. An online curriculum offers interactive case studies on topics like how to measure costs of care and how to order cost-effective medications. Faculty like Stacey Chang, the former health lead of the Palo Alto–based design firm IDEO teach them to apply design thinking. For example, one class created an educational program to teach parents of pediatric patients how to deliver medications to their children the right way.

Schuster, dean of the new Kaiser Permanente Medical School, seeks to teach students about the scope and delivery of care in medical and community settings. As much as they understand the physiology of high cholesterol, they should think about the barriers that patients face—and the supports that exist—in getting access to fresh fruits and vegetables.

Pay-for-value health care creates more demand for different kinds of clinicians. The United States is facing a significant nursing shortage, which is exacerbated by the shortage of doctorally prepared nurses who teach in nursing colleges. In 2018, nursing schools turned away more than 75,000 qualified applicants because of insufficient faculty and clinical preceptors. To encourage more doctors to become primary care clinicians and serve both in urban and in rural and underserved communities, the National Health Service Corps Loan Repayment Program forgives loans of $30,000 to $75,000 in exchange for two to three years of service in the areas of primary care, mental health, dental health, and substance use disorders in designated shortage areas. These programs need expanding. In a pay-for-results world, we also need more health professionals like physician assistants, medical assistants, social workers, community health workers, and others who can support team-based care, prevention, and home- and community-based care.

One part of the workforce that is bearing a disproportionate burden of care, without compensation, are family caregivers—the daughters, partners, sons-in-law, and parents who help family members get dressed, bathe, make medical appointments, drive them to those appointments, fill prescriptions, and more. Estimated to exceed 40 million in the United States in 2018, caregivers provide over $500 billion in uncompensated care. We need better aging-at-home strategies and more support for the caregivers who bear much of the responsibility.

The Most Powerful Drug: Coproducing Your Health

Every one of us has a role in the Long Fix—we are all soldiers in the war against disease. Sometimes we're the supporter, the caregiver, the cheerleader. We may take on the role of the community member—like the grandma who picks up donated books and hands them out to kids in her beauty salon, or the volunteer shuttle driver for seniors who need to pick up their medications. We may be the parent, the brother, the daughter-in-law, the next-door neighbor. Or we just may be the patient.

We are responsible for our share of coproducing our own health. We may need better leaders, but we also need to be better leaders. It's our money. It's our health. It's our future. It's our problem to fix. As Carolyn Clancy says, there's no drug as powerful as people engaged in their own health.

EPILOGUE

*COVID-19 has very much sharpened our focus on
what is of value in an economy.*

—Mariana Mazzucato, professor,
University College London

The first edition of this book was published in the midst of a global pandemic that caused more suffering and more deaths than any other outbreak since the 1918–1919 influenza pandemic. COVID-19 exposed shocking flaws of the US health care system—most of which are detailed in this book. Leading up to the pandemic, fee-for-service or pay-for-action payment models depleted resources for primary care and public health and instead overfed high-end specialty and procedure-based care. During the pandemic, specialty care centers emptied, and many hospitals nearly went broke. People without adequate health insurance avoided care, even when infected with the COVID-19 virus. All in all, the coronavirus pandemic ruined millions of families and cost trillions in lost productivity, and those economic losses, in turn, jeopardize the future financing of health care, social programs, and public health.

At the same time, the coronavirus crisis spurred some unexpected advances. For example, by the close of 2020, over a million Americans had already received approved vaccines that used novel technologies such as messenger RNA, a triumph of scientific collaboration and regulatory alacrity. After toppling decades-old regulatory barriers, the widespread deployment of telehealth meant that patients could safely communicate with doctors and nurses during the pandemic. Struggling hospitals and medical groups started championing new payment models—ones they had long resisted—because those models could provide more reliable funding, even if they capped profitability.

The COVID-19 pandemic has shown how vulnerable we are if we don't move forward with the commonsense solutions from *The Long Fix*. Among its most compelling eye-openers, the pandemic threw in sharp relief the gaping disparities in American health care. COVID-19 disproportionately struck the elderly, disenfranchised minorities, rural communities, the poor, and people with chronic conditions like diabetes, obesity, and pulmonary diseases. These groups have been among those with the poorest health and highest health care costs. With the pandemic, they are also the ones who have suffered the most. Let's start with the fastest growing demographic in the nation and in the world, seniors.

Loving Longevity

"In our country, we love longevity," says Terry Fulmer, president of the Hartford Foundation. "We love that in the 1900s we lived to be 40, and now we live to be 80." The trouble is, "we don't like taking care of older people." Instead of buttressing them so they can live in their homes, adds Fulmer, who is also a nurse and former dean of nursing at New York University, we offer medical services—mostly in institutional settings—and even then only if they are poor enough to qualify. Fulmer doesn't think much of how we warehoused 1.3 million seniors in nursing homes during the pandemic: "They look like prisons. Right now, they are prisons."

Despite efforts to keep them safe from potentially infected visitors, over 150,000 residents and staff of long-term care facilities had died of COVID-19 in the United States through the end of January 2021. They made up less than 1% of the population, over 5% of all COVID-19 cases, but about 36%

of all COVID-19 deaths. Rich Feifer, chief medical officer of the nation's largest for-profit nursing home company, Genesis Healthcare, defends his industry. He says the charge of "neglect" in nursing homes isn't fair because the real problem is that they are underresourced.

Howard Gleckman argues in *Forbes* that it's both. In his article "Why Are We so Shocked by COVID-19 Nursing Home Deaths? We Have Been Failing Our Frail Older Adults for Decades," he points out that we have a "profoundly flawed system of caring for older adults and younger people with disabilities." The challenges he points to are remarkably similar to the ones prisons faced as COVID-19 rapidly spread through their populations: they are densely populated, significantly underresourced, and not a priority.

COVID-19 has been devastating to nursing home residents. It's also crushing the business, because their most lucrative patients—seniors who use them as short-stay rehabilitation centers—have stayed away. Their bills are paid for by Medicare (for up to 100 days), and reimbursements are generous. During the pandemic, however, seniors put off all but the most necessary treatments and rarely got discharged from hospitals to nursing homes, preferring instead to go home.

They may be better off because moving patients from expensive hospital beds to less-expensive nursing homes hasn't been the most successful way of rehabilitating seniors. Without an electronic connection between the health records of the hospital and the nursing home, patients frequently arrive at nursing homes with very little information for their new care teams. They're missing a "warm" hand-off, a simple nurse-to-nurse call. "We're lucky to get a discharge summary rubber-banded to their chests or to their gurney," says Feifer. With incomplete information about their patients and fewer and fewer skilled staff, it's not surprising that up to one in four patients sent to nursing homes from a hospital are readmitted within a month. When Medicare started tying their payments to better performance in 2018, it penalized about 11,000 nursing homes and rewarded only 4,000. It was hard enough for the facilities to manage the reporting requirements for these programs, much less address the caliber of care.

During the pandemic, those remaining in nursing homes were mostly residents who had moved in for life. For them, Medicaid pays for their stays—*if* they are poor enough to qualify. The monthly income threshold varies by state; for liquid assets, all states set a limit of no more than $2,000. (A robust industry of consultants advises seniors on how to spend down their savings.) Because Medicaid reimburses nursing homes at about $200 per patient per day—less than the costs of providing care—these facilities must rely on low-cost labor. COVID-19 worsened the shortage of staff. Feifer says, "We have trouble when our staff can make more stocking shelves at Walmart."

With these models falling short, and with COVID-19 exploiting their weaknesses, how can we reimagine better systems for looking after seniors and paying for their care?

To start, we can help seniors age at home more independently. AARP says that about 7.2 million Americans have private long-term care (LTC) insurance they can use to cover the costs of care in the home. In 2019, the state of Washington took the first steps to making LTC a public benefit. It created an LTC fund from a 0.58% payroll tax. Beginning in 2025, eligible residents get a $100 per day allowance for nursing homes or in-home equipment and support. It can only be used for a year, but it's an important first step.

The government is also experimenting with new funding models for senior care. Federal waivers now allow Medicaid dollars to be spent for home and community-based services, not just nursing homes. Take, for example, the Community Aging in Place—Advancing Better Living for Elders (CAPABLE) program at the Johns Hopkins School of Nursing. It sends a registered nurse, occupational therapist, and licensed handyman to support seniors at home. In California, the Doctors Assisting Seniors at Home (DASH) initiative provides house calls for urgent care. Programs like these significantly lower costs, and they keep the elderly at home and out of hospitals.

Increasingly, Medicare Advantage programs like ChenMed and Iora Health are also allowed to spend their Medicare dollars on in-home services such as meal delivery and transportation. During the pandemic, ChenMed supplied seniors with digital tablets for telehealth visits, supported social workers who partnered with food banks to make sure patients had access to food, and converted mostly empty clinics into urgent care centers so seniors could stay out of emergency departments. In Albuquerque, Presbyterian Health Services found that most patients in its Complete Care program and Hospital at Home program preferred to stay put during the pandemic, even when they tested positive for COVID-19. Nancy Guinn, a family medicine physician and medical director, led an at-home COVID-19 monitoring program for members of their health plan across the state. Her team overnighted an oximeter and thermometer to them and used a smartphone app for regular check-ins. It took a lot more work than Guinn anticipated— nearly two-thirds of the people required some medical intervention, most often, supplemental oxygen. Yet with hundreds in the program, only six had been hospitalized by late summer 2020, and very few needed the emergency department.

New technologies like monitoring, assistive devices, and caregiver support can extend independent living at home for all seniors, including those with dementia. For example, smart home technologies can manage lighting, heating, the oven, and other appliances. They can readily connect family members via voice-activated virtual assistants. Telehealth apps and in-home medical monitoring obviate trips to the clinic and make it possible to detect impending illnesses early enough to allow prevention. In Japan, where there are already not enough people to look after the aging population, voice-activated robots and wheelchairs can help move individuals in the home. People who no longer can drive can use shared car services and perhaps soon, self-driving cars. These technologies keep aging seniors autonomous, and they can also keep people who live in remote communities connected.

The Swiss Army Knife of Medicine

About one in five or six Americans lives in a rural or frontier community. On average, they are older, have higher rates of underlying chronic diseases and disability, and are poorer and less likely to be insured. The coronavirus crisis highlighted the lack of rural health data to inform national policies and the need for more tailored solutions to benefit the 46 million people living in rural areas. Consider, for example, the shortage of doctors, nurses, and other clinicians.

Even though the number of doctors practicing in rural America is declining, Susan Anderson, a family medicine physician, says working with people in her hometown of Canistota, South Dakota (population 627)—such as her former science teacher and piano instructor—provides unrivaled satisfaction. If she had her way, Anderson, dean of rural medicine at the University of South Dakota's Sanford School of Medicine, would convince all her students to follow in her footsteps. For many, it won't take much persuading.

First-year medical student Alaire Buysse comes from a family of farmers in rural southwest Minnesota. Starting in high school, Buysse worked for five years as a nursing assistant in a nursing home while she also helped care for her grandmother with cancer. Buysse's grandma didn't drive, so she had to rely on family to bring her a couple of hours each way for her doctor's visits in Sioux Falls. Buysse says the telehealth COVID-19 has made commonplace would have been invaluable for her grandma. She imagines how her primary care doctor could have videoconferenced with her oncologist during her visits and how much better her life would have been with a completely redesigned clinic appointment.

The practice she describes sounds a lot like what ChenMed, Iora Health, Presbyterian Health Services, and others are delivering today: more time with patients to talk about their concerns and about important concepts like healthy eating, and partnering with nonprofit organizations like food banks and housing services. "It can't be done in the current fee-for-service system," Buysse tells me. Instead of "idolizing specialists . . . who use fancy technology," she thinks we should put more funding into primary care that will save money in the long run; by avoiding tests, procedures, and surgeries, "we'd save patients time and pain."

To expose more medical students like Buysse to the joys of rural medicine, the University of South Dakota has been sending 11 third-year medical students to rural South Dakota each year since 2012. I caught up with two students in the Frontier and Rural Medicine (FARM) program, Carl Lang and Riley Schaap, about halfway through their stay. They live in Winner, South Dakota (population 2,923), three hours west of Sioux Falls, and three hours east of Rapid City. What *is* nearby? The Rosebud Indian Reservation. "I'm learning so much from them," Schaap says of his patients, of whom "half are cowboys and the other half are Native Americans."

The Winner clinic provides much-needed supplemental resources for the reservation. One government report found that in 2017, the Indian Health Service spending on tribal members, on a per-person basis, was only one-half that of Medicaid, and less than one-third of Medicare. Members of these communities suffer from chronic conditions like obesity, diabetes, high blood pressure, lung diseases, substance use disorder, and mental disease, and they need more support, not less. With these vulnerabilities, they and Alaska Natives were infected with COVID-19 at a rate at least 3.5 times that of non-Hispanic Whites. Some predominantly Native American counties were at the top of the list of most affected in the United States.

Schaap and Lang work at Winner Regional Hospital—a 25-bed critical access hospital that is next door to a clinic and nursing home. Their mentors are the two family medicine doctors who have to be able to do a little of everything, including deliver babies. (Anderson says family medicine doctors are called "the Swiss Army knife of health care.")

The students get to practice medicine in ways that most medical students would envy. They see patients in the clinic, emergency department, hospital, and operating room, and often are in all those places the same day. Schaap estimates he's already helped deliver 30 babies. When Winner's one general surgeon operates, Lang or Schaap can serve as his first assist—an uncommon luxury; in most medical schools, residents and fellows occupy that coveted position.

Both students acknowledge that life isn't easy in Winner and that for their two family medicine mentors, it's probably not that fun to be on call every other night. But the work is fulfilling, intellectually and emotionally, and they love the autonomy and the chance to be vital members of a close-knit community. Both say their dream job is to become a family medicine doctor, just like their Winner instructors. And Buysse? She's readying her application to the FARM program.

Anderson and other medical school deans know that exposure to rural settings helps convince students and residents to practice there. Scholarship and incentive programs, like Title VII of the Public Health Service Act and the National Health Service Corps, increase practice in underserved areas, but both need more investment. To match the proportion of Americans living in rural communities, the number of rural medical students would have to quadruple. That hasn't been a goal of most medical schools, but it should be.

From Farm to Able

Having enough doctors is one challenge; having the hospitals for them to practice in is another. Each year, 10–15 rural hospitals in the United States close, which means more ailing people have to travel longer distances to see a doctor. Whether it's after an accident, heart attack, or stroke, these delays are costly. Rural and frontier hospitals are especially tough businesses to run. They rely heavily on government payers like Medicare and Medicaid, and they have fewer high-paying, commercially insured patients and many more uninsured patients. To make matters worse, most rural hospitals operate close to two-thirds empty. To offset some of these challenges, Medicare reimburses them more generously than most hospitals, but it still isn't enough.

Rural hospitals can build in more stability and durability by affiliating with a hospital or health system network and by connecting digitally. When I was at the University of Utah, 18 rural and community hospitals affiliated with our hospital and relied on our telehealth programs. For rural hospitals short on specialists, the university's intensive care unit (ICU) doctors provide overnight coverage. In this tele-ICU program, they watch over that community's sickest patients and communicate with their nurses overnight using remote-control robots—mobile cameras and screens on wheels—that can be guided from room to room.

Telehealth programs also mean that people who need emergency help can start vital treatment from a distance. One woman from southern Utah told me about the day her husband had a stroke—one side of his face started drooping and he couldn't speak normally. As soon as they got to the local hospital's emergency department, he underwent a CT scan of his brain. The images were transmitted immediately to the University of Utah (eight doctors provide 24-hour on-call service to 28 rural hospitals). Based on his scan, the doctors in his local hospital started infusing a critical clot-dissolving medication, and he was flown to the university hospital. Now he's fully recovered. By treating the patient as quickly as possible—"time is brain"—stroke patients in rural communities can do just as well as those who live near these hospitals. These same services have offered a critical safety net for people with other conditions, including severe COVID-19 infections.

Ember Alert

Across frontier communities and densely packed cities, over 90% of hospitalized COVID-19 patients and 84% of people who died from COVID-19 had one or more chronic medical conditions such as hypertension, type 2 diabetes, or obesity. Taken together, about 60% of all Americans have at least one of these conditions. They have become the rule, not the exception. Yet many of these conditions are preventable. With the right medications, they are treatable. But too many people aren't getting the treatment they need. For example, only half of those with high blood pressure are taking the medications that could save their lives. An increasing number of the 30 million Americans with diabetes can't afford their insulin medications because of rising costs.

Initially, the higher prevalence of these conditions among African Americans and Hispanics in the United States was blamed for their 4.5 and 3.5 times higher chances, respectively, of developing COVID-19 and also their increased risk of death. Selwyn Vickers, a pancreatic cancer surgeon and dean of the University of Alabama Birmingham's medical school, says that before the pandemic, these disparities had long been known. They're like a "smoldering ember. As long as it's not burning the house down, we live with it." Complications of these conditions, like heart attacks and strokes, usually took years to play out. But not in 2020. "COVID-19 has linked lethality with chronic disease in a specific population like we've never seen before," says Vickers.

Exacerbating these inequities has been the lack of health insurance. The Affordable Care Act of 2010 saw the percentage of Americans who were uninsured drop from 16% in 2010 to 10% in 2016. It also narrowed racial and ethnic disparities. But the pandemic erased those gains and widened the gap. The Commonwealth Fund's Biennial Health Insurance Survey found that in the first half of 2020, almost half of all working-age adults in the United States did not have stable health insurance. Among the most hard-hit were people of color, small business workers, people with low incomes, and young adults. Their health outcomes are getting worse. A closer look at those disparities offers valuable lessons for improving everyone's health.

Consider, for example, maternal mortality. In the United States, Black women are dying from pregnancy-related causes at a rate that is three to four times the rate for White women. Liz Howell, an obstetrician-gynecologist and chair of the Department of Obstetrics and Gynecology at the University of Pennsylvania, has shown that beyond issues of systemic racism, about half of the difference in deaths between Black and White women is simply because of differences in the quality of hospitals. About 75% of Black women deliver babies in minority-serving hospitals that, on average, had worse outcomes. Ashish Jha and colleagues found similar trends when looking at the elderly: hospital care for Black seniors is concentrated in a few hospitals that generally scored badly on quality measures. While these are not the only factors, improving hospital quality and safety would improve health for all, especially Black mothers and seniors.

Good for What Ails Us

Improving the health of our most frail, vulnerable, needy, and often most costly members of society is a critical component of *The Long Fix*. The same strategies to improve their health have the potential to lift us all, whether through the use of technologies to enable seniors to live longer, more independent lives; making sure all communities have enough doctors, nurses, and hospitals; providing better prevention and primary care to reduce chronic conditions; or ensuring better and safer hospitals. The COVID-19 pandemic also offers a few glimmers of encouragement for us to achieve these goals. Here are three valuable lessons:

1. How technologies like telehealth and digital health can improve health, provide greater access to care, and reduce costs
2. How shared learnings can accelerate our understanding of disease and improve the quality and consistency of care of patients
3. How paying for health outcomes instead of paying for action (or "fee for service") can create a more economically efficient, resilient, and just health system

Each lesson has been crucial for emerging from the crisis and may protect us against future ones, pandemics or otherwise.

#1: From Testing to Texting

For years, most insurers and government payers were unwilling to pay for anything other than in-person visits, fearing overuse of videoconferencing or texting could escalate rising health care costs. The exceptions were health systems that also managed the health insurance of many of their patients, like Kaiser Permanente. Then the pandemic changed everything.

Telehealth barriers that had been in place for decades fell overnight, and both clinicians and patients adapted quickly. Many found telehealth visits not only safer, but also more convenient and surprisingly effective. A Willis Tower Watson survey reported that about six months into the crisis, four out of five employees regarded virtual care as good as in-person, and one in four rated it better. Telehealth lends itself particularly well to mental and behavioral health. With rising rates of depression, anxiety, sleep disturbances, and other psychiatric issues, employers surveyed in 2020 reported that 91% would offer telemental health for their employees in 2021. At the same time, Medicare and others are more willing to pay for technology that can supplement the information a doctor gets from a video visit—like continuous glucose monitors for people with diabetes.

For these remote care technologies to work, access to broadband is vital. The Federal Communications Commission reported in 2016 that 34 million Americans didn't have adequate broadband. In urban areas, 97% have high-speed fixed broadband service, but the percentage drops to 65% in rural areas and 60% on tribal lands. The cost of addressing this crisis—an estimated $80 billion—is large, but a worthy infrastructure investment beyond health care, from education to employment.

Even without broadband, digital connections can be helpful. At Coastal Medical, an accountable care organization in Providence, Rhode Island, Ed McGookin, a physician and chief medical officer, and Meryl Moss, chief operating officer, tell me about how they shifted from phones to texting during the pandemic: Every morning at 9 a.m. they'd send out texts to about 200–300 patients recovering from COVID-19 at home. Within 10 minutes, 78% would have already responded. "We weren't having an army each call fifty patients for one minute," said McGookin. Both say that the direct messaging has great potential beyond the pandemic, whether it's reminding patients to undergo their mammogram or colon cancer screening test or getting the right blood tests. For medical practices like Coastal or ChenMed or Iora Health that are paid to keep their patients healthy, delivering care more cost-effectively helps them make more money in the long run. For clinics that practice fee-for-service (paying for action) medicine, the motivations aren't as clear.

For example, during the early days of the pandemic, I called a physician's office to schedule a family member's COVID-19 test. At the end of the call, the assistant said, "This call is going to be billed to your insurer as a telehealth visit." Before I could respond, she quickly reassured me, "Don't worry, you won't have to pay. It will be covered." Multiply that by hundreds of thousands of calls like this across the country each day, and it's easy to understand why insurance companies are beginning to push back on paying for telehealth visits. The country cannot afford to have telehealth recapitulate the trillion-dollar tug-of-war between insurers and health systems.

That's why Onduo, the digital health company I am responsible for at Verily, has taken a different approach. Instead of being paid each time a patient clicks on the app or texts with a health coach or doctor, Onduo is willing to get paid only when it has made people healthier—only when people with diabetes have lowered their blood sugar or people with hypertension have successfully gotten their blood pressure in normal range. That's how digital health technologies can redefine not only how health is coproduced with patients, but also how it's paid for.

#2: A Global Rapid-Response Team

In the early days, the novel coronavirus ruthlessly struck down its victims, and one in four hospitalized patients in New York City died from the disease. Each infected patient was studied as carefully as one of Ernest Amory Codman's surgical patients. Within months, the risk of death dropped to 7.6%. That improvement came, in part, because people sought care sooner and had lower viral loads thanks to masking and social distancing. Also, those infected later were younger and generally healthier than those in the first wave. But importantly, clinicians also learned how to provide better care, use more effective drugs, and improve safety in hospitals.

Those valuable lessons were made possible by the sharing and learning that took place through worldwide digital connections. Videoconferences sponsored by hospitals and medical associations brought together speakers from across the world. Social media outlets like Twitter became podiums for frontline clinicians to share lessons learned and for professors like Bob Wachter, chair of medicine at the University of California at San Francisco, to weave together observations from the anecdotal patient case to sophisticated clinical trials, propelling him to Twitter superstar status.

Supplemented by the rapid posting of research papers online (not always peer reviewed), the community came to understand how this coronavirus differed from the common cold or flu. It was killing people because it made them prone to clotting, it overexcited the immune system with proinflammatory cytokines, and it often targeted organs outside the lungs, like the heart, kidneys, and brain. With this hard-won knowledge, clinicians started using anticoagulation to prevent clots and steroids to suppress the immune system. They learned that flipping patients onto their stomachs could improve lung function so that fewer people needed a ventilator.

The research community took matters one step further, posting massive data sets online, including digital pathology images, genomic sequence data on the coronavirus, epidemiologic models about how it spread, and more. From the government and the private sector, domestic and international sources, these databases accelerated the discovery of new diagnostics, therapeutics, and vaccines.

James Fallows, writing in *The Atlantic*, triggered a national movement to build the same data sharing model for hospitals and health systems. In his article "The 3 Weeks That Changed Everything: Imagine if the National Transportation Safety Board Investigated America's Response to the Coronavirus Pandemic," he asked whether we were as prepared as a pilot readying for a flight: Did the United States have ample planning and early warning signs (a flight plan)? Was there adequate international coordination (air traffic controllers)? Did we use existing playbooks to guide our decision making (the emergency checklist)? And so on.

Taking his lead, Karen Feinstein, president and CEO of the Jewish Health Foundation in Pittsburgh, along with others, proposed a new federal agency, the National Patient and Provider Safety Authority, responsible for improving the safety and quality, modeled on the National Transportation Safety Board. Its primary functions would be to collect data from hospitals and health systems across the nation and make them available for research and policy decisions. It would be a modern, national, digitized End-Results system that Ernest Amory Codman would have adored.

#3: Axe or Scalpel?

Besides its crushing impact on hospitals and clinicians, COVID-19 also brutally exploited the failings of the business model of US health care. When patients avoided most medical routine appointments and operations, many of the hospitals and clinics dependent on a fee-for-service (pay-for-action) payments teetered on the brink of financial ruin. No services meant no fees. Even after over $175 billion was spent bailing out hospitals in mid-2020, one in four rural hospitals remained on the brink of bankruptcy. In April 2020—in the midst of a cataclysmic health crisis—over 1.4 million doctors and nurses were furloughed. The pay-for-action model proved more clearly than ever that it was bad for patients and bad for hospitals.

Beyond making millions of people sick, the coronavirus pandemic created an economic crisis with lasting health implications. Burdened with more debt than any time since 1945, the federal government will look to cutting health care to manage challenges like the imminent insolvency (in 2024) of Medicare Part A (the part that pays for hospital stays). When I talked with Liz Fowler, executive vice president for programs of the Commonwealth Fund, she said, "When you're talking about budget cuts, [Congress] take[s] a meat-axe approach to solving a problem rather than a scalpel."

Rather than across-the-board cuts that reduce benefits for seniors, the poor and disabled, and the already underserved, we'd rather neatly trim out the waste, improve safety, reduce the costs of mistakes, and spend more on prevention to stay healthier and save money in the long run. We'd also prefer to have more resilient health systems, like the Military Health System and Veterans Affairs Health System, and medical groups like Coastal, Presbyterian, and Iora Health that get paid for keeping their patients healthy, instead of getting paid for each service they provide. COVID-19 underscored that in these systems, clinicians can look after their patients better and withstand downturns in the economy. Digital health solutions and telehealth offer cheaper, more accessible, and more engaging care, and the data from those technologies can also enhance the analytic prowess of the proposed

National Patient and Provider Safety Authority to improve health, reduce mistakes, and help everyone get healthier.

The Long Fix highlights how these changes are critical for a healthier world, and now it's clear that they are essential for a more robust, equitable, and resilient future, too.

Accelerating the Long Fix

Fixing our health system will be expensive, but not fixing it will exact a much higher toll in costs, and in suffering and lives lost. It will be a key part of how we recover from this scourge, how we rebuild our economy, and how we revitalize our society. It will be a test of our commitment to our fellow citizens. Now is the time to make our nation's health better and our country stronger and ready for future challenges. It's time to accelerate the Long Fix.

DISCUSSION GUIDE

THE LONG FIX: SOLVING AMERICA'S HEALTH CARE CRISIS WITH STRATEGIES THAT WORK FOR EVERYONE, BY VIVIAN S. LEE, MD.

The Long Fix is structured as a series of twelve chapters and an epilogue that can be read and interpreted independently of each other. This Discussion Guide provides a sampling of questions for the entire book.

1. What about health care inspires you the most? Have you had a first-hand experience that has made you feel really positive about the care that was provided?

2. What about health care concerns you the most? Have you had a firsthand experience that has made you feel negative or concerned about the US health care system?

3. Digital health programs for people who have type-2 diabetes need

people to use their apps regularly to enter information about themselves—what they're eating, how they're exercising, what medications they are taking. Discuss how you feel about these programs. Do you think these kinds of programs might keep you healthier? What features would be important to you and why?

4. Have you ever tried to figure out in advance what your costs will be for health care? Share a story about whether you were able to determine those costs and whether the estimates proved to be accurate.

5. To make them more efficient and safe, hospitals can adopt lessons from manufacturing plants that make care more standard and reduce distractions. In what ways would you hope that your hospital would be more like a piano factory, and in what ways do you expect it to differ?

6. One of the points Dr. Lee makes in *The Long Fix* is that everyone is paying for health care—even in invisible ways (like the pay raises that should have happened but didn't because the money had to go to pay for mounting health care costs). Think about some examples in your own lives where you may have asked for care—a prescription, a test, or a referral to another doctor—that you might have skipped altogether, if you had thought you would be paying for it.

7. Whether it's exercising and eating healthily or managing medical conditions, everyone has a role to play in coproducing their health or the health of their loved ones. Discuss the balance of responsibility: an individual; the individual's family; the individual's doctor or nurse; the community; and others.

8. One of the challenges of using cost-effectiveness numbers to decide which drugs are "worth it" and which are not is coming up with a dollar amount for the "value" of a year of healthy life. In *The Long Fix*,

Dr. Lee offers a few possible numbers: $63,000 because that's the average annual household income in the United States, or $60,000 because that's the per capita gross domestic product. Others have used higher numbers like $100,000 or $150,000 per quality-adjusted life year (QALY). Discuss what this number should be in your view, and what it means.

9. In *The Long Fix*, Dr. Tom Delbanco champions the Open Notes movement. Discuss how you feel about being able to read the notes your doctors write about you. Do you want to read those notes? Would you feel comfortable correcting your doctor if he or she got something wrong? Would you like to be able to write your own section of these notes?

10. Employers, second only to the government, pay the largest chunk of America's health care bills. Why are they struggling with bringing costs down? Having read *The Long Fix*, what would you advise your business (or boss) to do differently?

11. Dr. Lee discusses the concept of "readiness" as a mandate for federal health administration. What does readiness mean to you, and how would this change the kinds of programs the government might support? How is your definition affected by the COVID-19 pandemic?

12. What three top takeaways would you cite from *The Long Fix*?

Individual chapter discussion guides, deep-dive activities for *The Long Fix*, and customized discussion guides for groups such as business and community leaders, business students, health care professionals, medical students, and social groups are available from the author at www .vivianleemd.com.

ACKNOWLEDGMENTS

Throughout my career, I have been fortunate to work with people who have a thirst for tackling difficult problems and the passion for improvement. Bob Grossman is one. At NYU Langone Medical Center, he has energetically demonstrated just how much difference a leader can make—first for the Department of Radiology, where I had the privilege of working with him as vice chair for research, and then as the dean and CEO of the Medical Center, where I served as vice dean and chief scientific officer. From Bob, I learned invaluable lessons about academic medicine, health care, and leadership. I would not have considered the CEO role at Utah were it not for his mentorship.

My six-year tenure leading University of Utah Health introduced me to a community committed to providing not just excellent, but exceptional care. Many of the cornerstone lessons of this book come from those experiences. Amy Albo, Joe Borgenicht, and their teams did a fine job documenting our initiatives, and together with our chief marketing officer, Dave Perry, and publicists Rimjhim Dey and Kavita Tomlinson of DEY, first encouraged me to consider writing a book based on my lectures for our students. I thank the University of Utah for supporting my sabbatical to conduct research for this project.

My colleagues at Verily, led by our visionary and fearless CEO Andy Conrad, approach the challenges of health care with a data-driven, technology-enabled, consumer (patient)-centered perspective that is as refreshing as it is bold. I am grateful for their support and encouragement to complete this book. Each day, I feel inspired by the talent, passion, and drive of our team members who are all committed to accelerating the long fix of health care. In Chapter 1, I acknowledge the critical role that Gregg Meyer played in the trajectory of my career leading to Utah. Serendipitously, he and his partner, Bonnie Blanchfield, also played an instrumental role in my introduction to Verily. For their friendship—and the impact it has had on my life—I will always be thankful.

Working in Boston, I have also felt fortunate that Jim Brink, chair of the Department of Radiology at Massachusetts General Hospital, and his colleague Bruce Rosen, director of the Martinos Center for Biomedical Imaging, have so kindly welcomed me into their department and to Harvard Medical School as a senior lecturer. I also thank Don Berwick and Derek Feeley of the Institute for Healthcare Improvement for my appointment as a Senior Fellow of IHI.

The Long Fix is an optimistic book about solving America's health care crisis. It reflects the strong collective commitment of leaders to make things better, and a growing clarity about how to do so. I am grateful for the many illuminating conversations I have had with colleagues at conferences, including the Snowbird Health Summit. I have also had the honor of working alongside many inspiring leaders while serving on boards and advisory committees such as the Board of the Commonwealth Fund and the Defense Health Board. I especially would like to thank the following individuals for agreeing to be interviewed for this book and for sharing their experiences and insights so candidly and insightfully: Marcia Angell, David Asch, Bonnie Blanchfield, David Blumenthal, Rob Califf, Carolyn Clancy, Ceci Connelly, Patrick Conway, David Cutler, Karen DeSalvo, Karen Feinstein, Rushika Fernandopulle, Terri Fulmer, Bob Galvin, Clif Gaus, Reshma Gupta, Clay Johnston, Ken Kim, Mike Leavitt, Jennifer Lee, Bruce Leff, Peter Margolis, Justin Masterson, Mark McClellan, Gregg Meyer, LaQuandra Nesbitt, Pamela Peele, Richard Platt, Karen Remley, Leonard Saltz, Mark Schuster, Tom Sequist, and Vindell Washington and a number of individuals at the University of Utah Health: Erin Fox, Cheri Hunter, Jim Livingston, Cary Martin, Charlton Park, Bob Pendleton, Brad Rockwell, Ming Tu, Russell Vinik, Peter Weir, Chad Westover, and Kip Williams.

Seeing successful models of care firsthand in beacon organizations across the country and world has been one of the highlights of this project. I am deeply indebted to the many who have welcomed me and who shared stories and learnings that enrich this work. I thank them and their staff for their generosity:

- Dan Lessler, Washington Health Authority, and Bob Mecklenburg, Bree Collaborative, Seattle, Washington
- Chris Chen, Stephen Greene, Carlos Perez, Sofia Recabarren, ChenMed, Miami, Florida
- Peter Margolis, Andy Beck, Anita Brentley, Rob Kahn, Cincinnati Children's Hospital, Cincinnati, Ohio
- Captain Juliann Althoff, Major General George Anderson, Vice Admiral Raquel Bono, Nancy Dickey, Commander Andrew Lin, Captain Greg Gorman, Defense Health Board and Military Health System, Falls Church, Virginia
- Clay Johnston, Kevin Bozic, Stacey Chang, Sue Cox, Martin Harris, Liz Jacobs, Mimi Kahlon, Chris Moriates, Beth Nelson, Lorrayne Ward, Dell Medical School, University of Texas, Austin
- Karen Feinstein, Judy Black, Robert Ferguson, David Golebiewski, Mara Leff, Megan Steinmetz, Nancy Zionts, Jewish Health Foundation in Pittsburgh
- Al Siu, Mount Sinai Health System, New York, New York
- John Wong, Song Chua, Keith Lim, Jason Phua, James Yip, National University Health System of Singapore
- Nancy Guinn, Jason Mitchell, Ries Robinson, Todd Sandman, Presbyterian Healthcare Services, Albuquerque, New Mexico
- Kara Wright, Midge Wilson, Tenderloin Community School, San Francisco, California

- Bob Mecklenburg, Andrew Kartunen, Sarah Patterson, Rebecca Pumpian, Bill Poppy, Rajiv Sethi, Virginia Mason Medical Center, Seattle, Washington

I admire the many who have devoted their lives to improving the health of others and have done my best to reflect their stories accurately. Any errors and shortcomings in this book are solely my own in reporting them.

An academic scientist trying to write a book on health care that is readable and engaging to the general public needs help from a lot of people.

I am especially thankful for the contributions of Bob Roe. With the intuition of a seasoned editor, Bob identified, culled, and reshaped the most compelling sections of my initial draft into a strong book proposal. Bob also introduced me to my wonderful agent, Kathy Robbins, who believed in this book from the beginning and has been an enthusiastic champion at every step of the process. Her conviction about the importance of identifying solutions to America's health care crisis was fortunately shared by John Glusman, editor-in-chief at W. W. Norton & Company, who decided to take a gamble on a (heavy sigh) "health care book." Then, in between our kids' hockey games and tournaments, Bob contributed a second round of his editorial prowess. He ruthlessly revised and sharpened the writing of the full draft manuscript and offered advice on how to mold the chapters into a book with a narrative arc that might be understandable—and maybe even appealing—to a broader readership.

Over the course of writing and revising, I burdened several busy friends and colleagues by asking them to provide feedback on the draft manuscript. Dan Costin and Tara Deal, dear friends from college, gave page-by-page detailed feedback and challenged many ideas in the book from their well-informed, nonmedical perspectives. A longtime colleague and friend from the MRI community, Margaret-Hall Craggs—who roped in her husband and lawyer–civil servant, Roland Green, to provide his own reading and comments—delivered fresh British perspectives that convinced me to share more lessons from outside our borders and helped me hone the overall recommendations. Bob Galvin read the book not once, but twice, and his expert insights about health care influenced much of the book, especially the employee health chapter. Danielle Sample did more than provide feedback from a careful reading of the book. Throughout the journey that led to this book being written, she left an indelible mark on much of its content through her irrepressible energy and passion to bring people together to work on big problems and to accomplish great things.

I am also thankful to Captain Greg Gorman and Major General George Anderson for their careful readings, especially of the military health chapter. I also appreciate the excellent work that two fact-checkers, Noah Flora and Sophie Kasakove, did to ensure that statistics and references properly reflected the publicly available sources.

This book is a tribute to those who hold the future of medicine in their hands—the students and trainees in the health professions who always give me reasons to feel optimistic, and to the patients and their families who, by entrusting us with their lives and health, add urgency to the long fix.

NOTES

Chapter 1: A Revolution of Common Sense

1 **Hal Belknap:** Harold (Hal) Belknap Jr. (1934–2008) was born and raised in Norman, Oklahoma. Having earned his MD at Tulane University, he joined the army and trained during his 3-year residency at US Army Medical Service at Fitzsimons General Hospital in Denver, Colorado, and served as chief resident. In 1967, he returned to Norman to become the town's first internal medicine specialist. His practice grew to become one of the largest physician practices in the area, Norman Clinic. Throughout his life he was passionate about the Boy Scouts Association and founded Troop 777 as well as the Medical Explorer Post 901 group for both girls and boys interested in medicine. Carol Cole-Frowe, "Longtime Norman Physician Hal Belknap Dies," *Norman Transcript*, April 21, 2008, https://www.normantranscript.com/news/local_news/longtime-norman-physician-hal-belknap-dies/article_7253e1ca-09d2-5f87-8f3d-59fc9e2ec3c4.html.

2 **magnetic resonance imaging:** MRI and CT were cited as among the most significant medical inventions of the 20th century. The invention of MRI earned Paul Lauterbur and Sir Peter Mansfield the Nobel Prize in Physiology or Medicine in 2003. Victor R. Fuchs and Harold C. Sox, "Physicians' Views of the Relative Importance of Thirty Medical Innovations," *Health Affairs* 20, no. 5 (Fall 2001), https://doi.org/10.1377/hlthaff.20.5.30.

3 **A series of widely cited reports:** For example, the landmark reports from the Institute of Medicine (now National Academy of Medicine): Committee on Quality of Health Care in America, *To Err is Human: Building a Safer Health System* (Washington, DC: Institute of Medicine, 1999), accessed October 27, 2019, http://www.nationalacademies.org/hmd/Reports/1999/To-Err-is-Human-Building-A-Safer-Health-System.aspx; Committee on Quality of Health Care in America, *Crossing the Quality Chasm: A New Health System for the 21st Century* (Washington, DC: Institute of Medicine, 2001), accessed October 27, 2019, http://www.nationalacademies.org/hmd/Reports/2001/Crossing-the-Quality-Chasm-A-New-Health-System-for-the-21st-Century.aspx; Commit-

tee on the Learning Health Care System in America, *Best Care at Lower Cost: The Path to Continuously Learning Health Care in America* (Washington, DC: National Academies Press, 2013), https://doi.org/10.17226/13444.

3 **Gregg Meyer:** In 2019, Meyer was the chief clinical officer of Partners Healthcare System and professor of medicine at Harvard Medical School. He practices medicine at the Massachusetts General Hospital. He was also interviewed by the author on October 12, 2017.

3 **Massachusetts General Hospital:** Since 2015, I have served on the Scientific Advisory Board of the Massachusetts General Hospital. Since December 2018, I have been a senior lecturer (uncompensated) at Harvard Medical School and at the Massachusetts General Hospital as well.

4 *Designing Care:* Richard M. J. Bohmer, *Designing Care: Aligning the Nature and Management of Health Care* (Brighton: Harvard Business Review Press, 2009).

4 **University of Utah ranked #1:** The year I joined the University of Utah, it was ranked #1 in quality and safety by University Healthsystem Consortium (now Vizient, Inc.), the organization of teaching hospitals in the United States. From 2011 to 2019, Utah remained in the top ten, reaching #1 again in 2016. The university is the research and training partner (and sometimes clinical rival) of Intermountain Healthcare.

6 **one of the best in the world:** *Scientific American* ranked the United States at the top of the list in overall innovation in 2016, followed by Singapore, Denmark, New Zealand, and Australia: "Worldview Scorecard," *Scientific American WorldVIEW*, accessed October 27, 2019, http://www.saworldview.com/scorecard/the-2016-scientific-american-worldview-overall-scores/; Aaron E. Carroll and Austin Frakt, "Can the U.S. Repair Its Health Care While Keeping Its Innovation Edge?," *New York Times*, October 9, 2017, https://www.nytimes.com/2017/10/09/upshot/can-the-us-repair-its-health-care-while-keeping-its-innovation-edge.html.

6 **one of the worst:** A number of comparisons of high-income nations conclude that health system performance is worst in the United States. For example: Eric C. Schneider et al., *Mirror, Mirror 2017: International Comparison Reflects Flaws and Opportunities for Better U.S. Health Care,* Commonwealth Fund, July 14, 2017, https://interactives.commonwealthfund.org/2017/july/mirror-mirror/; Bradley Sawyer and Daniel McDermott, "How Does the Quality of the U.S. Healthcare System Compare to Other Countries?," Peterson-Kaiser Health System Tracker, 2019, accessed October 27, 2019, https://www.healthsystemtracker.org/chart-collection/quality-u-s-healthcare-system-compare-countries/#item-start; Irene Papanicolas, Liana R. Woskie, and Ashish K. Jha, "Health Care Spending in the United States and Other High-Income Countries," *JAMA* 319, no. 10 (March 13, 2018): 1024–39, doi: 10.1001/jama.2018.1150.

6 **immune cells, engineered to attack cancer cells:** Carl H. June et al., "CAR T Cell Immunotherapy for Human Cancer," *Science* 359, no. 6382 (March 23, 2018): 1361–65, doi: 10.1126/science.aar6711.

6 **without opening the chest:** Gernot Wagner et al., "Comparison of Transcath-
eter Aortic Valve Implantation with Other Approaches to Treat Aortic Valve
Stenosis: A Systematic Review and Meta-Analysis," *Systematic Reviews* 8, no. 1
(February 2019): 44, https://doi.org/10.1186/s13643-019-0954-3.

6 **hepatitis C can now be cured:** Jeffrey A. Tice, Daniel A. Ollendorf, and Steven
D. Pearson, *The Comparative Clinical Effectiveness and Value of Simeprevir and
Sofosbuvir in the Treatment of Chronic Hepatitis C Infection* (Boston: Institute for
Clinical and Economic Review, 2014), accessed September 3, 2019, https://icer
-review.org/wp-content/uploads/2016/02/CTAF_Hep_C_Apr14_final.pdf.

6 **46% of US adults have high blood pressure:** Using the 2017 criteria that define
hypertension as a systolic blood pressure of 130 mm Hg or above or a diastolic
blood pressure of 80 mm Hg or above. Emelia J. Benjamin et al., "Heart Disease
and Stroke Statistics—2019 Update: A Report from the American Heart Association," *Circulation* 139, no. 10 (January 2019), e56–e528, https://doi.org/10
.1161/CIR.0000000000000659.

6 **aren't taking the life-saving pills:** This landmark study demonstrated that
about 50% of hypertensive patients had stopped taking their blood pressure
medications within one year: Bernard Vrijens et al., "Adherence to Prescribed
Antihypertensive Drug Treatments: Longitudinal Study of Electronically
Compiled Dosing Histories," *BMJ* 336 (May 2008): 1114, https://doi.org/10
.1136/bmj.39553.670231.25.

6 **nearly one-fifth of the US economy goes to pay for health:** The United States
spent $10,224 on health care per capita in 2017, compared to the next highest,
Switzerland, at $8,009. Germans spent $5,728, Canadians, $4,826, Japanese,
$4,717, Australians, $4,543, and the British, $4,246. Bradley Sawyer and Cyn-
thia Cox, "How Does Health Spending in the U.S. Compare to Other Countries?," Peterson-Kaiser Health System Tracker, 2019, accessed October 27,
2019, https://www.healthsystemtracker.org/chart-collection/health-spending
-u-s-compare-countries/#item-average-wealthy-countries-spend-half-much
-per-person-health-u-s-spends; Papanicolas, Woskie, and Jha, "Health Care
Spending in the United States and Other High-Income Countries."

6 **1 in 11 Americans don't have health insurance and can't afford care:** Edward
R. Berchick, Jessica C. Barnett, and Rachel D. Upton, *Health Insurance Coverage in the United States: 2018* (Suitland: United States Census Bureau, 2019),
accessed October 27, 2019, https://www.census.gov/content/dam/Census/
library/publications/2019/demo/p60-267.pdf.

Other surveys, such as the 2018 Commonwealth Fund's Biennial Health
Insurance Survey, found similar numbers, focusing just on nonelderly adults:
12.4% of adults ages 19–64 were uninsured (unchanged from 2016), while the
Kaiser Family Foundation survey of 2017 reported 10.2% (27.4 million) nonelderly adults were uninsured. Sara R. Collins, Herman K. Bhupal, and Michelle
M. Doty, *Health Insurance Coverage Eight Years after the ACA* (New York: Commonwealth Fund, 2019), https://www.commonwealthfund.org/publications/

issue-briefs/2019/feb/health-insurance-coverage-eight-years-after-aca; Rachel
Garfield, Kendal Orgera, and Anthony Damico, *The Uninsured and the ACA:
A Primer—Key Facts about Health Insurance and the Uninsured Amidst Changes
to the Affordable Care Act* (San Francisco: Kaiser Family Foundation, 2019),
accessed October 27, 2019, https://www.kff.org/report-section/the-uninsured
-and-the-aca-a-primer-key-facts-about-health-insurance-and-the-uninsured
-amidst-changes-to-the-affordable-care-act-how-many-people-are-uninsured/.

6 **diseases of despair:** Anne Case and Angus Deaton, "Mortality and Morbidity in the 21st Century," *Brookings Papers on Economic Activity* (Spring 2017):
397–476.

6 **34,768 life-saving organ transplants:** "Deceased Organ Donors in United
States Exceeded 10,000 for First Time in 2017," United Network for Organ
Sharing, accessed October 28, 2019, https://unos.org/news/deceased-organ
-donors-in-united-states-exceeded-10000-for-first-time-in-2017/.

6 **47,600 people to opioid overdoses . . . 47,174 to suicide:** "Drug Overdose
Deaths," Centers for Disease Control and Prevention, accessed October 27, 2019,
https://www.cdc.gov/drugoverdose/data/statedeaths.html; *Pain in the Nation
Update: While Deaths from Alcohol, Drugs, and Suicide Slowed Slightly in 2017,
Rates Are Still at Historic Highs* (Washington, DC: Trust for America's Health
and Well Being Trust), accessed September 3, 2019, https://www.tfah.org/wp
-content/uploads/2019/03/TFAH-2019-PainNationUpdateBrief-07.pdf.

7 **5.6 years less than those born in Japan:** "Health Status: Life Expectancy,"
OECD.Stat, accessed October 27, 2019, https://stats.oecd.org/index.aspx
?queryid=30114.

7 **Four out of ten adults are obese:** "Overweight & Obesity," Centers for Disease Control and Prevention, accessed August 15, 2019, https://www.cdc.gov/
obesity/data/adult.html.

7 **among young adults:** "Mental Illness," National Institute of Mental Health,
accessed September 3, 2019, https://www.nimh.nih.gov/health/statistics/
mental-illness.shtml.

7 **the most common reason being their weight:** Miriam Jordan, "Recruits' Ineligibility Tests the Military," *Wall Street Journal*, June 27, 2014, https://www.wsj
.com/articles/recruits-ineligibility-tests-the-military-1403909945?mod=e2tw.

7 **flat wages over the past 50 years:** Drew Desilver, *For Most U.S. Workers,
Real Wages Have Barely Budged in Decades* (Washington, DC: Pew Research
Center, 2018), accessed October 27, 2019, https://www.pewresearch.org/
fact-tank/2018/08/07/for-most-us-workers-real-wages-have-barely-budged
-for-decades/; Andrea Koncz, *Salary Trends through Salary Survey: A Historical Perspective on Starting Salaries for New College Graduates* (Bethlehem, PA:
NACE Center, 2016), accessed October 27, 2019, https://www.naceweb.org/
job-market/compensation/salary-trends-through-salary-survey-a-historical
-perspective-on-starting-salaries-for-new-college-graduates/.

7 **$275 billion in 2016 alone:** Alexis Pozen, "Five Myths about Health Insurance,"

Washington Post, June 30, 2017, https://www.washingtonpost.com/outlook/ five-myths/five-myths-about-health-insurance/2017/06/30/0136f34e-5cd2 -11e7-a9f6-7c3296387341_story.html?utm_term=.06c0cba3edb3.

7 **rapidly approaching $4 trillion per year:** The United States spent about $3.65 trillion on health care in 2018. *National Health Expenditure Projections 2018–2027* (Baltimore: Center for Medicare and Medicaid Services, 2019), accessed October 27, 2019, https://www.cms.gov/Research-Statistics-Data -and-Systems/Statistics-Trends-and-Reports/NationalHealthExpendData/ Downloads/ForecastSummary.pdf.

8 **we waste 30 cents of every dollar we spend on health care:** Institute of Medicine of the National Academies, *Best Care at Lower Cost: The Path to Continuously Learning Health Care in America* (Washington, DC: National Academies Press, 2013); Tanya G. K. Bentley et al., "Waste in the U.S. Health Care System: A Conceptual Framework," *Milbank Quarterly* 86, no. 4 (December 2008): 629–59, doi: 10.1111/j.1468-0009.2008.00537.x; William H. Shrank, Teresa L. Rogstad, and Natasha Parekh, "Waste in the US Health Care System: Estimated Costs and Potential for Savings," *JAMA* 322, no. 15 (October 2019): 1501–9, doi: 10.1001/jama.2019.13978.

8 **overdiagnosis and overtreatment:** For an excellent exploration of overdiagnosis and overtreatment, I recommend Shannon Brownlee, *Overtreated: Why Medicine Is Making Us Sicker and Poorer* (London: Bloomsbury, 2010).

8 **20% of all medical care was unnecessary:** Heather Lyu et al., "Overtreatment in the United States," *PLoS One* 12, no. 9 (September 6, 2017): e0181970, doi: 10.1371/journal.pone.0181970.

8 **behind only heart disease and cancer:** Martin A. Makary and Michael Daniel, "Medical Error—the Third Leading Cause of Death in the US," *BMJ* 353 (May 3, 2016): i2139, https://doi.org/10.1136/bmj.i2139.

8 **Physicians follow recommended guidelines:** Sanjaya Kumar and David B. Nash, "Health Care Myth Busters: Is There a High Degree of Scientific Certainty in Modern Medicine?," *Scientific American*, March 25, 2011, https://www .scientificamerican.com/article/demand-better-health-care-book/.

8 **spent on administration:** Papanicolas, Woskie, and Jha, "Health Care Spending in the United States and Other High-Income Countries."

8 **average US generalist physician makes about $218,000; specialists average $316,000:** Papanicolas, Woskie, and Jha, "Health Care Spending in the United States and Other High-Income Countries."

8 **overprescription of antibiotics:** Papanicolas, Woskie, and Jha, "Health Care Spending in the United States and Other High-Income Countries."

9 **sweets and drinks (spending $4 billion):** *High Fructose Corn Syrup Production Industry in the US—Market Research Report* (Los Angeles: IBISWorld, 2019), accessed September 3, 2019, https://www.ibisworld.com/industry -trends/specialized-market-research-reports/consumer-goods-services/food -production/high-fructose-corn-syrup-production.html.

9 **$200 billion for fast food**: Bernadette Keefe, "Fast Food Nation (Around the World)," accessed August 15, 2019, https://blog.centerforinnovation.mayo .edu/2016/04/07/fast-food-nation-around-the-world/.

9 **tobacco ($130 billion)**: Ian Tiseo, "Tobacco Market Value in the U.S. 2015–20," *Statista*, August 7, 2019, https://www.statista.com/statistics/491709/tobacco-united-states-market-value/.

9 **video gaming ($43 billion)**: Jonathan Shieber, "Video Game Revenue Tops $43 Billion in 2018, an 18% Jump from 2017," *TechCrunch*, January 22, 2019, https://techcrunch.com/2019/01/22/video-game-revenue-tops-43-billion-in -2018-an-18-jump-from-2017/.

9 **four out of five people would prefer to die at home**: Liz Hamel, Bryan Wu, and Mollyann Brodie, *Views and Experiences with End-of-Life Medical Care in the U.S.* (San Francisco: Kaiser Family Foundation, 2017), accessed October 27, 2019, https://www.kff.org/report-section/views-and-experiences-with-end-of -life-medical-care-in-the-us-findings/.

9 **Most people still die in a hospital or nursing home**: "Percent of Deaths Occurring in Hospital," Dartmouth Atlas of Health Care, accessed August 15, 2019, http://archive.dartmouthatlas.org/data/table.aspx?ind=15; "*QuickStats*: Percentage Distribution of Deaths, by Place of Death—United States, 2000–2014," *Morbidity and Mortality Weekly Report* 65, no. 357 (2016), doi: http://dx .doi.org/10.15585/mmwr.6513a6.

10 **shot up from $3 billion to $37 billion**: Office of Evaluation and Inspections, *Medicare Hospital Prospective Payment System: How DRG Rates Are Calculated and Updated* (Washington, DC: US Department of Health and Human Services, 2001), accessed July 4, 2019, https://oig.hhs.gov/oei/reports/oei-09-00 -00200.pdf.

10 **the figure was a stunning $308 billion**: Medicare Part A payments to hospitals totaled $308 billion of the $741 billion in total Medicare benefits paid in 2018: *Trustees Report & Trust Funds* (Baltimore, MD: Centers for Medicare & Medicaid Services, 2019), accessed October 27, 2019, https://www.cms .gov/Research-Statistics-Data-and-Systems/Statistics-Trends-and-Reports/ ReportsTrustFunds/index.html.

10 **Ceci Connelly**: Interview of Ceci Connelly by the author, August 2, 2019.

11 **how much health care her employees will need**: They don't have to accurately predict your health costs; they just have to be close with their prediction for the entire group. Their predictions are more accurate with larger numbers of employees.

11 **deductibles, co-payments, or coinsurance**: The deductible is the amount you pay for covered health services before the health insurance or benefit plan starts to pay. A co-payment or co-pay is a fixed amount that you pay for a covered service, while the remainder is paid by the plan. Coinsurance is the percentage of the costs of a covered service (20%, for example), after you've paid your deductible, and the balance is covered by the plan.

12 **rules of the market don't readily apply:** Kenneth J. Arrow, "Uncertainty and the Welfare Economics of Medical Care," *American Economic Review* 53, no. 5 (December 1963): 941–73.

12 **moderately healthy people are priced out:** In economic terms, this is referred to as adverse selection.

12 **"That's where we are in health care":** Saltz attributed this analogy to a friend of his. Interview of Leonard Saltz by the author, June 14, 2019.

12 **higher premiums for everyone next year:** This surf 'n' turf metaphor is also referred to as moral hazard in economic terms.

15 **disproportionately affected the poor:** "2018 Poverty Guidelines," Office of the Assistant Secretary for Planning and Evaluation, accessed October 19, 2019, https://aspe.hhs.gov/2018-poverty-guidelines.

15 **Rural Americans:** Much has been written about rural-urban disparities in care. For example: *Rural-Urban Disparities in Health Care in Medicare* (Baltimore, MD: Centers for Medicare & Medicaid Services, 2018) and *Access in Brief: Rural and Urban Health Care* (Washington, DC: Medicaid and CHIP Payment and Access Commission, 2018).

15 **Race and ethnicity:** The issues of racial and ethnic disparities in health and health care have been documented and studied extensively. Two helpful reviews are Wayne J. Riley, "Health Disparities: Gaps in Access, Quality and Affordability of Medical Care," *Transactions of the American Clinical and Climatological Association* 123 (2012): 167–74, PMID: 23303983; and John Z. Ayanian, "The Costs of Racial Disparities in Health Care," *New England Journal of Medicine Catalyst*, February 15, 2016, https://catalyst.nejm.org/the-costs-of-racial-disparities-in-health-care/.

One publication suggested that Medicare Advantage programs might be improving disparities (at least those programs in the West): John Z. Ayanian et al., "Racial and Ethnic Disparities among Enrollees in Medicare Advantage Plans," *New England Journal of Medicine* 371 (2014): 2288–97, doi: 10.1056/NEJMsa1407273.

15 **and more likely to die from them:** One study provocatively showed that physicians treated "patients" with the same chest pain (actors who followed the same script) differently depending on their race and gender. Doctors were 40% less likely to recommend a cardiac catheterization (a procedure for diagnosing and treating coronary artery disease) if the "patient" was black or a woman, and 60% less likely if she was both. Kevin A. Schulman et al., "The Effect of Race and Sex on Physicians' Recommendations for Cardiac Catheterization," *New England Journal of Medicine* 340, no. 8 (February 1999): 618–26, doi: 10.1056/NEJM199902253400806.

15 **More education:** Anne Case and Angus Deaton, *Mortality and Morbidity in the 21st Century* (Washington, DC: Brookings Institution, 2017), accessed November 11, 2019, http://www.princeton.edu/~accase/downloads/Mortality_and_Morbidity_in_21st_Century_Case-Deaton-BPEA-published.pdf.

Chapter 2: An Apple a Day Keeps the Patient Away

18   **Nancy Guinn:** Interview of Nancy Guinn, the medical director of Presbyterian Health Services' Healthcare at Home program, Albuquerque, New Mexico, by the author, August 30, 2018.

18   **his father's clinic in Miami:** This narrative is drawn from an interview of Chris Chen by the author, January 8, 2018, and a podcast: Chris Chen, "Running through Walls: Medicine Is a Family Affair," Venrock, accessed August 28, 2019, http://hwcdn.libsyn.com/p/d/0/a/d0a803bed4b762ca/RTW-0038-ChrisChen -ChenMed-BryanRoberts-m1_08a.mp3?c_id=18553240&cs_id=18553240&ex piration=1565991477&hwt=3bda781571dc55642db59dba79ba5da1.

20   **"You know what's going on in their lives":** Interview of Sofia Recabarren by the author, January 12, 2018.

21   **"minister for loneliness":** "PM Launches Government's First Loneliness Strategy," Gov.UK, last updated October 16, 2018, https://www.gov.uk/government/ news/pm-launches-governments-first-loneliness-strategy.

21   **lowered the number of days spent in the hospital by 38%:** Craig Tanio and Christopher Chen, "Innovations at Miami Practice Show Promise for Treating High-Risk Medicare Patients," *Health Affairs* 32, no. 6 (June 2013), https://doi .org/10.1377/hlthaff.2012.0201.

21   **California's CareMore Health:** Martha Hostetter, Sarah Klein, and Douglas McCarthy, "CareMore: Improving Outcomes and Controlling Health Care Spending for High-Needs Patients," Commonwealth Fund, March 28, 2017, https://www.commonwealthfund.org/publications/case-study/2017/mar/ caremore-improving-outcomes-and-controlling-health-care-spending.

21   **Chicago's Oak Street Health:** Griffin Myers and Thomas H. Lee, "Rebuilding Health Care as It Should Be: Personal, Equitable, and Accountable," *New England Journal of Medicine Catalyst*, August 3, 2018, https://catalyst.nejm.org/ rebuilding-health-care-oak-street-health/.

21   **Rhode Island's Coastal Medical:** Richard Salit, "R.I.'s Coastal Medical Gets National Recognition for New Care Model," *Providence Journal*, October 23, 2015, https://www.providencejournal.com/article/20151023/NEWS/151029591.

21   **the key challenges:** Interview of Rushika Fernandopulle by the author, February 22, 2018, and a podcast: Rushika Fernandopulle, "Episode 38: Iora Health—with Dr. Rushika Fernandopulle," Direct Primary Care Podcast, June 3, 2018, accessed October 5, 2019.

23   **Canceling annual electrocardiograms:** "American Academy of Family Physicians: Twenty Things Physicians and Patients Should Question," Choosing Wisely, last updated July 18, 2018, https://www.choosingwisely.org/societies/ american-academy-of-family-physicians/. The Choosing Wisely campaign keeps a website of care that is recommended and care that is deemed unnecessary. https://www.choosingwisely.org/.

24 **$43 billion a year on this pastime:** Jonathan Shieber, "Video Game Revenue Tops $43 Billion in 2018, an 18% Jump from 2017," *TechCrunch*, January 22, 2019, https://techcrunch.com/2019/01/22/video-game-revenue-tops-43-billion-in -2018-an-18-jump-from-2017/.

24 **Altizer shows me what he was thinking:** See also Peter Rosen, "Prescription to Play: U. Working to Improve Your Health with Apps, Games," KSL.com, March 17, 2017, https://www.ksl.com/article/43531850/prescription-to-play -u-working-to-improve-your-health-with-apps-games.

24 **Stephen King:** King was featured in this newspaper story: Andy Miller, "Managing Diabetes through a 'Virtual' Clinic," *Gwinnett Daily Post*, October 1, 2018, https://www.gwinnettdailypost.com/local/health/managing-diabetes -through-a-virtual-clinic/article_26868022-53f0-50b1-8328-08972004e54b .html.

24 **he was diagnosed with prediabetes:** Prediabetes affects about one in three Americans, 90% of whom don't know they have it. The diagnosis is based on elevated fasting blood sugars. The National Diabetes Prevention Program is effective at preventing the development of diabetics: "National Diabetes Prevention Program," Centers for Disease Control and Prevention, accessed September 3, 2019, https://www.cdc.gov/diabetes/prevention/index.html.

26 **substantially interfered with life activities:** "Results From the 2017 National Survey on Drug Use and Health: Detailed Tables," Rockville, MD: Substance Abuse and Mental Health Services Administration, 2017, accessed September 1, 2019, https://www.samhsa.gov/data/sites/default/files/cbhsq-reports/ NSDUHDetailedTabs2017/NSDUHDetailedTabs2017.pdf.

26 **extra spending was for medical services:** Stephen P. Melek, Doug T. Norris, and J. Paulus, *Economic Impact of Integrated Medical-Behavioral Healthcare: Implications for Psychiatry* (Denver, CO: Milliman, 2014), accessed September 1, 2019, https://www.integration.samhsa.gov/about-us/Milliman-Report -Economic-Impact-Integrated-Implications-Psychiatry.pdf.

26 **a doc-in-a-pocket of sorts:** David D. Luxton et al., "mHealth for Mental Health: Integrating Smartphone Technology in Behavioral Healthcare," *Professional Psychology: Research and Practice* 42, no. 6 (2011): 505–12, doi: 10.1037/ a0024485; Hannah E. Payne et al., "Behavioral Functionality of Mobile Apps in Health Interventions: A Systematic Review of the Literature," *Journal of Medical Internet Research* 3, no. 1 (Spring 2015): e20, doi: 10.2196/mhealth.3335.

27 **physician-to-physician videoconferencing:** Sanjeev Arora et al., "Outcomes of Treatment for Hepatitis C Virus Infection by Primary Care Providers," *New England Journal of Medicine* 364 (June 2011): 2199–207, doi: 10.1056/ NEJMoa1009370.

27 **"teach-a-man-to-fish":** This refers to the proverb: Give a man a fish and you feed him for a day; teach a man to fish and you feed him for a lifetime.

28 **telehealth has been routine:** Mary E. Reed et al., "Real-Time Patient–Provider

Video Telemedicine Integrated with Clinical Care," *New England Journal of Medicine* 379 (October 2018): 1478–79, doi: 10.1056/NEJMc1805746.

29 **14.3 million American households reported "food insecurity":** "Food Security in the U.S.," USDA Economic Research Service, accessed October 5, 2019, https://www.ers.usda.gov/topics/food-nutrition-assistance/food-security-in-the-us/key-statistics-graphics.aspx.

29 **difficulty managing their blood sugars:** "Fresh Food Farmacy: Stories," Geisinger Health System, accessed July 28, 2019, https://www.geisinger.org/freshfoodfarmacy/stories.

29 **"Have we asked the families?":** Interview of Anita Brentley by the author, March 6, 2018.

30 *Why Spending More Is Getting Us Less:* Elizabeth Bradley and Lauren A. Taylor, *The American Health Care Paradox: Why Spending More Is Getting Us Less* (New York: Public Affairs, 2013).

30 **partnership with community programs:** The Commonwealth Fund built a return on investment calculator to help health systems build business plans to support social services for high-need, high-cost patients. "Welcome to the Return on Investment (ROI) Calculator for Partnerships to Address the Social Determinants of Health," Commonwealth Fund, accessed September 2, 2019, https://www.commonwealthfund.org/roi-calculator.

30 **manage their blood pressure better:** Antoinette M. Schoenthaler et al., "Cluster Randomized Clinical Trial of FAITH (Faith-Based Approaches in the Treatment of Hypertension) in Blacks," *Circulation: Cardiovascular Quality and Outcomes* 11 (October 2018): e004691, https://doi.org/10.1161/CIRCOUTCOMES.118.004691.

31 **Jewish Healthcare Foundation:** Interview of Karen Feinstein by the author, April 12, 2018.

31 **Stanley:** Not his real name. This story is from an interview with Al Siu by the author, February 26, 2018.

32 **Hospital at Home model:** Interview of Bruce Leff by the author, April 2, 2018.

32 **caring for patients at home is a sensible strategy:** Michael Montalto, "The 500-Bed Hospital that Isn't There: The Victorian Department of Health Review of the Hospital in the Home Program," *Medical Journal of Australia* 193, no. 10 (November 2010): 598–601, doi: 10.5694/j.1326-5377.2010.tb04070.x; Geraldine A. Lee and Karen Titchener, "The Guy's and St. Thomas's NHS Foundation Trust @Home Service: An Overview of a New Service," *London Journal of Primary Care* 9, no. 2 (March 2017): 18–22, doi: 10.1080/17571472.2016.1211592; Sarah Klein, " 'Hospital at Home' Programs Improve Outcomes, Lower Costs but Face Resistance from Providers and Payers," Commonwealth Fund, accessed September 3, 2019, https://www.commonwealthfund.org/publications/newsletter-article/hospital-home-programs-improve-outcomes-lower-costs-face-resistance.

32 **5% of patients acquire a serious infection:** *Current HAI Progress Report: 2017 National and State Healthcare-Associated Infections Progress Report* (Atlanta, GA: Centers for Disease Control and Prevention, 2017), accessed December 10, 2017, https://www.cdc.gov/hai/data/archive/2017-HAI-progress-report.html.

32 **severe confusion or delirium:** Tamara G. Fong, Samir R. Tulebaev, and Sharon K. Inouye, "Delirium in Elderly Adults: Diagnosis, Prevention, and Treatment," *Nature Reviews Neurology* 5 (2009): 210–20, https://doi.org/10.1038/nrneurol.2009.24.

33 **Nancy Guinn:** Interview of Nancy Guinn by the author, August 30, 2018.

Chapter 3: At Your Health's Expense

36 **Secretary Alex M. Azar II:** From his speech: Alex M. Azar II, "Remarks on Value-Based Transformation to the Federation of American Hospitals," (speech, Washington DC, March 5, 2018), US Department of Health and Human Services, https://www.hhs.gov/about/leadership/secretary/speeches/2018-speeches/remarks-on-value-based-transformation-to-the-federation-of-american-hospitals.html?new.

37 **solutions to their unintelligible bills:** Elisabeth Rosenthal subsequently wrote a superb book, *An American Sickness: How Healthcare Became Big Business and How You Can Take It Back* (New York: Penguin Press, 2017) that built upon this work and elucidates the many causes of excessive health care costs in the United States and what consumers can do about them.

37 **journalist Steve Brill:** Brill subsequently also wrote an excellent book, *America's Bitter Pill: Money, Politics, Backroom Deals, and the Fight to Fix Our Broken Healthcare System* (New York: Random House, 2015) about how the Affordable Care Act became law.

37 **$1.3 trillion in bills to Medicare and Medicaid in 2017:** "NHE Fact Sheet," Centers for Medicare & Medicaid Services, accessed August 29, 2019, https://www.cms.gov/research-statistics-data-and-systems/statistics-trends-and-reports/nationalhealthexpenddata/nhe-fact-sheet.html.

38 **agreed-upon prices are secret:** Sometimes the secrets can be revealed. Many states have created "All Payers Claims Databases," where pooled anonymized data enable analysts to view the prices that health care facilities and professionals have charged payers. Employers have also pooled claims data for their employees (again anonymously) to compare the rates that they are paying (through their insurance administrator) with others. See this RAND report, as an example: Chapin White and Christopher Whaley, *Prices Paid to Hospitals by Private Health Plans Are High Relative to Medicare and Vary Widely* (Santa Monica, CA: RAND Corporation, 2019), accessed August 26, 2019, https://www.rand.org/pubs/research_reports/RR3033.html.

38 **overusing mental health care:** Richard G. Frank and Rachel L. Garfield, "Managed Behavioral Health Care Carve-Outs: Past Performance and Future

Prospects," *Annual Review of Public Health* 28 (2007): 303–20, doi: 10.1146/annurev.publhealth.28.021406.144029.

38 **separate networks of mental health clinicians:** Daria Pelech and Tamara Hayford, "Medicare Advantage and Commercial Prices for Mental Health Services," *Health Affairs* 38, no. 2 (February 2019), https://doi.org/10.1377/hlthaff.2018.05226.

39 **from signing up:** Frank and Garfield, "Managed Behavioral Health Care Carve-Outs."

39 **means significantly higher out-of-pocket costs:** This study by Milliman drew from medical claims records for 42 million adults in preferred provider organization health plans:. Stephen P. Melek, Daniel Perlman, and Stoddard Davenport, *Addiction and Mental Health vs. Physical Health: Analyzing Disparities in Network Use and Provider Reimbursement Rates* (Seattle: Milliman, 2017), accessed September 1, 2019, https://www.milliman.com/uploadedFiles/insight/2017/NQTLDisparityAnalysis.pdf.

39 **Intermountain Healthcare, explained:** Melinda Beck, "Here's What Your Operation Will Really Cost," *Wall Street Journal*, November 17, 2013, https://www.wsj.com/articles/here8217s-what-your-operation-will-really-cost-1384548628.

40 **A 2016 article:** Ge Bai and Gerard F. Anderson, "US Hospitals Are Still Using Chargemaster Markups to Maximize Revenues," *Health Affairs* 35, no. 9 (September 2016), https://doi.org/10.1377/hlthaff.2016.0093.

40 **three times the Medicare rates:** White and Whaley, "Prices Paid to Hospitals."

40 **"prospective payment system":** Stuart Guterman and Allen Dobson, "Impact of the Medicare Prospective Payment System for Hospitals," *Health Care Financing Review* 7, no. 3 (Spring 1986).

40 **referred to as ICD-10 codes:** The alphanumeric codes derive from the World Health Organization's International Statistical Classification of Diseases and Related Health Problems (ICD). In 2015, the United States adopted the 10th revision of ICD, referred to as "ICD-10" codes.

40 **another opportunity to increase the bill to Medicare:** A case study on medical coding using ICD-10 diagnostic codes: "ICD-10 Documentation Example," AAPC, accessed July 20, 2019, https://www.aapc.com/icd-10/icd-10-documentation-example.aspx.

41 **Medicare-Severity Diagnosis Related Groups or MS-DRGs:** *Design and Development of the Diagnosis Related Group (DRG)* (Baltimore, MD: Centers for Medicare & Medicaid Services, October 1, 2016), accessed July 14, 2019, https://www.cms.gov/ICD10Manual/version34-fullcode-cms/fullcode_cms/Design_and_development_of_the_Diagnosis_Related_Group_(DRGs)_PBL-038.pdf.

41 **the disease-related group multiplier:** Other factors include a geographic factor (reflecting local wages), a quality and patient satisfaction score, and two significant multipliers if the hospital also teaches residents or cares for indigent patients.

41 **its multiplier is 1.9898:** Note, in a feat of circular logic, the calculations of DRG weights are made each year by Medicare based on the prior year's data on hospital charges. The charges include those billed to Medicare as well as those to the uninsured or out-of-network patients taken from the chargemasters. The Centers for Medicare & Medicaid Services uses a correction factor, called a cost-to-charge ratio, that is intended to estimate the real "cost." For example, the labor and delivery cost-to-charge ratio is 44.5%, which means that annually when Medicare reviews a hospital's bills, a bill for $1,000 in labor and delivery would be multiplied to arrive at $445 as the true cost of caring for that patient. Simcha B. Rimler, Brian D. Gale, and Deborah L. Reede, "Diagnosis-Related Groups and Hospital Inpatient Federal Reimbursement," *RadioGraphics* 35 (2015): 1825–34, doi: 10.1148/rg.2015150043.

42 **for "professional" services:** Physicians use an entirely different set of codes—called the American Medical Association's Current Procedural Terminology (CPT) codes—for both inpatient and outpatient care. For outpatient care, hospitals use yet another billing and coding system, called Ambulatory Payment Classifications (APC). APCs and physician CPT codes are mapped to Medicare's outpatient billing system called Healthcare Common Procedure Coding System codes (HCPCS codes).

43 **Alliance of Community Health Plans:** Interview of Ceci Connelly by the author, August 2, 2019.

44 **is doubtful:** Leemore Dafny, Kate Ho, and Robin S. Lee, "The Price Effects of Cross-Market Hospital Mergers" (NBER Working Paper no. 22106, Cambridge, MA: National Bureau of Economic Research, revised October 2018), https:// www.nber.org/papers/w22106; Paul B. Ginsburg, "Health Care Market Consolidations: Impacts on Costs, Quality and Access," Brookings, March 16, 2016, https://www.brookings.edu/testimonies/health-care-market-consolidations -impacts-on-costs-quality-and-access/.

44 **Operating margins for nonprofit hospitals ... 1.6%–2.5% in 2017:** Moody's Investor Services reported a median operating margin of 1.6% for nonprofit hospitals. Alex Kacik, "Operating Margins Stabilize, but Not-For-Profit Hospitals Still Vulnerable," *Modern Healthcare*, April 26, 2019, https://www .modernhealthcare.com/providers/operating-margins-stabilize-not-profit -hospitals-still-vulnerable.

A Navigant study found nonprofit hospitals averaged a 2.53% operating margin while for profits averaged 3.38%, for an overall operating margin of 2.56%. Jeff Goldsmith, Rulon Stacey, Alex Hunter, and Navigant, *Stiffening Headwinds Challenge Health Systems to Grow Smarter* (Chicago: Navigant Consulting, September 2018), accessed November 2, 2019, http://images.e-navigant.com/Web/ NavigantConsultingInc/%7B7900bba7-87bd-4a9b-9cec-54cf0b6ea9d4%7D_ HC_HealthSystemFinancialAnalysis_TL_0818_REV08.pdf.

44 **losses from Medicare:** On average, hospitals have negative 10% margins (–10%) with Medicare patients. *A Data Book: Health Care Spending and the Medicare*

Program (Washington, DC: Medicare Payment Advisory Commission, June 2019), accessed November 2, 2019, p. 71, http://www.medpac.gov/docs/default -source/data-book/jun19_databook_entirereport_sec.pdf?sfvrsn=0.

44 **profit margin of 2.4% ... lowering profit:** *U.S. Health Insurance Industry: 2018 Annual Results* (Kansas City: National Association of Insurance Commissioners, 2018), accessed November 2, 2019, https://naic.org/documents/ topic_insurance_industry_snapshots_2018_health_ins_ind_report.pdf.

44 **is spent on administration:** David U. Himmelstein et al., "A Comparison of Hospital Administrative Costs in Eight Nations: US Costs Exceed all Others by Far," *Health Affairs* 33, no. 9 (September 2014): 1586–94, doi: 10.1377/ hlthaff.2013.1327.

44 **1%–3% in OECD nations:** Irene Papanicolas, Liana R. Woskie, and Ashish K. Jha, "Health Care Spending in the United States and Other High-Income Countries," *JAMA* 319, no. 10 (March 13, 2018): 1024–39, doi: 10.1001/ jama.2018.1150.

44 **work of a primary care physician:** Duke has a single office to handle billing for all the physicians and hospital staff. This is unusual; most large facilities have separate offices for each physician group and hospital. Phillip Tseng et al., "Administrative Costs Associated with Physician Billing and Insurance-Related Activities at an Academic Health Care System," *JAMA* 319, no. 7 (February 2018): 691–97, doi: 10.1001/jama.2017.19148.

44 **electronic health record system:** Vivian S. Lee and Bonnie B. Blanchfield, "Disentangling Health Care Billing for Patients' Physical and Financial Health," *JAMA* 319, no. 7 (February 2018): 661–63, doi: 10.1001/jama.2017.19966.

45 **from around 14% to 6% or less:** Sara R. Collins, "Testimony: Status of U.S. Health Insurance Coverage and the Potential of Recent Congressional Health Reform Bills to Expand Coverage and Lower Consumer Costs," Commonwealth Fund, April 30, 2019, https://www.commonwealthfund.org/ publications/2019/apr/testimony-health-insurance-recent-congressional -reform-bills.

45 **consumers to play their role:** The challenges of a market approach to health care are well described in this article: Kenneth J. Arrow, "Uncertainty and the Welfare Economics of Medical Care," *American Economic Review* 53, no. 5 (Dec 1963): 941–73.

45 **the costs of his own care:** Azar, "Remarks on Value-Based Transformation to the Federation of American Hospitals."

46 **an online price estimator:** "Estimate Your Out-Of-Pocket Costs," University of Utah Health, accessed October 5, 2019, https://healthcare.utah.edu/ pricing/.

47 **American household had $11,700 in savings:** Kathleen Elkins, "Here's How Much Money Americans Have in Savings at Every Income Level," CNBC Make It, September 27, 2018, https://www.cnbc.com/2018/09/27/heres-how-much -money-americans-have-in-savings-at-every-income-level.html.

47 **hard for people to choose the right plan:** Keith M. Marzilli Ericson and Amanda Starc, "How Product Standardization Affects Choice: Evidence from the Massachusetts Health Insurance Exchange" (NBER Working Paper no. 19527, Cambridge, MA: National Bureau of Economic Research, 2013), accessed August 26, 2019, https://papers.ssrn.com/sol3/papers.cfm?abstract_id=2338898.

47 **without leaving the initial screen:** Douglas Jacobs, "CMS' Standardized Plan Option Could Reduce Discrimination," *Health Affairs*, January 6, 2016, https://www.healthaffairs.org/do/10.1377/hblog20160106.052546/full/.

49 **coronary artery bypass grafting, and stroke:** Bundled Payments for Care Improvement Advanced and Centers for Medicare & Medicaid Services, "Model Overview," April, 2019, https://innovation.cms.gov/Files/slides/bpciadvanced-my3-modeloverview-slides.pdf.

49 **the responsibility for keeping costs down:** Seema Verma, "More ACOs Taking Accountability under MSSP through 'Pathways to Success,'" *Health Affairs*, July 17, 2019, https://www.healthaffairs.org/do/10.1377/hblog20190717.482997/full/.

49 **with a similar approach:** "Medicaid Managed Care Market Tracker," Kaiser Family Foundation, accessed August 29, 2019, https://www.kff.org/data-collection/medicaid-managed-care-market-tracker/.

Chapter 4: Manufacturing Out the Mishaps

52 **Sarah Patterson:** Interview of Sarah Patterson by the author, January 23, 2018.

53 **in her father's arms:** This story is modified from one that I heard a hospital executive tell at a conference on health care.

53 ***To Err is Human: Building a Safer Health System:*** Committee on Quality of Health Care in America, *To Err is Human: Building a Safer Health System* (Washington, DC: Institute of Medicine, November 1999), accessed November 2, 2019, http://www.nationalacademies.org/hmd/~/media/Files/Report%20Files/1999/To-Err-is-Human/To%20Err%20is%20Human%201999%20%20report%20brief.pdf.

53 **killed annually by medical errors:** John T. James, "A New, Evidence-Based Estimate of Patient Harms Associated with Hospital Care," *Journal of Patient Safety* 9, no. 3 (September 2013): 122–28, doi: 10.1097/PTS.0b013e3182948a69.

53 **medical mistakes the third-leading cause of death:** According to this article, heart disease (611,000 deaths per year), cancer (585,000 deaths per year) and chronic obstructive pulmonary disease (149,000 deaths per year) are some of the other leading causes of death in the United States: Martin A. Makary and Michael Daniel, "Medical Error––the Third Leading Cause of Death in the US," *BMJ* 353 (May 2016): i2139, https://doi.org/10.1136/bmj.i2139.

53 **probably ten times as large:** Danielle Ofri, "Ashamed to Admit It: Owning Up to Medical Error," *Health Affairs* 29, no. 8 (August 2010): 1549–51, https://doi.org/10.1377/hlthaff.2009.0946.

54 **over $55 billion:** Michelle M. Mello et al., "National Costs of the Medical Liability System," *Health Affairs* 29, no. 9 (September 2010): 1569–77, https://doi.org/10.1377/hlthaff.2009.0807.

54 **surgical "never events":** *Eliminating Serious, Preventable, and Costly Medical Errors—Never Events* (Baltimore: Centers for Medicare & Medicaid Services, May 2006), accessed November 2, 2019, https://www.cms.gov/newsroom/fact-sheets/eliminating-serious-preventable-and-costly-medical-errors-never-events.

54 **congressman John Murtha in 2010:** Mark Roth, "Gallbladder Surgery Problems More Common in Older Patients," *Pittsburgh Post-Gazette*, February 4, 2010, http://old.post-gazette.com/pg/10035/1033474-454.stm.

54 **4,000 or more surgical "never events" in the United States each year:** Winta T. Mehtsun et al., "Surgical Never Events in the United States," *Surgery* 153, no. 4 (April 2013): 465–72, https://doi.org/10.1016/j.surg.2012.10.005.

55 **A 2015 National Academy of Medicine report:** *Improving Diagnosis in Health Care* (Washington, DC: National Academies of Sciences, Engineering, and Medicine, September 2015), accessed November 2, 2019, http://www.nationalacademies.org/hmd/Reports/2015/Improving-Diagnosis-in-Healthcare.

55 **30% of abnormal findings on an exam are missed:** Cindy S. Lee et al., "Cognitive and System Factors Contributing to Diagnostic Errors in Radiology," *American Journal of Roentgenology* 201, no. 3 (September 2013): 611–17, doi: 10.2214/AJR.12.10375.

55 **four different medications:** Robert Preidt, "Americans Taking More Prescription Drugs than Ever," WebMD, August 3, 2017, https://www.webmd.com/drug-medication/news/20170803/americans-taking-more-prescription-drugs-than-ever-survey.

55 **Seattle Children's Hospital:** This story has been detailed in the media. For example: JoNel Aleccia, "Nurse's Suicide Highlights Twin Tragedies of Medical Errors," *NBC News*, June 27, 2011, http://www.nbcnews.com/id/43529641/ns/health-health_care/t/nurses-suicide-highlights-twin-tragedies-medical-errors/.

56 **at least one clinical error:** Mary A. Blegen, "Chapter 37: Medication Administration Safety," in *Patient Safety and Quality: An Evidence-Based Handbook for Nurses*, ed. Ronda G. Hughes (Rockville, MD: Agency for Healthcare Research and Quality, 2008); Kenneth N. Barker et al., "Medication Errors Observed in 36 Health Care Facilities," *Archives of Internal Medicine* 162, no. 16 (September 2002): 1897–903, doi: 10.1001/archinte.162.16.1897; Johanna I. Westbrook et al., "Association of Interruptions with an Increased Risk and Severity of Medication Administration Errors," *Archives of Internal Medicine* 170, no. 8 (April 2010): 683–90, doi: 10.1001/archinternmed.2010.65.

56 **one medication error per day:** Institute of Medicine, *Preventing Medication Errors* (Washington, DC: National Academies Press, 2007).

56 **look-alike or sound-alike drug names:** "FDA and ISMP Lists of Look-Alike Drug Names with Recommended Tall Man Letters," Institute for Safe Medication Practices, accessed July 31, 2019, https://www.ismp.org/sites/default/files/attachments/2017-11/tallmanletters.pdf.

56 **handwritten prescriptions by medical residents had an error:** Allen F. Shaughnessy and Ronald O. Nickel, "Prescription-Writing Patterns and Errors in a Family Medicine Residency Program," *Journal of Family Practice* 29, no. 3 (September 1989): 290–95.

57 **happen all the time in health care:** Suzanne Beyea, "Interruptions and Distractions in Health Care: Improved Safety with Mindfulness," Agency for Healthcare Research and Quality Patient Safety Network, February 2014, https://psnet.ahrq.gov/perspective/interruptions-and-distractions-health -care-improved-safety-mindfulness; "Side Tracks on the Safety Express. Interruptions Lead to Errors and Unfinished . . . Wait What Was I Doing?," Institute for Safe Medication Practices, November 29, 2012, https://www.ismp.org/resources/side-tracks-safety-express-interruptions-lead-errors-and-unfinished -wait-what-was-i-doing.

57 **about once every two to five minutes:** Eileen Relihan et al., "The Impact of a Set of Interventions to Reduce Interruptions and Distractions to Nurses during Medication Administration," *Quality and Safety in Health Care* 19, no. 5 (May 2010): e52.

57 **These lead to slips and lapses:** Richard N. Keers et al., "Causes of Medication Administration Errors in Hospitals: A Systematic Review of Quantitative and Qualitative Evidence," *Drug Safety* 36, no. 11 (August 2013): 1045–67, doi: 10.1007/s40264-013-0090-2.

57 **numbers are on the rise:** Lotte N. Dyrbye et al., "Burnout among Health Care Professionals," *National Academy of Medicine*, July 5, 2017, https://nam.edu/wp-content/uploads/2017/07/Burnout-Among-Health-Care-Professionals -A-Call-to-Explore-and-Address-This-Underrecognized-Threat.pdf; Tait D. Shanafelt et al., "Burnout and Satisfaction with Work-Life Balance among US Physicians Relative to the General US Population," *Archives of Internal Medicine* 172, no. 18 (October 2012): 1377–85, doi: 10.1001/archinternmed.2012.3199.

57 **twice as high as for other professionals:** Pauline Anderson, "Physicians Experience Highest Suicide Rate of Any Profession," *Medscape*, May 7, 2018, https://www.medscape.com/viewarticle/896257.

58 **second leading cause of death among all residents:** Nicholas A. Yaghmour et al., "Causes of Death of Residents in ACGME-Accredited Programs 2000 through 2014: Implications for the Learning Environment," *Academic Medicine* 92, no. 7 (July 2017): 976–83, doi: 10.1097/ACM.0000000000001736.

58 **15% suffered from alcoholism:** Michael R. Oreskovich et al., "Prevalence of Alcohol Use Disorders among American Surgeons," *Archives of Surgery* 147, no. 2 (February 2012): 168–74, doi: 10.1001/archsurg.2011.1481.

58 **health care–associated infections in their patients:** Jeannie P. Comiotti et

al., "Nurse Staffing, Burnout, and Health Care–Associated Infection," *American Journal of Infection Control* 40, no. 6 (August 2012): 486–90, https://doi .org/10.1016/j.ajic.2012.02.029.

58 **serious shortages in the United States:** Rebecca Grant, "The U.S. Is Running Out of Nurses," *The Atlantic*, February 3, 2016, https://www.theatlantic.com/ health/archive/2016/02/nursing-shortage/459741/.

58 **disclose errors to their patients:** American Medical Association Council on Ethical and Judicial Affairs, *Code of Medical Ethics: Current Opinions with Annotations*, section 8.12.125.3 (Chicago: American Medical Association, 1997), accessed August 28, 2019, https://openlibrary.org/books/OL24203632M/ Code_of_medical_ethics; American College of Physicians, "Ethics Manual. Fourth Edition. American College of Physicians," *Annals of Internal Medicine* 128, no. 7 (April 1998): 576–94, PMID: 9518406.

58 **admitting a mistake began to gain acceptance:** Steve S. Kraman and G. Hamm, "Risk Management: Extreme Honesty May Be the Best Policy," *Annals of Internal Medicine* 131, no. 12 (December 1999): 963–67, doi: 10.7326/0003-4819-131 -12-199912210-00010; Allen Kachila, "Liability Claims and Costs before and after Implementation of a Medical Error Disclosure Program," *Annals of Internal Medicine*, August 17, 2010, https://annals.org/aim/article-abstract/745972/ liability-claims-costs-before-after-implementation-medical-error-disclosure -program?doi=10.7326%2f0003-4819-153-4-201008170-00002.

58 **prevent apologies from being used in litigation as evidence of fault:** Thomas H. Gallagher, David Studdert, and Wendy Levinson, "Disclosing Harmful Medical Error to Patients," *New England Journal of Medicine* 356, no. 26 (2007): 2713–19, PMID: 17664451.

59 **advanced radiologic imaging may be unnecessary:** Patricia E. Litkowski et al., "Curing the Urge to Image," *American Journal of Medicine* 129, no. 10 (October 2016): 1131–35, https://doi.org/10.1016/j.amjmed.2016.06.020.

59 **defensive spending:** Mello et al., "National Costs of the Medical Liability System."

59 **would have his fingers cut off:** Allen D. Spiegel, "Hammurabi's Managed Health Care—circa 1700 B.C.," *Managed Care*, May 1, 1997, https://www .managedcaremag.com/archives/1997/5/hammurabis-managed-health-care -circa-1700-bc.

59 **huge payouts ($5.72 billion per year):** Mello et al., "National Costs of the Medical Liability System."

59 **medical malpractice "no-fault" system:** "No-Fault Compensation in New Zealand: Harmonizing Injury Compensation, Provider Accountability, and Patient Safety," Commonwealth Fund, February 24, 2006, https://www .commonwealthfund.org/publications/journal-article/2006/feb/no-fault -compensation-new-zealand-harmonizing-injury.

59 **with an average payout of $30,000:** Olga Pierce and Marshall Allen, "How Denmark Dumped Medical Malpractice and Improved Patient Safety," *Pro-*

Publica, December 31, 2015, https://www.propublica.org/article/how-denmark
-dumped-medical-malpractice-and-improved-patient-safety.

60 **Florida enacted similar no-fault programs:** Jill Horwitz and Troyen A. Brennan, "No-Fault Compensation for Medical Injury: A Case Study," *Health Affairs*
14, no. 4 (Winter 1995), https://doi.org/10.1377/hlthaff.14.4.164.

60 **substantially lower for no-fault than tort law:** The total cost for administering a claim, including attorneys' fees for both sides, was $18,000. In contrast,
in the tort system, attorneys' fees and litigation costs in Florida comprised 57%
of total insurance costs (claimant payments were 43%). Horwitz and Brennan,
"No-Fault Compensation for Medical Injury."

60 **states that eased medical tort laws didn't make medicine less safe:** Daniel P.
Kessler, "Evaluating the Medical Malpractice System and Options for Reform,"
Journal of Economic Perspectives 25, no. 2 (Spring 2011): 93–110; Michael Frakes
and Anupam B. Jena, "Does Medical Malpractice Law Improve Health Care
Quality?," *Journal of Public Economics* 143 (September 2016): 142–58, doi:
10.1016/j.jpubeco.2016.09.002.

61 **typically below 10,000 feet:** "14 CFR § 121.542—Flight Crewmember
Duties," Cornell Law School, accessed November 2, 2019, https://www.law
.cornell.edu/cfr/text/14/121.542.

61 **while they dispense medications:** Johanna I. Westbrook et al., "Effectiveness of a 'Do Not Interrupt' Bundled Intervention to Reduce Interruptions
during Medical Administration: A Cluster Randomised Controlled Feasi-
bility Study," *BMJ Quality & Safety* 26, no. 9 (2017): 734–42, doi: 10.1136/
bmjqs-2016-006123.

61 **a simple five-step checklist:** Peter Pronovost et al., "An Intervention to Decrease
Catheter-Related Bloodstream Infections in the ICU," *New England Journal of
Medicine* 355 (December 2006): 2725–32, doi: 10.1056/NEJMoa061115.

61 **the central line infection rate declined by two-thirds:** Peter J. Pronovost
et al., "Sustaining Reductions in Catheter Related Bloodstream Infections
in Michigan Intensive Care Units," *BMJ* 340 (February 2010): c309, doi:
10.1136/bmj.c309.

61 **death rates were cut in half:** Alex B. Haynes et al., "A Surgical Safety Checklist
to Reduce Morbidity and Mortality in a Global Population," *New England Journal of Medicine* 360 (January 2009): 491–99, doi: 10.1056/NEJMsa0810119.

62 **350 hospitals had violations:** Stephanie Armour, "Hospital Watchdog Gives
Seal of Approval, Even after Problems Emerged," *Wall Street Journal*, September 8, 2017, https://www.wsj.com/articles/watchdog-awards-hospitals-seal-of
-approval-even-after-problems-emerge-1504889146.

62 **almost all remain accredited:** The Centers for Medicare and Medicaid Services made public the database of serious safety violations at over 1,000 hospitals since 2011, which is available on a website: "Search Hospital Inspections,"
Association of Health Care Journalists, accessed August 28, 2019, http://www
.hospitalinspections.org/.

62 **248 had it revoked:** "U.S. Medical Regulatory Trends and Actions 2018," Federation of State Medical Boards of the United States, accessed August 1, 2019, https://www.fsmb.org/siteassets/advocacy/publications/us-medical-regulatory -trends-actions.pdf. For details of why they were disciplined: James Morrison and Peter Wickersham, "Physicians Disciplined by a State Medical Board," *JAMA* 279, no. 23 (June 1998): 1889–93, doi: 10.1001/jama.279.23.1889.

62 **moved to another state and kept working:** John Fauber and Matt Wynn, "7 Takeaways from Our Year-Long Investigation into the Country's Broken Medical License System," *USA Today*, November 30, 2018, https://www.usatoday .com/story/news/2018/11/30/medical-board-license-discipline-failures-7 -takeaways-investigation/2092321002/.

62 **accidentally left inside a patient:** Catharine Paddock, "Medicare Will Not Pay for Hospital Mistakes and Infections, New Rule," *Medical News Today*, August 20, 2007, https://www.medicalnewstoday.com/articles/80074.php.

63 **far fewer patients suffered:** Harlan M. Krumholz et al., "Mortality, Hospitalizations, and Expenditures for the Medicare Population Aged 65 Years or Older, 1999–2013," *JAMA* 314, no. 4 (July 2015): 355–65, doi: 10.1001/ jama.2015.8035.

63 **"Hospital-acquired conditions":** "AHRQ National Scorecard on Hospital-Acquired Conditions Updated Baseline Rates and Preliminary Results 2014– 2017," Agency for Healthcare Research and Quality, accessed August 1, 2019, https://www.ahrq.gov/sites/default/files/wysiwyg/professionals/quality -patient-safety/pfp/hacreport-2019.pdf.

63 **rather than developing a culture of safety:** Helen Lester et al., "The Impact of Removing Financial Incentives from Clinical Quality Indicators: Longitudinal Analysis of Four Kaiser Permanente Indicators," *BMJ* 340 (May 2010): c1898, https://doi.org/10.1136/bmj.c1898.

63 **patients are *really* sick:** Michael Geruso and Timothy Layton, *Upcoding: Evidence from Medicare on Squishy Risk Adjustment* (Cambridge, MA: National Bureau of Economic Research, 2018), accessed August 28, 2018, doi: 10.3386/ w21222; Bruce E. Landon and Robert E. Mechanic, "The Paradox of Coding: Policy Concerns in the Move to Risk-Based Provider Contracts," *New England Journal of Medicine* 377, no. 13 (May 2018): 1211–13, doi: 10.1056/ NEJMp1708084.

65 **"Made in USA":** Mark Magnier, "Rebuilding Japan with the Help of 2 Americans," *Los Angeles Times*, October 25, 1999, http://articles.latimes.com/1999/ oct/25/news/ss-26184.

65 **W. Edwards Deming:** Magnier, "Rebuilding Japan with the Help of 2 Americans."

65 **revitalize an entire nation:** Jim L. Smith, "Management: The Lasting Legacy of the Modern Quality Giants," *Quality Magazine*, October 6, 2011, https:// www.qualitymag.com/articles/88493-management--the-lasting-legacy-of-the -modern-quality-giants.

65 **Sarah Patterson:** Interview of Sarah Patterson by the author, October 26, 2017, and January 23, 2018.

66 **Lean manufacturing worked in his health system:** David Leonhardt, "Making Health Care Better," *New York Times Magazine,* November 3, 2009, https://www.nytimes.com/2009/11/08/magazine/08Healthcare-t.html.

66 **"impeccable patient experience.":** Interview of Rajiv Sethi by the author, January 24, 2018.

66 **the science of quality improvement:** I joined the Institute for Healthcare Improvement as a Senior Fellow in 2017 (uncompensated).

Chapter 5: Learning to Deliver Perfect Care

70 **Ernest A. Codman:** Richard A. Brand, "Ernest Amory Codman, MD, 1869–1940," *Clinical Orthopaedics and Related Research* 467, no. 11 (August 2009): 2763–65, doi: 10.1007/s11999-009-1047-8; William J. Mallon, *Ernest Amory Codman: The End Result of a Life in Medicine* (Philadelphia: WB Saunders, 2000).

70 **the beginning of modern surgery:** Francis D. Moore, "John Collins Warren and His Act of Conscience: A Brief Narrative of the Trial and Triumph of a Great Surgeon," *Annals of Surgery* 229, no. 2 (1999): 187–96.

   For a detailed account of the inventorship feuds over ether as an anesthetic, Chaturvedi and Gogna offer a revealing account: Ravindra Chaturvedi, RL Gonga, "Ether Day: An Intriguing History," *Medical Journal Armed Forces India* 67, no. 4 (October 2011): 306–8, doi: 10.1016/S0377-1237(11)60098-1.

71 **Nightingale reduced mortality rates from 42.7% to only 2.2%:** I. Bernard Cohen, "Florence Nightingale," *Scientific American* 250, no. 3 (March 1984): 128–37.

71 **tumors of the bone:** As an aside, every student of medicine is familiar with at least one of Codman's eponyms—key parts of anatomy or medical observations or treatments that bear his name: Codman's triangle, Codman's tumor, Codman's sign, Codman's paradox, Codman's bursa, Codman's exercises.

72 **how much good they were doing for patients:** Caitlin W. Hicks and Martin A. Makary, "A Prophet to Modern Medicine: Ernest Amory Codman," *BMJ* 347 (December 2013): f7368, https://doi.org/10.1136/bmj.f7368; Mallon, *Ernest Amory Codman.*

72 **"he is really justified in having":** Mallon, *Ernest Amory Codman.*

72 **judge their abilities by their End Results:** Joel Howell and John Ayanian, "Ernest Codman and the End Result System: A Pioneer of Health Outcomes Revisited," *Journal of Health Services Research & Policy* 21, no. 4 (May 2016): 279–81, https://doi.org/10.1177/1355819616648984.

72 *First Five Years of Private Hospital:* Ernest Amory Codman, "The Classic: A Study in Hospital Efficiency: As Demonstrated by the Case Report of First Five Years of Private Hospital," *Clinical Orthopaedics and Related Research* 471,

no. 6 (June 2013): 1778–83, doi: 10.1007/s11999-012-2751-3. This excerpt was reprinted from Ernest Amory Codman, *A Study in Hospital Efficiency: As Demonstrated by the Case Report of First Five Years of Private Hospital* (Boston: Thomas Todd, 1918), 4–10, 108, 162.

72 **a missed stomach ulcer:** Mallon, *Ernest Amory Codman.*

73 **According to his biographer Bill Mallon:** Mallon, *Ernest Amory Codman.*

73 **"he tilted but never managed to topple":** One wintry night in 1915, at the Suffolk Medical Society of Boston, Codman managed to capture the attention of the entire Boston medical community and turn most of it against him. In a room filled with the most distinguished leaders in Boston, he unveiled a large triptych cartoon he had commissioned called "The Back Bay Golden Goose Ostrich." It depicted an ostrich burying its head in the sand (prosperous Beacon Hill) while grasping gold from wealthy patients. The image was a not-so-subtle metaphor for the unethical fee-for-service system making doctors and hospitals rich through poor-quality care, while members of the board turned a blind eye. Codman was forced to resign his position as chair of the society and subsequently also relinquished his academic position at Harvard Medical School. (Hicks and Makary, "A Prophet to Modern Medicine").

Codman died in 1940; his ashes were buried in his wife's family plot without a personal marker—that is, until Massachusetts General Hospital surgeon Andy Warshaw raised $20,000 in 2014 to dedicate a granite and bronze memorial in his honor. Nevertheless, Codman inspired a few important people who have shaped the standards of quality in medicine. One of those people was Dr. William J. Mayo, who went on to start the Mayo Clinic in Rochester, Minnesota: Lawrence K. Altman, "The Doctor's World; A Reformer's Battle," *New York Times*, June 12, 1984, https://www.nytimes.com/1984/06/12/science/the-doctor-s-world-a-reformer-s-battle.html.

73 **the Joint Commission on Accreditation of Healthcare Organizations:** Hicks and Makary, "A Prophet to Modern Medicine."

74 **dropped from 4.2% to 2.5%:** Mark R. Chassin, Edward L. Hannan, and Barbara A. DeBuono, "Benefits and Hazards of Reporting Medical Outcomes Publicly," *New England Journal of Medicine* 334, no. 6 (February 8, 1996): 394–98, doi: 10.1056/NEJM199602083340611.

74 **rate had fallen to 1.6%:** "State Department of Health Issues Report on Adult Cardiac Surgery and Angioplasty Procedures In-Hospital and Thirty-Day Valve and Combined Valve Bypass Mortality Rate at All-Time Low," New York State Department of Health, October 15, 2012, https://www.health.ny.gov/press/releases/2012/2012-10-15_cardiac_reports_released.htm.

74 **a few years later in Pennsylvania:** Eric C. Schneider and Arnold M. Epstein, "Influence of Cardiac-Surgery Performance Reports on Referral Practices and Access to Care. A Survey of Cardiovascular Specialists," *New England Journal of Medicine* 335, no. 4 (July 25, 1996): 251–56, doi: 10.1056/NEJM1996072533504.

75 **Daniel Pink:** Daniel Pink, *Drive: The Surprising Truth about What Motivates Us* (New York: Riverhead Books, 2009).

76 **crowd out intrinsic motivation:** Emad H. Atiq, "Why Motives Matter: Reframing the Crowding Out Effect of Legal Incentives," *Yale Law Journal* 123, no. 4 (January 2014): 862–1117.

77 **its specialized nurses and therapists:** With the department's excellent reputation (Olympic athletes and Utah Jazz basketball team seek their care, for example), the Utah surgeons were in high demand, and their patients frequently overflowed into beds outside of the orthopedic ward. After failing to meet this component of Perfect Care—care on the orthopedic ward—the orthopedic surgeons convinced hospital leaders to convert a general surgery ward into an orthopedic unit.

77 **patients with blockages in their coronary arteries:** Ronald A. Paulus, Karen Davis, and Glenn D. Steele, "Continuous Innovation in Health Care: Implications of the Geisinger Experience," *Health Affairs* 27, no. 5 (2008): 1235–45, doi: 10.1377/hlthaff.27.5.1235.

77 **saved about $1,300 per patient:** "Health Care Insider: Health Care with a Warranty? That's ProvenCare," University of Utah Health, accessed August 15, 2019, https://healthcare.utah.edu/the-scope/shows.php?shows=0_xmqu3uf9.

78 **"We shouldn't get paid if we don't do the right thing":** Peter Carbonara, "Geisinger Health System's Plan to Fix America's Health Care," *Fast Company*, October 1, 2008, https://www.fastcompany.com/1007043/geisinger-health -systems-plan-fix-americas-health-care.

78 **Medicare's primary care scorecard:** "Consensus Core Set: ACO and PCMH/ Primary Care Measures Version 1.0," Centers for Medicare & Medicaid Services, accessed August 29, 2019, https://www.cms.gov/Medicare/Quality -Initiatives-Patient-Assessment-Instruments/QualityMeasures/Downloads/ ACO-and-PCMH-Primary-Care-Measures.pdf.

78 **preventive care guidelines:** Kimberly S. H. Yarnall et al., "Family Physicians as Team Leaders: 'Time' to Share the Care," *Preventing Chronic Disease* 6, no. 2 (April 2009): A59, PMID: 19289002; Kimberly S. H. Yarnall et al., "Primary Care: Is There Enough Time for Prevention?," *American Journal of Public Health* 93, no. 4 (April 2003): 635–41, PMID: 12660210; Truls Østbye et al., "Is There Time for Management of Patients with Chronic Diseases in Primary Care?," *Annals of Family Medicine* 3, no. 3 (May 2005): 209–14, PMID: 15928223; Justin Altschuler et al., "Estimating a Reasonable Patient Panel Size for Primary Care Physicians with Team-Based Task Delegation," *Annals of Family Medicine* 10, no. 5 (Fall 2012): 396–400, doi: 10.1370/afm.1400.

78 **Tom Sequist:** Interview of Tom Sequist by the author, December 13, 2017.

79 **American College of Cardiology's online risk prediction calculator:** "Heart Risk Calculator," ACC/AHA, accessed August 27, 2019, http://www .cvriskcalculator.com/.

79 **ten-minute adaptive questionnaire:** Joshua Biber et al., "Patient Reported

Outcomes—Experiences with Implementation in a University Health Care Setting," *Journal of Patient-Reported Outcomes* 2, no. 34 (December 2018), doi: 10.1186/s41687-018-0059-0.

80 **End Results for heart surgery available to the public:** Edward L. Hannan et al., "Public Release of Cardiac Surgery Outcomes Data in New York: What Do New York State Cardiologists Think of It?," *American Heart Journal* 134, no. 6 (December 1997): 1120–28, doi: 10.1016/s0002-8703(97)70034-6.

80 **Medicare has a website, www.medicare.gov/hospitalcompare:** "Hospital Compare," Medicare.gov, accessed August 15, 2019, www.medicare.gov/hospitalcompare.

81 **scorecards all differ:** Karl Y. Bilimoria et al., "Rating the Raters: An Evaluation of Publicly Reported Hospital Quality Rating Systems," *New England Journal of Medicine Catalyst*, August 14, 2019, https://catalyst.nejm.org/evaluation-hospital-quality-rating-systems/.

82 **Singers Have Coaches. Should You?:** Atul Gawande, "Personal Best: Top Athletes and Singers Have Coaches. Should You?," *New Yorker*, September 26, 2011, https://www.newyorker.com/magazine/2011/10/03/personal-best.

83 **founded a company called QURE:** John W. Peabody et al., "Measuring the Quality of Physician Practice by Using Clinical Vignettes: A Prospective Validation Study," *Annals of Internal Medicine* 141, no. 10 (November 2004): 771–80, doi: 10.7326/0003-4819-141-10-200411160-00008. I have no financial relationship or interests with QURE.

84 **perform better in actual practice:** John W. Peabody et al., "Comparison of Vignettes, Standardized Patients, and Chart Abstraction," *JAMA* 283, no. 13 (April 2000): 1715–22, doi: 10.1001/jama.283.13.1715; Timothy R. Dresselhaus et al., "An Evaluation of Vignettes for Predicting Variation in the Quality of Preventive Care," *Journal of General Internal Medicine* 19, no. 10 (October 2004), doi: 10.1007/s11606-004-0003-2; Timothy Kubal et al., "Longitudinal Cohort Study to Determine Effectiveness of a Novel Simulated Case and Feedback System to Improve Clinical Pathway Adherence in Breast, Lung, and GI Cancers," *BMJ Open* 6, no. 9 (2016): e012312, doi: 10.1136/bmjopen-2016- 012312.

84 **have had the scan so far:** Ahmedin Jemal and Stacey A. Fedewa, "Lung Cancer Screening with Low-Dose Computed Tomography in the United States—2010 to 2015," *JAMA Oncology* 3, no. 9 (September 1, 2017): 1278–81, doi: 10.1001/jamaoncol.2016.6416.

84 **do it more reliably:** Among radiologists interpreting CT scans for lung nodules, interobserver agreement is low: Sarah J. van Riel et al., "Observer Variability for Classification of Pulmonary Nodules on Low-Dose CT Images and Its Effect on Nodule Management," *Radiology* 277, no. 3 (May 2015), https://doi.org/10.1148/radiol.2015142700.

85 **relieves them of tedious work:** Matthew Brown, "Integration of Chest CT CAD into the Clinical Workflow and Impact on Radiologist Efficiency," *Academic Radiology* 26, no. 5 (May 2019): 626–31, doi: 10.1016/j.acra.2018.07.006;

Mingzhu Liang et al., "Low-Dose CT Screening for Lung Cancer: Computer-Aided Detection of Missed Lung Cancers," *Radiology* 281, no. 1 (October 2016): 279–88, doi: 10.1148/radiol.2016150063.

Chapter 6: The Price Isn't Right

87   **Michael E. Porter and Thomas H. Lee:** Michael E. Porter and Thomas H. Lee, "The Strategy That Will Fix Health Care," *Harvard Business Review*, October 2013, https://hbr.org/2013/10/the-strategy-that-will-fix-health-care.

87   *Utah System Is Trying to Learn:* Gina Kolata, "What Are a Hospital's Costs? Utah System Is Trying to Learn," *New York Times*, September 8, 2015. https://www.nytimes.com/2015/09/08/health/what-are-a-hospitals-costs-utah-system-is-trying-to-learn.html.

90   **"transforming the economics of health care":** Robert S. Kaplan and Michael E. Porter, "The Big Idea: How to Solve the Cost Crisis in Health Care," *Harvard Business Review*, September 2011, https://hbr.org/2011/09/how-to-solve-the-cost-crisis-in-health-care.

90   **Charlton Park:** Interview of Charlton Park by the author, February 15, 2018.

90   **Cheri Hunter:** Interview of Cheri Hunter by the author, February 15, 2018.

90   **Cary Martin:** Interview of Cary Martin by the author, February 20, 2018.

90   **Jim Livingston:** Interview of Jim Livingston by the author, February 20, 2018.

91   **Bob Pendleton:** Interview of Bob Pendleton by the author, February 15, 2018.

91   **"Value Driven Outcomes":** Kensaku Kawamoto et al., "Value Driven Outcomes (VDO): A Pragmatic, Modular, and Extensible Software Framework for Understanding and Improving Health Care Costs and Outcomes," *Journal of the American Medical Informatics Association* 22, no. 1 (January 2015): 223–5, https://doi.org/10.1136/amiajnl-2013-002511.

92   **opportunity costs:** Ronald D. Shippert, "A Study of Time-Dependent Operating Room Fees and How to Save $100 000 by Using Time-Saving Products," *American Journal of Cosmetic Surgery* 22, no. 1 (March 2005): 25–34, https://doi.org/10.1177/074880680502200104.

94   **reducing costs by more than 10%:** Because the hospital was reimbursed by Medicare using disease-related groups (DRGs, discussed in Chapter 3), reductions in days spent in the hospital meant lower expenses for the hospital while the payment from Medicare was constant, resulting in higher operating margins. Vivian S. Lee et al., "Implementation of a Value-Driven Outcomes Program to Identify High Variability in Clinical Costs and Outcomes and Association with Reduced Cost and Improved Quality," *JAMA* 316, no. 10 (September 2016): 1061–72, doi: 10.1001/jama.2016.12226.

  For the accompanying editorial: Michael E. Porter and Thomas H. Lee, "From Volume to Value in Health Care: The Work Begins," *JAMA* 316, no. 10 (September 2016): 1047–48, doi: 10.1001/jama.2016.11698.

95   **in simple terms:** For a detailed description of how Kaplan came up with these

calculations, see Kaplan and Porter, "The Big Idea: How to Solve the Cost Crisis in Health Care."

96 **$0.37 per minute:** This method of estimating labor costs per minute by taking overall compensation and dividing by 100,000 is based on personal communication, November 9, 2019. The numbers used to illustrate the approach are based on approximate average salaries in the United States. For example, median annual salary for a registered nurse, according to the US Bureau of Labor Statistics, was $71,730 in 2017, and adding 15% for benefits, results in a total compensation of about $82,000. "Occupational Employment and Wages, May 2017," US Department of Labor Bureau of Labor Statistics, accessed November 16, 2019, https://www.bls.gov/oes/2017/may/oes319092.htm. Data from the same source indicate that medical assistants garner around $33,580 ($16.15 per hour). With 10% benefits, total compensation would add up to $37,000. An estimate of physician compensation comes from the American Medical Group Association's 2018 Compensation and Productivity Survey (a standard in the profession), which showed that cardiothoracic surgeons made a median of $734,299. With 20% benefits, total compensation would be over $880,000: Daniel Allar, "Cardiothoracic Surgeons' Salaries Up 23% since 2015," *Cardiovascular Business*, August 3, 2018, https://www.cardiovascularbusiness.com/topics/healthcare-economics/cardiothoracic-surgeons-salaries-23-2015.

96 **important medical inventions of the prior century:** Victor R. Fuchs and Harold C. Sox Jr., "Physicians' Views of the Relative Importance of Thirty Medical Innovations," *Health Affairs* 20, no. 5 (Fall 2001): 30–42, PMID: 11558715.

97 **mostly through reduced payments:** Direct Research and Medical Imaging & Technology Alliance, *Imaging Today: Medical Imaging Trends in Medicare* (Arlington, VA: Medical Imaging & Technology Alliance, 2012).

97 **CT scanner costs:** Yoshimi Anzai et al., "Dissecting Costs of CT Study: Application of TDABC (Time-Driven Activity-Based Costing) in a Tertiary Academic Center," *Academic Radiology* 24, no. 2 (February 2017): 200–208, doi: 10.1016/j.acra.2016.11.001.

97 **$5.80 per minute:** The American Medical Group Association's survey of physicians' salaries reported the median radiologist's compensation dropped 3% in 2017 to $487,239. With 20% benefits, total compensation would run around $580,000 on average: Richard Dargan, "Survey Shows Radiology Salaries Dipped Slightly in 2017," *RSNA News*, August 14, 2018, https://www.rsna.org/en/news/2018/october/radiology-salaries-2017.

98 **the average generalist physician in the United States made $218,173 a year:** Irene Papanicolas, Liana R. Woskie, and Ashish K. Jha, "Health Care Spending in the United States and Other High-Income Countries," *JAMA* 319, no. 10 (March 13, 2018): 1024–39, doi: 10.1001/jama.2018.1150.

98 **compared to $42,000–$65,000:** Papanicolas, Woskie, and Jha, "Health Care Spending in the United States and Other High-Income Countries."

98 **2% to total national health care spending:** Uwe E. Reinhardt et al., "What

Doctors Make, and Why (6 Letters)," *New York Times*, August 5, 2007, https://
www.nytimes.com/2007/08/05/opinion/l05doctors.html.

98 **professional liability insurance:** José R. Guardado, *Policy Research Perspectives. Medical Professional Liability Insurance Premiums: An Overview of the Market from 2008 to 2017* (Chicago: American Medical Association, 2018), accessed
July 10, 2019, https://www.ama-assn.org/sites/ama-assn.org/files/corp/media
-browser/public/government/advocacy/policy-research-perspective-liability
-insurance-premiums.pdf.

98 **$20,000 to $40,000, depending on the state:** Malpractice cases in most
countries outside of the United States are decided by judges and result in significantly lower awards, and some countries, like New Zealand, have no malpractice insurance business because the country has a no-fault insurance program
run by the government.

99 **the median amount of debt was $200,000 in 2018:** Association of American
Medical Colleges, "An Exploration of the Recent Decline in the Percentage of U.S.
Medical School Graduates with Education Debt," *Analysis in Brief* 18, no. 4 (September 2018), accessed July 10, 2019, https://www.aamc.org/system/files/reports/1/
september2018anexplorationoftherecentdeclineinthepercentageofu..pdf.

99 **for private schools, it's $322,767:** When New York University announced
its students would all receive full tuition scholarships (covering the $55,000
annual tuition, leaving $27,000 per year for room and board and fees), it became
the first top-ranked medical school in the nation to do so: David W. Chen,
"Surprise Gift: Free Tuition for All N.Y.U. Medical Students," *New York Times*,
August 16, 2018, https://www.nytimes.com/2018/08/16/nyregion/nyu-free
-tuition-medical-school.html.

99 **shortage of doctors in the United States:** Association of American Medical Colleges, *New Research Reaffirms Physician Shortage* (Washington, DC:
Association of American Medical Colleges, 2017), accessed August 21, 2019,
https://www.aamc.org/news-insights/press-releases/new-findings-confirm
-predictions-physician-shortage.

100 **saved about 7% in costs:** Personal communication, November 19, 2019, and
John E. L. Wong, *Engaging Physicians Using Value Management Tools—NUHS
Experience* (Orlando, FL: Institute for Healthcare Improvement National
Forum, December 11, 2018).

Chapter 7: From Caring to Coproducing

102 **Justin Masterson:** Interview of Justin Masterson by the author, August 22,
2018.

102 **suffered a kidney stone:** Personal communication provided by Lorris and Ann
Betz, February 21, 2018.

105 **top 1 percentile in patient satisfaction:** Patient satisfaction is derived from
Press Ganey surveys.

106 **"Dr. Scaife was awesome":** "Courtney L. Scaife, MD," University of Utah Health, accessed September 3, 2019, https://healthcare.utah.edu/fad/mddetail .php?physicianID=u0102229&name=courtney-l-scaife.

107 **After the scores were posted:** For a full account of the Exceptional Patient Experience journey and its consequences, see Vivian S. Lee et al., "Creating the Exceptional Patient Experience in One Academic Health System," *Academic Medicine* 91, no. 3 (March 2016): 338–44, doi: 10.1097/ACM.0000000000001007.

107 **top ten in quality and safety:** In 2010, the University of Utah was ranked #1 among all teaching hospitals by University Healthsystem Consortium (now Vizient). Since then, it has remained in the top ten (returning to #1 in 2016). "Vizient, Inc. Presents the Bernard A. Birnbaum, MD, Quality Leadership Award to 27 Top-Performing Academic Medical Centers and Community Hospitals," Vizient, September 30, 2016, https://newsroom.vizientinc.com/ press-release/vizient/vizient-inc-presents-bernard-birnbaum-md-quality -leadership-award-27-top-perfo.

108 **They point to medical literature:** I review some of the literature for the interested reader: Lee et al. "Creating the Exceptional Patient Experience."

108 **subsequent addiction crisis:** See, for example: Jerome Adams, Gregory H. Bledsoe, and John H. Armstrong, "Are Pain Management Questions in Patient Satisfaction Surveys Driving the Opioid Epidemic?," *American Journal of Public Health* 106, no. 6 (June 2016): 985–86, doi: 10.2105/AJPH.2016.303228; David W. Baker, "History of the Joint Commission's Pain Standards: Lessons for Today's Prescription Opioid Epidemic," *JAMA* 317, no. 11 (2017): 1117–18, accessed August 29, 2019, doi: 10.1001/jama.2017.0935.

108 **HCAHPS surveys in October 2019:** "What's New," Hospital Consumer Assessment of Healthcare Providers and Systems, accessed August 26, 2019, https://www.hcahpsonline.org/en/whats-new/.

108 **University of Utah:** Lee et al., "Creating the Exceptional Patient Experience."

108 **Harvard study:** Ashish K. Jha et al., "Patients' Perception of Hospital Care in the United States," *New England Journal of Medicine* 359 (October 2008): 1921–31, doi: 10.1056/NEJMsa0804116.

108 **researchers at Duke University:** Matthew P. Manary et al., "The Patient Experience and Health Outcomes," *New England Journal of Medicine* 368, no. 3 (January 2013): 201–3, doi: 10.1056/NEJMp1211775.

109 **"crowd out" the intrinsic motivation to be a great doctor:** Emad H. Atiq, "Why Motives Matter: Reframing the Crowding Out Effect of Legal Incentives," *Yale Law Journal* 123, no. 4 (January 2014): 862–1117.

110 **remind patients of a boutique hotel:** Some organizations have taken this a step further. At Leon Medical Center in Miami, the reception area sits in front of a sky-high atrium with gently bubbling fountains and glass-walled elevators. The receptionists and staff don't wear medical badges; they have lapel name tags. ChenMed, the Miami-based network of clinics serving elderly Medicare

Advantage patients, hired one clinic manager from a Courtyard Marriott hotel and also appointed a board member from Ritz Carlton.

110 **Justin Masterson's daughter:** Interview of Justin Masterson by the author, August 22, 2018. Also, their story was published here: Shahd Husein, "The Effort to Make Type 1 Diabetes Care More Human-Centric in Design," *T1D Exchange,* January 7, 2019, https://myglu.org/articles/the-effort-to-make-type -1-diabetes-care-more-human-centric-in-design.

112 **"Walk a Mile":** Available for purchase at WalkAMileCards.com.

112 **noted Stanford economist Victor Fuchs:** Victor Fuchs, *The Service Economy* (Cambridge: National Bureau of Economic Research, 1968).

113 **coproduction:** Maren Batalden et al., "Coproduction of Healthcare Service," *BMJ Quality & Safety* 25, no. 7 (2016): 509–17, http://dx.doi.org/10.1136/ bmjqs-2015-004315.

113 **"What matters to you?":** Michael J. Barry and Susan Edgman-Levitan, "Shared Decision Making—The Pinnacle of Patient-Centered Care," *New England Journal of Medicine* 366 (March 2012): 780–81, doi: 10.1056/NEJMp1109283.

114 **in ways he never imagined:** Interview of Peter Margolis by the author, February 19, 2018.

115 **"Lead User innovator":** Eric von Hippel, "Lead Users: A Source of Novel Product Concepts," *Management Science* 32, no. 7 (July 1986): 791–806, https://doi .org/10.1287/mnsc.32.7.791.

Chapter 8: Pharmaceuticals: A Web of Vested Interests

117 **Frederick Banting:** "Insulin Patent Sold for $1," Banting House, December 14, 2018, https://bantinghousenhsc.wordpress.com/2018/12/14/insulin-patent -sold-for-1/.

117 **7.4 million people in the United States:** William T. Cefalu et al., "Insulin Access and Affordability Working Group: Conclusions and Recommendations," *Diabetes Care* 41, no. 6 (June 2018): 1299–311, https://doi.org/10.2337/ dci18-0019.

117 **150 million to 200 million globally:** Satish K. Garg, Amanda H. Rewers, and Halis Kaan Akturk, "Ever-Increasing Insulin-Requiring Patients Globally," *Diabetes Technology & Therapeutics* 20, no. 2 (June 2018), https://doi.org/10 .1089/dia.2018.0101.

117 **from $21 per vial in 1996 to $275 in 2017:** Nathaniel Weixel, "Skyrocketing Insulin Prices Provoke New Outrage," *The Hill,* June 21, 2018, https://thehill .com/policy/healthcare/393378-skyrocketing-insulin-prices-provoke-new -outrage.

118 **skipped to save money:** On the problem of patients skipping doses of medications to save money: Jay Hancock, "Americans Ready to Crack Down on Drug Prices that Force Some to Skip Doses," *Kaiser Health News,* March 1, 2019,

https://khn.org/news/americans-ready-to-crack-down-on-drug-prices-that
-force-some-to-skip-doses/.

118 **because of its high cost:** Darby Herkert et al., "Cost-Related Insulin Under-
use among Patients with Diabetes," *JAMA Internal Medicine* 179, no. 1 (January
2019): 112–14, doi: 10.1001/jamainternmed.2018.5008.

118 **dying because they can't afford their insulin:** Ken Alltucker, "Struggling
to Stay Alive: Rising Insulin Prices Cause Diabetics to Go to Extremes,"
USA Today, March 27, 2019, https://www.usatoday.com/in-depth/
news/50-states/2019/03/21/diabetes-insulin-costs-diabetics-drug-prices
-increase/3196757002/; Bram Sable-Smith, "Insulin's High Cost Leads to
Lethal Rationing," *National Public Radio*, September 1, 2018, https://www
.npr.org/sections/health-shots/2018/09/01/641615877/insulins-high-cost
-leads-to-lethal-rationing.

118 **It's not so much because Americans are taking more drugs:** Shannon
Brownlee and Judith Garber, "Overprescribed: High Cost Isn't America's Only
Drug Problem," *STAT*, April 2, 2019, https://www.statnews.com/2019/04/02/
overprescribed-americas-other-drug-problem/.

118 **A 2018 US Senate report:** Claire McCaskill, *Manufactured Crisis: How Devastat-
ing Drug Price Increases Are Harming America's Seniors* (Washington, DC: Senate
Homeland Security & Governmental Affairs Committee, Minority Office, 2018),
accessed August 22, 2019, https://www.hsgac.senate.gov/imo/media/doc/
Manufactured%20Crisis%20-%20How%20Devastating%20Drug%20Price%20
Increases%20Are%20Harming%20America's%20Seniors%20-%20Report.pdf.

118 **to pay for prescription drugs:** Rabah Kamal, Cynthia Cox, and Daniel
McDermott, *What Are the Recent and Forecasted Trends in Prescription Drug
Spending?* (San Francisco: Peterson-Kaiser Health System Tracker, 2019),
accessed June 1, 2019, https://www.healthsystemtracker.org/chart-collection/
recent-forecasted-trends-prescription-drug-spending/; Nancy L. Yu, Pres-
ton Atteberry, and Peter B. Bach, "Spending on Prescription Drugs in the US:
Where Does All the Money Go?," *Health Affairs*, July 31, 2018, https://www
.healthaffairs.org/do/10.1377/hblog20180726.670593/full/.

118 **more on drugs than on inpatient hospital stays:** The study estimated that
in 2018, 23.2% of insurance premiums went to pay for prescription drugs,
while 40.2% went to clinic visits (about half to pay for the doctors), and 20%
for inpatient stays: Sara Heath, "High Drug Prices Account for One-Quarter
of Patient Insurance Costs," *PatientEngagementHIT*, May 23, 2018, https://
patientengagementhit.com/news/high-drug-prices-account-for-one-quarter
-of-patient-insurance-costs.

118 **Prescription drug spending will continue to rise:** "Accuracy Analysis of
the Short-Term (10-Year) National Health Expenditure Projections," Office
of the Actuary at the Centers for Medicare & Medicaid Services, February 14, 2018, https://www.cms.gov/Research-Statistics-Data-and-Systems/
Statistics-Trends-and-Reports/NationalHealthExpendData/Downloads/

ProjectionAccuracy.pdf. These data apply to outpatient medications and do not include those administered in the hospital or clinic.

118 **Some pharmaceutical CEOs:** The annual Gallup Poll of Business and Industry Sectors in 2019 showed that across 25 different business sectors, the pharmaceutical industry placed last (only just worse than the federal government), with 27% of Americans having a positive view of drug makers, 15% feeling neutral, and 58% having a negative view. (Note that the healthcare industry was only marginally better, with 38%, 14%, and 48%, respectively). "Business and Industry Sector Ratings," Gallup News, accessed September 14, 2019, https://news.gallup.com/poll/12748/business-industry-sector-ratings.aspx.

119 **stratospheric $75,000:** After its CEO was convicted of securities fraud, Turing renamed itself Vyera Pharmaceuticals and then optimistically renamed itself again as Phoenixus. Tori Marsh, "The 20 Most Expensive Prescription Drugs in the U.S.A.," *GoodRx*, July 17, 2019, https://www.goodrx.com/blog/20-most-expensive-drugs-in-the-usa/

119 **remained one of the 20 most expensive drugs:** Tori Marsh, "The 20 Most Expensive Prescription Drugs in the U.S.A."

119 **they cost $600:** Mylan made further news when it agreed to a $465 million settlement with the US Attorney's Office for misclassifying its branded EpiPen as a generic to avoid having to pay higher rebates to the Medicaid program: Katie Thomas, "Mylan to Settle EpiPen Overpricing Case for $465 Million," *New York Times*, October 7, 2016, https://www.nytimes.com/2016/10/08/business/epipen-mylan-justice-department-settlement.html; "Mylan Agrees to Pay $465 Million to Resolve False Claims Act Liability," US Department of Justice, August 17, 2017, https://www.justice.gov/usao-ma/pr/mylan-agrees-pay-465-million-resolve-false-claims-act-liability.

119 **"All I care about is our shareholders":** Bethany McLean, "The Valeant Meltdown and Wall Street's Major Drug Problem," *Vanity Fair*, June 5, 2016, https://www.vanityfair.com/news/2016/06/the-valeant-meltdown-and-wall-streets-major-drug-problem.

119 **"zero-gravity economics":** Stephen S. Hall, "The Cost of Living," *New York*, October 18, 2013, http://nymag.com/news/features/cancer-drugs-2013-10/.

119 **Independent researchers calculate that it's closer to $648 million:** Joseph A. DiMasi, Henry G. Grabowski, and Ronald W. Hansen, "Innovation in the Pharmaceutical Industry: New Estimates of R&D Costs," *Journal of Health Economics* 47 (May 2016): 20–33, https://doi.org/10.1016/j.jhealeco.2016.01.012; Vinay Prasad and Sham Mailankody, "Research and Development Spending to Bring a Single Cancer Drug to Market and Revenues after Approval," *JAMA Internal Medicine* 177, no. 11 (November 2017): 1569–75, doi: 10.1001/jamainternmed.2017.3601.

120 **one in ten:** Chi Heem Wong, Kien Wei Siah, and Andrew W Lo, "Estimation of Clinical Trial Success Rates and Related Parameters," *Biostatistics* 20, no. 2 (April 2019): 273–86, https://doi.org/10.1093/biostatistics/kxx069; Derek

Lowe, "In the Pipeline: A New Look at Clinical Success Rates," *American Association for the Advancement of Science*, February 2, 2018, https://blogs.sciencemag.org/pipeline/archives/2018/02/02/a-new-look-at-clinical-success-rates.

120 **Rob Califf:** Interview of Robert Califf by the author, September 17, 2019.

120 **were introducing about twice as many drugs to the market as American companies:** David Michels and Aimison Jonnard, *Review of Global Competitiveness in the Pharmaceutical Industry* (Washington, DC: US International Trade Commission, 1999), accessed August 22, 2019, https://www.usitc.gov/publications/332/pub3172.pdf.

121 **exceeding sales milestones:** "Royalty Pharma Acquires a Portion of New York University's Royalty Interest in Remicade for $650 Million," Royalty Pharma, May 4, 2007, https://www.royaltypharma.com/royalty-pharma-acquires-a-portion-of-new-york-universitys-royalty-interest-in-remicade-for-650-million/.

121 **a boon for many universities:** The Association of University Technology Managers reported that in 2017, American universities were issued 7,459 patents, produced 755 new products, and collected $3.14 billion in licensing fees. While generating more than $1 million in revenue from a single license is a rare event (less than 1% in 2017), the lure of licensing revenue has led to new innovation centers in just about all university medical centers. *AUTM 2017 Licensing Activity Survey* (Oakbrook Terrace, IL: Association of University Technology Managers, 2017), accessed November 9, 2019, https://autm.net/AUTM/media/SurveyReportsPDF/AUTM_2017_US_Licensing_Survey_no_appendix.pdf.

121 **$250 million in licensing revenue:** Maryann P. Feldman, Alessandra Colaianni, and Connie Kang Liu, "Lessons from the Commercialization of the Cohen-Boyer Patents: The Stanford University Licensing Program," in *Intellectual Property Management in Health and Agricultural Innovation: A Handbook of Best Practices*, ed. Anatole Krattiger et al. (Oxford: MIHR, 2007), 1797–807, http://www.iphandbook.org/handbook/resources/Publications/links/ipHandbook%20Volume%201.pdf.

121 **Lyrica (pregabalin, Pfizer) for $700 million:** Goldie Blumenstyk, "Northwestern U. Sells Royalty Rights from Blockbuster Drug for $700-Million," *Chronicle of Higher Education*, December 19, 2007, https://www.chronicle.com/article/Northwestern-U-Sells-Royalty/342.

121 **specifically, breast cancer genes:** The Supreme Court's decision in Association of Molecular Pathology v. Myriad Genetics, Inc in 2013 about whether the BRCA1 and BRCA2 breast cancer genes could be patented was a unanimous "no" for the patenting of genes, based on the exception to Section 101 of the Patent Act that excludes "Laws of nature, natural phenomena, and abstract ideas," although the Supreme Court did rule that the synthesized complementary DNA fragments (cDNA) were patentable: Tobin Klusty and Richard Weinmeyer, "Supreme Court to Myriad Genetics: Synthetic DNA Is Patentable but Isolated Genes Are Not," *AMA Journal of Ethics* 17, no. 9 (September 2015): 849–53, doi: 10.1001/journalofethics.2015.17.9.hlaw1-1509.

121 **at least one license from a university:** Stephen Ezell, "The Bayh-Dole Act's Vital Importance to the U.S. Life-Sciences Innovation System," *Information Technology & Innovation Foundation*, March 4, 2019, https://itif.org/publications/2019/03/04/bayh-dole-acts-vital-importance-us-life-sciences-innovation-system.

122 **taxpayer-funded federal grants:** According to the National Institutes of Health (NIH) website, in 2019 alone, June's lab received over $13.3 million from the NIH for research. "NIH RePORTER," US Department of Health & Human Services, accessed November 10, 2019, https://projectreporter.nih.gov/.

122 **B-cell acute lymphoblastic leukemia:** Denise Grady, "F.D.A. Approves First Gene-Altering Leukemia Treatment, Costing $475,000," *New York Times*, August 30, 2017, https://www.nytimes.com/2017/08/30/health/gene-therapy-cancer.html.

122 **stands to profit handsomely:** Björn Jürgens and Nigel S. Clarke, "Evolution of CAR T-Cell Immunotherapy in Terms of Patenting Activity," *Nature Biotechnology* 37 (April 2019): 370–75, https://doi.org/10.1038/s41587-019-0083-5.

122 **costs easily exceed $1 million:** Jo Cavallo, "Weighing the Cost and Value of CAR T-Cell Therapy," *ASCO Post*, May 25, 2018, https://www.ascopost.com/issues/may-25-2018/weighing-the-cost-and-value-of-car-t-cell-therapy/.

122 **to about 46% in 2014:** Andrew Pollack, "Sales of Sovaldi, New Gilead Hepatitis C Drug, Soar to $10.3 Billion," *New York Times*, February 3, 2015, https://www.nytimes.com/2015/02/04/business/sales-of-sovaldi-new-gilead-hepatitis-c-drug-soar-to-10-3-billion.html.

122 **at a bargain basement $26,400:** Julia Kollewe, "Non-Profit's $300 Hepatitis C Cure as Effective as $84,000 Alternative," *Guardian*, April 12, 2018, https://www.theguardian.com/science/2018/apr/12/non-profits-300-hepatitis-c-cure-as-effective-as-84000-alternative.

122 **hepatitis C drugs:** Corie Lok, "Gilead to Make Generic Hepatitis C Drugs and Cut Prices Up to 75%," *EXOME*, September 24, 2018, https://xconomy.com/san-francisco/2018/09/24/gilead-to-make-generic-hepatitis-c-drugs-and-cut-prices-up-to-75/.

123 **Specialty drugs:** Specialty drugs were defined by Medicare in 2019 as costing more than $670 per month. Stacie Dusetzina et al., "Improving the Affordability of Specialty Drugs by Addressing Patients' Out-Of-Pocket Spending," *Health Affairs*, March 15, 2018, https://www.healthaffairs.org/do/10.1377/hpb20180116.800715/full/HPP_2018_CMWF_01_W.pdf.

123 **cost more than $100,000 per year:** *High-Priced Drugs: Estimates of Annual Per-Patient Expenditures for 150 Specialty Medications* (Washington, DC: America's Health Insurance Plans, April 2016), https://www.ahip.org/wp-content/uploads/2016/04/HighPriceDrugsReport.pdf.

123 **Hatch-Waxman Act of 1984:** The Drug Price Competition and Patent Term Restoration Act of 1984, sponsored by Senator Orrin Hatch (Republican from Utah) and Representative Henry Waxman (Democrat from California).

123 **up to five years:** Jonathan J. Darrow and Aaron S. Kesselheim, "Prescription Drug Pricing: Policy Options Paper," *Health Affairs*, March 15, 2018, https://www.healthaffairs.org/do/10.1377/hpb20180116.967310/full/HPP_2018_CMWF_02_W.pdf.

123 **The Biologics Price Competition and Innovation Act of 2009:** Center for Drug Evaluation and Research, *Reference Product Exclusivity for Biological Products Filed under Section 351(a) of the PHS Act* (Silver Spring, MD: US Food and Drug Administration, 2014), accessed August 23, 2019, https://www.fda.gov/media/89049/download.

123 **from 8 years to over 14 years:** NIHCM Foundation, *Prescription Drugs and Intellectual Property Protection* (Washington, DC: National Institute for Health Care Management Foundation, 2000), accessed November 10, 2019, https://nihcm.org/pdf/prescription.pdf.

123 **31 years after its introduction:** Christopher Rowland, "Drug Executives Grilled in Senate over High Prices," *Washington Post*, February 26, 2019, https://www.washingtonpost.com/business/economy/drug-executives-grilled-in-senate-over-high-prices/2019/02/25/abc89c04-393f-11e9-aaae-69364b2ed137_story.html?noredirect=on&utm_term=.5b5bd8263872.

124 **they represented nearly 90%:** "Prescription Drug Pricing: Biosimilars," *Health Affairs*, July, 2017, https://www.healthaffairs.org/do/10.1377/hpb201 70721.487227/full/healthpolicybrief_169.pdf.

124 **"bioequivalence" to existing drugs:** There have been a number of instances where manufacturers have obtained bioequivalence data fraudulently, as chronicled in the 2019 whistleblower's tale by Katherine Eban, *Bottle of Lies: The Inside Story of the Generic Drug Boom* (New York: HarperCollins).

124 **as much as the branded drug:** Presentation by Kimberly W. Raines, *A Primer on Generic Drugs and Bioequivalence: An Overview of the Generic Drug Approval Process* (Silver Spring, MD: US Food and Drug Administration, n.d.), accessed August 23, 2019, https://www.fda.gov/media/89135/download.

124 **one-fifth or less of the price:** *Generic Competition and Drug Prices* (Silver Spring, MD: US Food and Drug Administration), last modified November 20, 2017, https://www.fda.gov/about-fda/center-drug-evaluation-and-research/generic-competition-and-drug-prices.

124 **substitute generic drugs for branded products:** Yan Song and Douglas Barthold, "The Effects of State-Level Pharmacist Regulations on Generic Substitution of Prescription Drugs," *Health Economics*, July 10, 2018, https://onlinelibrary.wiley.com/doi/pdf/10.1002/hec.3796?casa_token=jqguQ6pfwHsAAAAA:cD9-x8jsAoJKk5FrnN20_8ruxM9sro4PZKJFvNPqeFoe2yFnYrmsc0s5g0rO7l9qsUgN_BcvgvCuzw.

125 **the hypothetical case of Bob:** Patterned after Neeraj Sood et al., *The Flow of Money through the Pharmaceutical Distribution System* (Los Angeles: USC Schaeffer, 2017), accessed August 23, 2019, https://healthpolicy.usc.edu/wp

-content/uploads/2017/06/USC_Flow-of-MoneyWhitePaper_Final_Spreads
.pdf; Yu, Atteberry, and Bach, "Spending on Prescription Drugs."

125 **almost 12 times as much:** Sood et al., *Flow of Money.*

126 **manage their out-of-pocket costs:** Consider how it might work for a diabetic patient, a hypothetical patient Nina, who has a Medicare Part D prescription plan with a $435 deductible. First, she pays for the full costs of the insulin for January (typically about $400 per vial, and she needs two kinds of insulin, so her monthly bill is $800). Having reached the deductible, she has a co-pay of $48 for each, or $96 per month. By May, when total drug costs (to Nina and to the plan) reach an "initial coverage limit" of $4,020, Nina has reached the "donut hole" for the Medicare prescription plan. Now, she has to start paying 25% of the costs for the insulin, or about $200 per month. In August, she and her health plan hit a new threshold, the "catastrophic threshold" (costs to the plan and Nina totaled over $6,350). At that point, Medicare will cover 80%, the plan 15%, and the enrollee's share drops to 5% of list price, or about $40 per month for the rest of the year.

    Figures are based on Medicare Part D amounts for 2020. "2020 Medicare Part D Outlook," Q1Medicare.com, accessed November 10, 2019, https://q1medicare.com/PartD-The-2020-Medicare-Part-D-Outlook.php.

126 **the impact of rising drug costs:** Gary Claxton et al., "Increases in Cost-Sharing Payments Continue to Outpace Wage Growth," Peterson-Kaiser Health System Tracker, 2018, accessed November 10, 2019, https://www.healthsystemtracker.org/brief/increases-in-cost-sharing-payments-have-far-outpaced-wage-growth/#item-start.

126 **Leonard Saltz:** Interview of Leonard Saltz by the author, June 14, 2019.

126 **overseeing these infusions:** Most patients are shielded from these Medicare Part B costs. While they would typically be expected to pay 20% out of pocket, about 85% of members have extra insurance to cover this benefit, either through a supplemental insurance plan called "Medigap," or through Medicaid or an employer-sponsored plan: Peter B. Bach, "New Math on Drug Cost-Effectiveness," *New England Journal of Medicine* 373 (November 2015): 1797–99, doi: 10.1056/NEJMp1512750.

127 **specifically Section 340B:** Sunita Desai and J. Michael McWilliams, "Consequences of the 340B Drug Pricing Program," *New England Journal of Medicine* 378 (February 2018): 539–48, doi: 10.1056/NEJMsa1706475.

127 **Over one-third of US hospitals qualify for the 340B program:** MEDPAC reported that 45% of all Medicare acute care hospitals participated in the 340B program. Medicare Payment Advisory Commission, *Report to the Congress: Overview of the 340B Drug Pricing Program* (Washington, DC: Medicare Payment Advisory Commission, 2015), p. vii. And since 2014, the number of facilities has increased by more than half. Debra A. Draper, *Drug Discount Program: Status of Agency Efforts to Improve 340B Program Oversight* (Washington, DC: US Government Accountability Office, 2018). While the program benefits hospitals that

care for a disproportionate share of low-income patients, it does not provide direct incentives for hospitals to use the savings to invest in care for the poor: Rena M. Conti and Peter B. Bach, "Cost Consequences of the 340B Drug Discount Program," *JAMA* 309, no. 19 (May 2013): 1995–96, doi: 10.1001/jama.2013.4156.

127 **$1 million in profit:** Andrew Pollack, "Dispute Develops over Discount Drug Program," *New York Times*, February 12, 2013, https://www.nytimes .com/2013/02/13/business/dispute-develops-over-340b-discount-drug-program .html?emc=eta1 https://www.ncbi.nlm.nih.gov/pmc/articles/PMC4036617/.

127 **David Cutler:** Interview of David Cutler by the author, February 18, 2018.

128 **better manage patients' pain:** Joan Stephenson, "Veterans' Pain a Vital Sign," *JAMA* 281, no. 11 (March 1999): 978, doi: 10.1001/jama.281.11.978.

128 **thrilled to see profits boom:** Scott Higham, Sari Horwitz, and Steven Rich, "76 Billion Opioid Pills: Newly Released Federal Data Unmasks the Epidemic," *Washington Post*, July 16, 2019, https://www.washingtonpost.com/ investigations/76-billion-opioid-pills-newly-released-federal-data-unmasks -the-epidemic/2019/07/16/5f29fd62-a73e-11e9-86dd-d7f0e60391e9_story .html; Automated Reports and Consolidated Ordering System, "ARCOS Retail Drug Summary Reports," Springfield, VA: US Department of Justice and Drug Enforcement Administration, accessed September 2, 2019, https://www .deadiversion.usdoj.gov/arcos/retail_drug_summary/.

128 **addicted to opioids:** "Opioid Overdose Crisis," National Institute of Drug Abuse, revised January 2019, https://www.drugabuse.gov/drugs-abuse/opioids/ opioid-overdose-crisis.

128 **130 died of overdoses *every day* in 2019:** National Institute of Drug Abuse, "Opioid Overdose Crisis."

128 **cardiovascular agents:** "Drug Shortages List," ASHP, accessed September 15, 2019, https://www.ashp.org/Drug-Shortages/Current-Shortages/Drug -Shortages-List?page=CurrentShortages. The FDA also keeps its own website: "FDA Drug Shortages," FDA, accessed July 26, 2019, https://www.accessdata .fda.gov/scripts/drugshortages/default.cfm.

128 **Pharmacist Erin Fox:** Interview of Erin Fox by the author, January 22, 2019.

128 **lead to shortages:** *Report on Drug Shortages for Calendar Year 2017* (Silver Spring, MD: US Food and Drug Administration, 2017), accessed November 10, 2019, https://www.fda.gov/media/113991/download.

128 **Civica Rx:** Marc Harrison, "How the Not-For-Profit Civica Rx Will Disrupt the Generic Drug Industry," *STAT*, March 14, 2019, https://www.statnews .com/2019/03/14/how-civica-rx-will-disrupt-generic-drug-industry/; Mark Terry, "Civica Rx Starting with 20 Generic Drugs for Hospitals, Plans to Expand to 100+," *BioSpace*, January 25, 2019, https://www.biospace.com/ article/-civica-rx-starting-with-20-generic-drugs-plans-to-expand-to-100-/.

129 **"fair system that rewards innovation":** Robert M. Califf and Andrew Slavitt, "Lowering Cost and Increasing Access to Drugs without Jeopardizing Innovation," *JAMA* 321, no. 16 (April 2019): 1571–73, doi: 10.1001/jama.2019.3846.

129　**Mark McClellan agrees:** Interview of Mark McClellan by the author, October 17, 2019.

129　**whether to include drugs on their formularies:** Fiona M. Clement et al., "Using Effectiveness and Cost-Effectiveness to Make Drug Coverage Decisions," *JAMA* 302, no. 13 (October 2009): 1427–43, doi: 10.1001/jama.2009.1409.

129　**year of high-quality life:** R. Kirkdale et al., "The Cost of a QALY," *QJM* 103, no. 9 (September 2010): 715–20, doi: 10.1093/qjmed/hcq081; Luis Prieto and José A Sacristán, "Problems and Solutions in Calculating Quality-Adjusted Life Years (QALYs)," *Health and Quality of Life Outcomes* 1, no. 80 (December 2003), doi: 10.1186/1477-7525-1-80.

129　**a figure it reaffirmed in 2015:** Karl Claxton et al., Methods for the Estimation of the NICE Cost Effectiveness Threshold (York: The University of York and CHE, 2013), accessed August 26, 2019, https://www.york.ac.uk/media/che/documents/reports/resubmitted_report.pdf; *Carrying NICE Over the Threshold* (London: National Institute for Health and Care Excellence, 2015), accessed November 10, 2019, https://www.nice.org.uk/news/blog/carrying-nice-over-the-threshold; "Consultation on Changes to Technology Appraisals and Highly Specialised Technologies," NICE, accessed August 26, 2019, https://www.nice.org.uk/about/what-we-do/our-programmes/nice-guidance/nice-technology-appraisal-guidance/consultation-on-changes-to-technology-appraisals-and-highly-specialised-technologies.

130　**no agreed-upon number:** Douglas K. Owens, "Interpretation of Cost-Effectiveness Analyses," *Journal of General Internal Medicine* 13, no. 10 (October 1998): 716–17, doi: 10.1046/j.1525-1497.1998.00211.x.

130　**median annual household income (about $63,000 in 2019):** Income, Poverty and Health Insurance Coverage in the United States: 2018 (Suitland, MD: United States Census Bureau, 2019).

130　**$60,000 in the United States in 2017:** "GDP per Capita (Current US$)," World Bank, accessed June 8, 2019, https://data.worldbank.org/indicator/NY.GDP.PCAP.CD?locations=US.

130　**include in its formulary:** Ed Silverman, "CVS and the $100,000 QALY," *Managed Care*, November 24, 2018, https://www.managedcaremag.com/archives/2018/12/cvs-and-100000-qaly.

130　**monetary value on a year of life:** William S. Smith, "The U.S. Shouldn't Use the 'QALY' in Drug Cost-Effectiveness Reviews," *STAT*, February 22, 2019, https://www.statnews.com/2019/02/22/qaly-drug-effectiveness-reviews/.

130　**by able-bodied individuals:** Ari Ne'eman, "Formulary Restrictions Devalue and Endanger the Lives of Disabled People," *Health Affairs*, October 29, 2018, https://www.healthaffairs.org/do/10.1377/hblog20181025.42661/full/.

130　**but what society can afford:** Peter J. Neumann and Joshua T. Cohen, "QALYs in 2018—Advantages and Concerns," *JAMA* 319, no. 24 (June 2018): 2473–74, doi: 10.1001/jama.2018.6072.

130 **"direct importance to patients":** "What Is PCORI's Official Policy on Cost and
     Cost-Effectiveness Analysis?," Patient-Centered Outcomes Research Institute,
     accessed June 9, 2019, https://help.pcori.org/hc/en-us/articles/213716587
     -What-is-PCORI-s-official-policy-on-cost-and-cost-effectiveness-analysis-.

130 **A 2015 Reuters study:** Ben Hirschler, "How the U.S. Pays 3 Times More for
     Drugs," *Reuters*, October 13, 2015, https://www.scientificamerican.com/
     article/how-the-u-s-pays-3-times-more-for-drugs/.

131 **His Drug Pricing Lab:** "Our Work," DrugPricing Lab, accessed June 8, 2019,
     https://drugpricinglab.org/our-work/.

131 **despite working no better:** Zaltrap (ziv-aflibercept) increased survival by less
     than 1.5 months. Eric Van Cutsem et al., "Addition of Aflibercept to Fluoroura-
     cil, Leucovorin, and Irinotecan Improves Survival in a Phase III Randomized
     Trial in Patients with Metastatic Colorectal Cancer Previously Treated with an
     Oxaliplatin-Based Regimen," *Journal of Clinical Oncology* 30, no. 28 (October
     2012): 3499–506, doi: 10.1200/JCO.2012.42.8201.

131 *New York Times* **op-ed:** Peter B. Bach, Leonard B. Saltz, and Robert E. Wittes,
     "In Cancer Care, Cost Matters," *New York Times*, October 14, 2012, https://
     www.nytimes.com/2012/10/15/opinion/a-hospital-says-no-to-an-11000-a
     -month-cancer-drug.html.

131 **50% rebates to doctors:** For a detailed analysis of who did and did not ben-
     efit from the rebate and why: Rena M. Conti and Ernst Berndt, "Winners
     and Losers from the Zaltrap Price Discount: Unintended Consequences?,"
     Health Affairs, February 20, 2013, https://www.healthaffairs.org/do/10.1377/
     hblog20130220.028367/full/.

132 **save $2.8 billion per year:** "McCaskill Report Shows Medicare Could Save
     Billions with Negotiation on Prescription Drug Prices," Homeland Security
     and Governmental Affairs, August 1, 2018, https://www.hsgac.senate.gov/
     media/minority-media/breaking-mccaskill-report-shows-medicare-could
     -save-billions-with-negotiation-on-prescription-drug-prices-.

132 **Rushika Fernandopulle:** Interview of Rushika Fernandopulle by the author,
     February 22, 2018.

132 **take at least five prescription drugs:** Dima M. Qato et al., "Changes in Pre-
     scription and Over-the-Counter Medication and Dietary Supplement Use
     among Older Adults in the United States, 2005 vs 2011," *JAMA Internal Medi-
     cine* 176, no. 4 (April 2016): 473–82, doi: 10.1001/jamainternmed.2015.8581;
     Daniel S. Budnitz et al., "Emergency Hospitalizations for Adverse Drug Events
     in Older Americans," *New England Journal of Medicine* 365 (November 2011):
     2002–12, doi: 10.1056/NEJMsa1103053.

133 **HIV medications and antianxiety medication:** Dawn Hoeft, "An Overview
     of Clinically Significant Drug Interactions between Medications used to Treat
     Psychiatric and Medical Conditions," *Mental Health Clinician* 4, no. 3 (2014):
     118–30, https://doi.org/10.9740/mhc.n197904.

133 **Reducing unnecessary medications:** Qato et al., "Changes in Prescription."

133   **75% to 98.4% in one year:** Mitesh S. Patel et al., "Generic Medication Prescription Rates after Health System-Wide Redesign of Default Options within the Electronic Health Record," *JAMA Internal Medicine* 176, no. 6 (June 2016): 847–48, doi: 10.1001/jamainternmed.2016.1691.

133   **one-fifth to two-fifths in just four weeks:** M. Kit Delgado et al., "Association between Electronic Medical Record Implementation of Default Opioid Prescription Quantities and Prescribing Behavior in Two Emergency Departments," *Journal of General Internal Medicine* 33, no. 4 (April 2018): 409–11, https://doi.org/10.1007/s11606-017-4286-5.

133   **Jennifer Lee:** Personal communication, October 21, 2019.

134   **five million Americans bought medications internationally, either in person or online:** Pharmacy Checker.com, "PharmacyChecker.com Public Comments on FDA's Proposed Regulations to Implement Section 708 of the Food and Drug Administration Safety and Innovation Act (FDASIA)," White Plains, NY: PharmacyChecker.com, 2014.

134   **into the United States for personal use:** The FDA website does offer exceptions to this rule: "Personal Importation," US Food and Drug Administration, accessed November 10, 2019, https://www.fda.gov/industry/import-basics/personal-importation.

134   **Pharmacy Tourism Program:** Utah's "Pharmacy Tourism Program," PEHP Health & Benefits, accessed November 10, 2019, https://www.pehp.org/members/prescription-drug-benefit/pharmacy-tourism-program.

134   **not under US FDA surveillance:** The US FDA does also include in its surveillance program foreign drug manufacturing facilities that produce goods that will be sold in the United States: "Statement From FDA Commissioner Scott Gottlieb, M.D., on the Agency's Global Efforts to Help Assure Product Quality and Transparency at Foreign Drug Manufacturing Facilities," White Oak, NY: US Food and Drug Administration, September 5, 2018, accessed November 10, 2019, https://www.fda.gov/news-events/press-announcements/statement-fda-commissioner-scott-gottlieb-md-agencys-global-efforts-help-assure-product-quality-and.

134   **certified online pharmacies:** "Verify a CIPA Pharmacy Website," Canadian International Pharmaceutical Association, accessed August 29, 2019, https://www.cipa.com/certified-safe-online-pharmacies/.

134   **frequently lower in the United States than in Canada:** "Generic Drugs 68% Cheaper in U.S. than from Canada," *Pharmacy Checker*, May 22, 2019, https://www.pharmacychecker.com/news/generic-drugs-cheaper-in-united-states-not-canada/.

Chapter 9: Big Data Dreams

138   **President Barack Obama:** Danny Bradbury, "Obama and E-Health Records: Can He Really?," *Guardian*, March 18, 2009, https://www.theguardian.com/society/2009/mar/18/electronic-medical-records.

138   **LaQuandra Nesbitt:** Interview of LaQuandra Nesbitt by the author, February 18, 2018.

140   **one of his top health advisors during his campaign, David Blumenthal:** Interview of David Blumenthal by the author, August 2, 2019.

140   **Homer Warner:** Interview of Homer Warner at a University of Utah Dean's Round Table (for university medical students) by the author, November 9, 2012. "Dean's Roundtable 2012," University of Utah Health, accessed November 10, 2019, https://medicine.utah.edu/alumni/deans_roundtable/2012.php.

140   **cardiovascular lab:** Homer Warner's cardiovascular lab was established at Latter Day Saints Hospital in Salt Lake City. It later became a part of the Intermountain Healthcare system, and Warner's computer systems laid the foundation for the electronic health records systems that enabled Intermountain and the University of Utah to build advanced electronic data warehouses and analytics capabilities that were among the most advanced in the nation.

140   **a basic electronic system:** Zach Winn, "Is the HITECH Act Working? A Summary of Its Effect on Healthcare," January 31, 2018, https://www.campussafetymagazine.com/hospital/hitech-act-summary-healthcare-compliance/. Most of Europe, New Zealand and Australia had electronic health records in their primary care offices by 2009: Ashish K. Jha et al., "Use of Electronic Health Records in U.S. Hospitals," *New England Journal of Medicine* 360 (April 2009): 1628–38, doi: 10.1056/NEJMsa0900592.

140   **Veterans Health Administration hospitals:** Two sources that provide more color on the history of the VA's electronic health system: Arthur Allen, "A 40-Year 'Conspiracy' at the VA," *The Agenda*, March 19, 2017, https://www.politico.com/agenda/story/2017/03/vista-computer-history-va-conspiracy-000367; Phillip Longman, *Best Care Anywhere: Why VA Health Care Is Better than Yours* (San Francisco: Berrett-Koehler, 2012).

140   **(HITECH) Act in 2009:** The HITECH Act was part of the American Recovery and Reinvestment Act of 2009.

140   **the circulatory system of modern medicine:** David Blumenthal, "Launching HITECH," *New England Journal of Medicine* 362, no. 5 (February 2010): 382–85.

141   **$18,000 per doctor:** The incentives were designed to diminish over time, declining to $2,000 by the fifth year, and penalties kicked in after that: David Blumenthal, "Implementation of the Federal Health Information Technology Initiative," *New England Journal of Medicine* 365 (December 2011): 2426–31, doi: 10.1056/NEJMsr1112158.

141   **increasing from 20% to 39%:** Blumenthal, "Implementation of the Federal Health Information Technology Initiative."

141   **96% of hospitals in the United States had an electronic health record:** The Office of the National Coordinator for Health Information Technology (IT) manages an online dashboard to track the progress of health IT in the United States: "Quick Stats," Office of the National Coordinator for Health Informa-

tion Technology, last updated June 17, 2019, https://dashboard.healthit.gov/quickstats/quickstats.php.

141 **following recommended guidelines like cancer screenings:** The governmental office responsible for health quality, the Agency for Health Research and Quality, summarizes the electronic health record impact on health outcomes: "Electronic Health Records," AHRQ, last updated January 2019, https://psnet.ahrq.gov/primers/primer/43/Electronic-Health-Records.

The federal government's website, HealthIT.gov, offers a number of case studies to demonstrate benefits of the electronic health record—"Case Studies," HealthIT.gov, accessed August 29, 2019, https://www.healthit.gov/case-studies.

A number of studies have shown not much significant improvement in health outcomes after electronic health record implementation: Senthil Selvaraj et al., "Association of Electronic Health Record Use with Quality of Care and Outcomes in Heart Failure: An Analysis of Get with the Guidelines—Heart Failure," *Journal of the American Heart Association* 7 (March 2018): e008158, https://doi.org/10.1161/JAHA.117.008158; Swati Yanamadala et al., "Electronic Health Records and Quality of Care: An Observational Study Modeling Impact on Mortality, Readmissions, and Complications. Medicine," *Medicine* 95, no. 19 (May 2016): e3332, doi: 10.1097/MD.0000000000003332.

A review of 47 different publications that looked at electronic health records and impact on health care quality: Paolo Campanella et al., "The Impact of Electronic Health Records on Healthcare Quality: A Systematic Review and Meta-Analysis," *European Journal of Public Health* 26, no. 1 (February 2016): 60–64, https://doi.org/10.1093/eurpub/ckv122.

141 **result in higher reimbursements:** The electronic health records increase the fraction of patients who are assigned to higher paying disease-related groups (DRGs, see Chapter 3), Bingyang Li, *Cracking the Codes: Do Electronic Medical Records Facilitate Hospital Revenue Enhancement?* (Evanston, IL: Kellogg School of Management, Northwestern University, 2013), https://pdfs.semanticscholar.org/d760/513ccf240bff1d60412898307fca3d4c1dbf.pdf.

141 **$1 billion to $16 billion for large health systems:** "11 Statistics on EMR Costs at Community Hospitals," Chicago: Becker's Health IT & CIO, November 4, 2013, accessed November 10, 2019, https://www.beckershospitalreview.com/healthcare-information-technology/11-statistics-on-emr-costs-at-community-hospitals.html. Just to implement the electronic medical record across their health system, it cost more than $1.2 billion for the Partners Health System in Massachusetts, where Blumenthal returned after serving as national coordinator. Priyanka Dayal McCluskey, "Partners' $1.2B Patient Data System Seen as Key to Future," *Boston Globe,* May 31, 2015, https://www.bostonglobe.com/business/2015/05/31/partners-launches-billion-electronic-health-records-system/oo4nJJW2rQyfWUWQlvydkK/story.html.

For the Veterans Health Administration's conversion from their home-grown system to a commercial electronic health record the budget is exceeding $16 billion, see Lily Lieberman, "VA Pushes Estimated Cost for Cerner EHR Revamp Past $16B," *Kansas City Business Journal*, November 19, 2018, https://www.bizjournals.com/kansascity/news/2018/11/19/va-cerner-ehr -modernization-cost-estimate.html.

142 **physicians log, on average, 86 minutes:** Sara Berg, "Family Doctors Spend 86 Minutes of 'Pajama Time' with EHRs Nightly," American Medical Association, September 11, 2017, https://www.ama-assn.org/practice-management/ digital/family-doctors-spend-86-minutes-pajama-time-ehrs-nightly.

142 **US physicians reported feeling burned out in 2017:** Marcela G. del Carmen et al., "Trends and Factors Associated with Physician Burnout at a Multispecialty Academic Faculty Practice Organization," *JAMA Network Open* 2, no. 3 (March 2019): e190554, doi: 10.1001/jamanetworkopen.2019.0554; Tait D. Shanafelt et al., "Burnout and Satisfaction with Work-Life Balance among US Physicians Relative to the General US Population," *JAMA Internal Medicine* 172, no. 6 (October 2012): 1377–85, doi: 10.1001/archinternmed.2012.3199.

142 **"I have become the typist":** Thomas Bodenheimer and Christine Sinsky, "From Triple to Quadruple Aim: Care of the Patient Requires Care of the Provider," *Annals of Family Medicine* 12, no. 6 (November 2014): 573–76, doi: 10.1370/afm.1713.

142 **"Every Hour of Direct Patient Care":** Christine Sinsky et al., "Physicians Spend Two Hours on EHRs and Desk Work for Every Hour of Direct Patient Care," *Annals of Internal Medicine* 165, no. 11 (September 2016): 753–60; Brian G. Arndt et al., "Tethered to the EHR: Primary Care Physician Workload Assessment Using EHR Event Log Data and Time-Motion Observations," *Annals of Family Medicine* 15, no. 5 (Fall 2017): 419–26, doi: 10.1370/afm.2121.

142 **nation's triple aim of health care priorities:** The Triple Aim, originally defined by Don Berwick and the Institute for Healthcare Improvement, includes (1) improving the patient experience of care (including quality and satisfaction), (2) improving the health of populations, and (3) reducing the per capita cost of health care: Donald M. Berwick, Thomas W. Nolan, and John Whittington, "The Triple Aim: Care, Health, and Cost," *Health Affairs* 27, no. 3 (Spring 2008): 759–69, doi: 10.1377/hlthaff.27.3.759.

143 **inpatient hospital rooms:** See, for example: Jennifer Bresnick, "How Big Data Analytics Can Improve Patient Utilization Rates," *Health IT Analytics*, August 16, 2016, https://healthitanalytics.com/news/how-big-data-analytics-can-improve -patient-utilization-rates; Xiruo Ding et al., "Designing Risk Prediction Models for Ambulatory No-Shows across Different Specialties and Clinics," *Journal of the American Medical Informatics Association* 25, no. 8 (August 2018): 924–30, https://doi.org/10.1093/jamia/ocy002.

143 **US e-commerce market in 2018:** Emily Dayton, "Amazon Statistics You Should Know: Opportunities to Make the Most of America's Top Online Marketplace," *Big Commerce*, accessed August 26, 2019, https://www.bigcommerce .com/blog/amazon-statistics/.

143 **2.4 billion monthly active users in 2019:** Adam D. I. Kramer, Jamie E. Guillory, and Jeffrey T. Hancock, "Experimental Evidence of Massive-Scale Emotional Contagion through Social Networks," *Proceedings of the National Academy of Sciences* 111, no. 24 (June 2014): 8788–90; "Facebook: Number of Monthly Active Users Worldwide 2008–2019," J. Clement, *Statista*, last edited August 9, 2019, https://www.statista.com/statistics/264810/number-of-monthly-active-facebook-users-worldwide/.

143 **extraordinary accuracy and success:** N. Venkat Venkatraman, "Netflix: A Case of Transformation for the Digital Future," *Medium*, April 16, 2017, https://medium.com/@nvenkatraman/netflix-a-case-of-transformation-for-the-digital-future-4ef612c8d8b.

143 **predictive analytics applied to health care:** David Blumenthal, "Realizing the Value (and Profitability) of Digital Health Data," *Annals of Internal Medicine* 166, no. 11 (June 2017): 842–43.

Another excellent review: Erika Fry and Sy Mukherjee, "Tech's Next Big Wave: Big Data Meets Biology," *Fortune*, March 19, 2018, https://fortune.com/2018/03/19/big-data-digital-health-tech/.

143 **$8.1 billion investment in 2018:** Sean Day and Megan Zweig, "2018 Year End Funding Report: Is Digital Health in a Bubble?," Rock Health, accessed August 30, 2019, https://rockhealth.com/reports/2018-year-end-funding-report-is-digital-health-in-a-bubble/.

144 **only 10% of inpatient safety events are detected:** Voluntary reporting captured only about 10% of all adverse events when compared with a chart review called the Global Trigger Tool method. Among 795 patient reviews, 393 adverse events were detected by at least one of three methods, whereas 354 or 90% were identified by the Global Trigger method. One of the national methods studied detected only 5.6%: David C. Classen et al., " 'Global Trigger Tool' Shows that Adverse Events in Hospitals May Be Ten Times Greater than Previously Measured," *Health Affairs* 30, no. 4 (2011): 581–89, doi: 10.1377/hlthaff.2011.0190.

144 **automatically prevent them:** Institute of Medicine, *Health IT and Patient Safety: Building Safer Systems for Better Care* (Washington, DC: National Academies Press, 2012), https://doi.org/10.17226/13269.

144 **health care–associated infection:** "Healthcare-Associated Infections," Centers for Disease Control and Prevention, accessed August 26, 2019, https://www.cdc.gov/hai/data/index.html; Nasia Safdar et al., "The Evolving Landscape of Healthcare-Associated Infections: Recent Advances in Prevention and a Road Map for Research," *Infection Control & Hospital Epidemiology* 35, no. 5 (May 2014): 480–93, doi: 10.1086/675821.

144 **on prophylactic antibiotics for too long:** R. Scott Evans et al., "Computer Surveillance of Hospital-Acquired Infections and Antibiotic Use," *JAMA* 256, no. 8 (August 1986): 1007–11, doi: 10.1001/jama.1986.03380080053027.

One of the earliest reports of an electronic health record described the University of Utah's system: T. Allan Pryor et al., "The HELP System," *Jour-*

nal of Medical Systems 7, no. 2 (April 1983): 87–102, https://doi.org/10.1007/BF00995116.

144 **saving lives and considerable staff time:** Lindsay Steele, Emma Orefuwa, and Petra Dickmann, "Drivers of Earlier Infectious Disease Outbreak Detection: A Systematic Literature Review," *International Journal of Infectious Diseases* 53 (December 2016): 15–20, https://doi.org/10.1016/j.ijid.2016.10.005; Phillip L. Russo et al., "The Impact of Electronic Healthcare-Associated Infection Surveillance Software on Infection Prevention Resources: A Systematic Review of the Literature," *Journal of Hospital Infection* 99, no. 1 (May 2018): 1–7, doi: 10.1016/j.jhin.2017.09.002.

144 **patient safety organization, Pascal Metrics:** David Classen et al., "An Electronic Health Record-Based Real-Time Analytics Program for Patient Surveillance and Improvement," *Health Affairs* 37, no. 11 (November 2018), https://doi.org/10.1377/hlthaff.2018.0728.

144 **the Global Trigger Tool:** The Global Trigger Tool was developed by the Institute for Healthcare Improvement. (Disclosure: I am affiliated with the Institute for Healthcare Improvement as a senior fellow, noncompensated). "IHI Global Trigger Tool for Measuring Adverse Events," Institute for Healthcare Improvement, accessed August 27, 2019, http://www.ihi.org/resources/Pages/Tools/IHIGlobalTriggerToolforMeasuringAEs.aspx.

145 **symptoms until the late stages:** "Kidney Disease: The Basics," National Kidney Foundation, accessed November 10, 2019, https://www.kidney.org/news/newsroom/factsheets/KidneyDiseaseBasics.

145 **experiences acute kidney injury:** Henry E. Wang et al., "Acute Kidney Injury and Mortality in Hospitalized Patients," *American Journal of Nephrology* 35, no. 4 (April 2012): 349–55, doi: 10.1159/000337487.

145 **two days before the usual laboratory values start changing:** Google's artificial intelligence team, Deep Mind, developed this algorithm. (Deep Mind was best known for defeating the world's champion of the board game Go.) Nenad Tomašev et al., "A Clinically Applicable Approach to Continuous Prediction of Future Acute Kidney Injury," *Nature* 572 (August 2019): 116–19, https://doi.org/10.1038/s41586-019-1390-1.

145 **reduce the death rate by half:** Sharad Manaktala and Stephen R. Claypool, "Evaluating the Impact of a Computerized Surveillance Algorithm and Decision Support System on Sepsis Mortality," *Journal of the American Medical Informatics Association* 24, no. 1 (January 2017): 88–95, https://doi.org/10.1093/jamia/ocw056; Evelyn M. Olenick et al., "Predicting Sepsis Risk Using the 'Sniffer' Algorithm in the Electronic Medical Record," *Journal of Nursing Care Quality* 32, no. 1 (Spring 2017): 25–31, doi: 10.1097/NCQ.0000000000000198.

145 **doubles every eight to nine years:** The statement assumes that you believe the rate of publications mirrors the development of new knowledge. Lutz Bornmann and Rüdiger Mutz, "Growth Rates of Modern Science: A Bibliometric Analysis Based on the Number of Publications and Cited References," *Journal*

of the Association for Information Science and Technology 66, no. 11 (November 2015): 2215–22, https://doi.org/10.1002/asi.23329.

146 **"Dr. Google":** Robert H. Shmerling, "Dr. Google: The Top 10 Health Searches in 2017," *Harvard Health Publishing*, February 21, 2018, https://www.health .harvard.edu/blog/google-top-10-health-searches-2017-2018022113300.

146 **Paul Chang:** Personal communication, November 3, 2019.

147 **the "OpenNotes" movement:** The organization Delbanco coleads, Open-Notes (www.opennotes.org), provides maps to help you find which hospitals are sharing. Tom Delbanco et al., "Inviting Patients to Read Their Doctors' Notes: A Quasi-Experimental Study and a Look Ahead," *Annals of Internal Medicine* 157, no. 7 (October 2012): 461–70, doi: 10.7326/0003-4819-157-7-201210020-00002; Tobias Esch et al., "Engaging Patients through Open Notes: An Evaluation Using Mixed Methods," *BMJ Open* 6, no. 1 (January 2016): e010034, http://dx.doi.org/10.1136/bmjopen-2015-010034.

147 **reported the greatest benefit:** Jan Walker et al., "OpenNotes After 7 Years: Patient Experiences with Ongoing Access to Their Clinicians' Outpatient Visit Notes," *Journal of Medical Internet Research* 21, no. 5 (June 2019): e13876, doi: 10.2196/13876.

148 **application programming interfaces:** William Gordon, Aneesh Chopra, and Adam Landman, "Patient-Led Data Sharing—a New Paradigm for Electronic Health Data," *New England Journal of Medicine Catalyst*, November 21, 2018, https://catalyst.nejm.org/patient-led-health-data-paradigm/.

148 **using Apple's health app:** "Empower Your Patients with Health Records on iPhone," Apple, accessed November 10, 2019, https://www.apple.com/healthcare/health-records/.

149 **hypertensive medications:** Patrick Ryan, Martijn Shuemie, and Marc Suchard, "Large-Scale Evidence Generation and Evaluation in a Network of Databases (LEGEND)," *Observational Health Data Sciences and Informatics*, October 12, 2018, accessed November 10, 2019, https://www.ohdsi.org/wp-content/uploads/2018/10/OHDSI-2018-Symposium-LEGEND-HTN-Ryan-12oct2018 .pdf; Seng Chan You et al., "Comparison of Combination Treatment in Hypertension," *Observational Health Data Sciences and Informatics*, accessed August 30, 2019, https://www.ohdsi.org/wp-content/uploads/2017/10/OHDSI_HTN_combi.pdf; George Hripcsak et al., "Characterizing Treatment Pathways at Scale Using the OHDSI Network," *Proceedings of the National Academy of Sciences* 113, no. 27 (July 2016): 7329–36, https://doi.org/10.1073/pnas.1510502113.

149 **it's a lot cheaper than those clinical trials:** Miguel A. Hernán and James M. Robins, "Using Big Data to Emulate a Target Trial when a Randomized Trial Is Not Available," *American Journal of Epidemiology* 183, no. 8 (April 2016): 758–64, doi: 10.1093/aje/kwv254.

149 **risk of heart attacks and strokes:** Snigdha Prakash and Vikki Valentine, "Timeline: The Rise and Fall of Vioxx," *National Public Radio*, November 10, 2007, https://www.npr.org/templates/story/story.php?storyId=5470430.

149   **A *Lancet* article:** David J. Graham et al., "Risk of Acute Myocardial Infarction
       and Sudden Cardiac Death in Patients Treated with Cyclooxygenase 2 Selec-
       tive and Non-Selective Non-Steroidal Anti-Inflammatory Drugs: Nested Case-
       Control Study," *Lancet* 365, no. 9458 (February 2005): 475–81, https://doi
       .org/10.1016/S0140-6736(05)17864-7.

150   **led to more people getting sicker:** Richard Platt et al., "The FDA Sentinel
       Initiative—An Evolving National Resource," *New England Journal of Medicine*
       379, no. 22 (November 2018): 2091–93.

150   **"Absolutely!":** Interview of Richard Platt by the author, August 27, 2018, and
       personal communication November 16, 2019.

151   **behaviors and medical risks:** Carrot Health is a software-as-a-service com-
       pany focused on collecting information it refers to as "social determinants of
       health," and 23andMe and Ancestry are two of the widely available home DNA
       testing companies, for example.

151   **communities that needed the most help:** Shelby Livingston, "Social Deter-
       minants Are Core of North Carolina's Medicaid Overhaul," *Modern Health-
       care*, August 3, 2018, https://www.modernhealthcare.com/article/20180803/
       TRANSFORMATION01/180809944/social-determinants-are-core-of
       -north-carolina-s-medicaid-overhaul.

          The map is here: "North Carolina Health Atlas," North Carolina Depart-
       ment of Health and Human Services, accessed August 27, 2019, https://schs
       .dph.ncdhhs.gov/data/hsa/.

Chapter 10: Employer, Heal Thyself

154   **Uwe Reinhardt:** Uwe E. Reinhardt, "The Culprit behind High U.S. Health
       Care Prices," *New York Times*, June 7, 2013, https://economix.blogs.nytimes
       .com/2013/06/07/the-culprit-behind-high-u-s-health-care-prices/?_r=0.

154   **found himself running a business:** Carl Kjeldsberg was interviewed in 2018
       about his career and the founding of ARUP: Carl Kjeldsberg, "An Interview
       with Dr. Carl Kjeldsberg (Part 1): Founding and the Early Shaping of ARUP,"
       July 6, 2018, https://www.listennotes.com/podcasts/labmind/an-interview
       -with-dr-carl-4MIgpZ9-kAN/.

155   **to control wages during World War II:** Institute of Medicine, "Origins and
       Evolution of Employment-Based Health Benefits," in *Employment and Health
       Benefits: A Connection at Risk*, ed. Marilyn J. Field and Harold T. Shapiro
       (Washington, DC: National Academies Press, 1993); Thomas C. Buchmueller
       and Alan C. Monheit, "Employer-Sponsored Health Insurance and the Prom-
       ise of Health Insurance Reform," *Journal of Health Care Organization, Provision,
       and Financing* 46, no. 2 (2009): 187–202; Melissa A. Thomasson, "The Impor-
       tance of Group Coverage: How Tax Policy Shaped U.S. Health Insurance"
       (NBER Working Paper no. 7543, Cambridge, MA: National Bureau of Eco-
       nomic Research, 2000); Melissa A. Thomasson, "From Sickness to Health: The

Twentieth-Century Development of U.S. Health Insurance," *Explorations in Economic History* 39, no. 3 (July 2002): 233–53, doi: 10.1006/exeh.2002.0788; Melissa A. Thomasson, "The Importance of Group Coverage: How Tax Policy Shaped U.S. Health Insurance," *American Economic Review* 93, no. 4 (September 2003): 1373–84, doi: 10.1257/000282803769206359; George B. Moseley III, "The U.S. Health Care Non-System, 1908–2008," *Virtual Mentor* 10, no. 5 (May 2008): 324–31, doi: 10.1001/virtualmentor.2008.10.5.mhst1-0805; David Rook, "How We Got to Now: A Brief History of Employer-Sponsored Healthcare," JP Griffin Group, August 17, 2015, https://www.griffinbenefits .com/employeebenefitsblog/history-of-employer-sponsored-healthcare.

156 **an employer-sponsored plan:** Edward R. Berchick, Emily Hood, and Jessica C. Barnett, *Health Insurance Coverage in the United States: 2017* (Washington, DC: US Government Printing Office, 2018), accessed August 27, 2019, https:// www.census.gov/library/publications/2018/demo/p60-264.html.

156 **nine out of ten government workers:** US Bureau of Labor Statistics, *National Compensation Survey: Employee Benefits in the United States, March 2018* (Washington, DC: US Department of Labor, 2018), accessed August 27, 2019, https:// www.bls.gov/ncs/ebs/benefits/2018/employee-benefits-in-the-united-states -march-2018.pdf.

156 **82% of the costs for individuals:** Gary Claxton et al., "Health Benefits in 2018: Modest Growth in Premiums, Higher Worker Contributions at Firms with More Low-Wage Workers," *Health Affairs* 37, no. 11 (October 2018), https://doi.org/10.1377/hlthaff.2018.1001; Kaiser Family Foundation, *2018 Employer Health Benefits Survey* (San Francisco: Henry J. Kaiser Family Foundation, 2018), accessed September 3, 2019, https://www.kff.org/health-costs/ report/2018-employer-health-benefits-survey/.

156 **massive health expenditures:** Kimberly Amadeo, "Auto Industry Bailout: Was the Big 3 Bailout Worth It?," *The Balance*, June 25, 2019, https://www.thebalance .com/auto-industry-bailout-gm-ford-chrysler-3305670; Brian Pascus, "GM, Ford, and Chrysler almost Died a Decade Ago during the Financial Crisis— Here's How the Auto Giants Have Changed Since," *Business Insider Australia*, September 16, 2018, https://www.businessinsider.com.au/gm-ford-chrysler -almost-died-during-financial-crisis-changes-since-2018-9?r=US&IR=T.

156 **while Toyota was spending $47:** Igor Volsky, "The Auto Makers and the Health Care Crisis," *Think Progress*, November 18, 2008, https://thinkprogress .org/the-auto-makers-and-the-health-care-crisis-55282007c3de/.

156 **"an auto company attached":** Ron French, "GM on a Crash Course with Health Care Costs," *San Jose Mercury News*, October 1, 2006, http://www.pnhp .org/news/2006/october/gm_on_a_crash_course.php.

156 **about one-third (36%):** Brendan McFarland and Steve Nyce, "Shifts in Benefit Allocations among U.S. Employers," *Willis Towers Watson*, July 14, 2017, https://www.willistowerswatson.com/en-US/Insights/2017/07/shifts-in -benefit-allocations-among-us-employers.

157 **180,000 people calling in sick every day:** Aligning Forces for Quality, *Reform in Action: How Employers Can Improve Value and Quality in Health Care* (Princeton, NJ: Robert Wood Johnson Foundation, 2013), accessed September 3, 2019, https://www.pcpcc.org/sites/default/files/resources/rwjf403361.pdf.

157 **"a health care administrator":** George Will, "More Health Care in GM Car than Steel," *The Ledger*, May 1, 2005, https://www.theledger.com/article/LK/20050501/news/608108105/LL.

157 **"self-insure":** Patricia McDonnell et al., "Self-Insured Health Plans," *Health Care Financing Review*. 8, no. 2 (Winter 1986): 1–16, PMID: 10312008.

157 **the figure was over 85%:** "2018 Employer Health Benefits Survey," Kaiser Family Foundation, October 3, 2018, https://www.kff.org/report-section/2018-employer-health-benefits-survey-section-10-plan-funding/.

157 **Weir, a family medicine physician:** Interview of Peter Weir by the author, January 6, 2018.

158 **stroke over the next ten years:** Here's the American College of Cardiology and American Heart Association's online tool: ACC/AHA, "Heart Risk Calculator," http://www.cvriskcalculator.com/.

158 **even the top bosses:** The relationship between ERISA and HIPAA regulations is carefully analyzed in this article: Jamie Lund, "ERISA Enforcement of the HIPAA Privacy Rules," *Chicago Unbound*, accessed August 27, 2019, https://chicagounbound.uchicago.edu/cgi/viewcontent.cgi?article=5346&context=uclrev.

160 **anecdotal success stories:** Steven A. Burd, "How Safeway Is Cutting Health-Care Costs," *Wall Street Journal*, June 12, 2009, https://www.wsj.com/articles/SB124476804026308603.

160 **some encouraging early publications:** Katherine Baicker, David Cutler, and Zirui Song, "Workplace Wellness Programs Can Generate Savings," *Health Affairs* 29, no. 2 (February 2010), https://doi.org/10.1377/hlthaff.2009.0626.

160 **weren't getting good results:** John P. Caloyeras et al., "Managing Manifest Diseases, but Not Health Risks, Saved PepsiCo Money over Seven Years," *Health Affairs* 33, no. 1 (January 2014), https://doi.org/10.1377/hlthaff.2013.0625.

160 **McKinsey consultants:** Stefan Brandt, Jan Hartmann, and Steffen Hehner, "How to Design a Successful Disease-Management Program," New York: McKinsey & Company, October 2010, accessed November 11, 2019, https://www.mckinsey.com/industries/healthcare-systems-and-services/our-insights/how-to-design-a-successful-disease-management-program.

161 **high-deductible plan in 2019:** In 2019, the US Internal Revenue Service defined a high-deductible plan as a deductible of at least $1,350 for an individual and $2,700 for a family (either in cash or through health savings accounts): *2019 Employer Health Benefits Survey* (San Francisco: Kaiser Family Foundation, 2019), accessed October 27, 2019, https://www.kff.org/report-section/ehbs-2019-section-8-high-deductible-health-plans-with-savings-option/.

161 **less than 15% in 1999:** Ezekiel J. Emanuel, Aaron Glickman, and David John-

son, "Measuring the Burden of Health Care Costs on Families: The Affordability Index," *JAMA* 318, no. 19 (November 2017): 1863–64, doi: 10.1001/jama.2017.15686.

162 **a family on a traditional plan:** Joseph P. Newhouse et al., "Some Interim Results from a Controlled Trial of Cost Sharing in Health Insurance," *New England Journal of Medicine* 305, no. 25 (December 1981): 1501–7, doi: 10.1056/NEJM198112173052504.

162 **high-deductible plans:** Jack Burke and Rob Pipich, *Consumer-Driven Impact Study* (Seattle: Milliman, 2008), accessed August 27, 2019.

162 **cost-sharing changed people's behaviors:** Karen Davis, "Consumer-Directed Health Care: Will It Improve Health System Performance?," *Health Services Research* 39, no. 4, pt. 2 (August 2004): 1219–34, doi: 10.1111/j.1475-6773.2004.00284.x.

162 **they were more likely to die earlier:** Edith Rasell, "Cost Sharing in Health Insurance—a Reexamination," *New England Journal of Medicine* 332 (April 1995): 1164–68, doi: 10.1056/NEJM199504273321711; Robert H. Brook et al., "Does Free Care Improve Adults' Health?—Results from a Randomized Controlled Trial," *New England Journal of Medicine* 309 (December 1983): 1426–34, doi: 10.1056/NEJM198312083092305.

162 **patients didn't fill their prescriptions:** Haiden A. Huskamp et al., "The Effect of Incentive-Based Formularies on Prescription-Drug Utilization and Spending," *New England Journal of Medicine* 349 (December 2003): 2224–32.

162 **didn't take their sick children to get care:** Kathleen N. Lohr, "Use of Medical Care in the RAND HIE," *Medical Care* 24, no. 9 (1986): S1–87.

162 **Bob Mecklenburg:** Interviews of Bob Mecklenburg by the author, November 2, 2017 and January 23–24, 2018.

164 **most commonly performed imaging procedures in the United States:** Jeffrey G. Jarvik et al., "Rapid Magnetic Resonance Imaging vs Radiographs for Patients with Low Back Pain: A Randomized Controlled Trial," *JAMA* 289, no. 21 (June 2003): 2810–18, doi: 10.1001/jama.289.21.2810.; Jeffrey G. Jarvik et al., "Association of Early Imaging for Back Pain with Clinical Outcomes in Older Adults," *JAMA* 313, no. 11 (March 2015): 1143–53, doi: 10.1001/jama.2015.1871.

164 **one in six are prescribed antibiotics:** James M. Chamberlain et al., "Practice Pattern Variation in the Care of Children with Acute Asthma," *Academic Emergency Medicine*, accessed August 30, 2019, doi: 10.1111/acem.12857.

165 **Virginia Mason Medical Center would have to meet:** Robert S. Mecklenburg, "What Employers Can Do to Accelerate Health Care Reform," *Harvard Business Review*, October 16, 2015, https://hbr.org/2015/10/what-employers-can-do-to-accelerate-health-care-reform.

167 **Raj Sethi:** Interview of Rajiv Sethi by the author, January 24, 2018.

168 **Bob Galvin:** Interview of Bob Galvin by the author, December 19, 2017.

170 **Bree Collaborative:** Public meeting of the Bree Collaborative on January 24, 2018. I attended in person.

170 **Centers of Excellence:** Jonathan R. Slotkin et al., "Why GE, Boeing, Lowe's, and Walmart Are Directly Buying Health Care for Employees," *Harvard Business Review*, June 8, 2017, https://hbr.org/2017/06/why-ge-boeing-lowes-and -walmart-are-directly-buying-health-care-for-employees.

171 **"wrong pocket" problem:** Interview of Karen DeSalvo by the author, February 18, 2019.

171 **stayed with the same employer for an average of 4.2 years:** *Employee Tenure Summary* (Washington, DC: US Department of Labor, 2018), accessed September 2, 2019, https://www.bls.gov/news.release/pdf/tenure.pdf.

171 **Rushika Fernandopulle, CEO of Iora Health:** Interview of Rushika Fernandopulle by the author, February 22, 2018.

Chapter 11: Restoring Readiness: Battle-Tested Care

176 **Major General George Anderson:** Interview of General Anderson by the author, April 27, 2018.

176 **an annual budget of about $50 billion a year:** *Military Medical Care: Frequently Asked Questions* (Washington, DC: Congressional Research Service, 2018), accessed August 31, 2019, https://fas.org/sgp/crs/misc/R45399.pdf.

176 **served at least 20 years of service:** Terri Tanielian and Carrie Farmer, "The US Military Health System: Promoting Readiness and Providing Health Care," *Health Affairs* 38, no. 8 (August 2019): 1259–67, https://doi.org/10.1377/ hlthaff.2019.00239; Phillip M. Lurie, Richard R. Bannick, and Elder Granger, *The Department of Defense's TRICARE Health Benefits Program as a Critical Plank in the Federal Platform for Health Care Reform* (Alexandria, VA: Institute for Defense Analyses, 2009), accessed August 31, 2019, https://www.ida.org/ -/media/feature/publications/i/id/ida-nsd3960-the-department-of-defenses -tricare-health-benefits-program-as-a-critical-plank-in-the-fe/ida-document -ns-d-3960.ashx; Phillip M. Lurie, *Comparing the Costs of Military Treatment Facilities with Private Sector Care* (Alexandria, VA: Institute for Defense Analyses, 2016), https://www.ida.org/research-and-publications/publications/all/c/ co/comparing-the-costs-of-military-treatment-facilities-with-private-sector -care, accessed August 31, 2019.

176 **a critical fourth, improved readiness:** Note that this fourth differs from the civilian fourth aim proposed by Christine Sinsky and Thomas Bodenheimer: improving the work life of clinicians and staff, as discussed in Chapter 7.

177 **including 177 overseas:** *Approaches to Changing Military Health Care* (Washington, DC: Congressional Budget Office, 2017), accessed August 31, 2019, https://www.cbo.gov/system/files/115th-congress-2017-2018/reports/53137 -approachestochangingmilitaryhealthcare.pdf; *Defense Primer: Military Health System* (Washington, DC: Congressional Research Service, 2018), accessed August 31, 2019, https://fas.org/sgp/crs/natsec/IF10530.pdf.

177 **$720 per year for families:** Congressional Research Service, *Military Medical Care: Frequently Asked Questions.*

177 **$5,800 less:** Defense Health Agency, *Evaluation of the TRICARE Program: Fiscal Year 2019 Report to Congress* (Washington, DC: US Department of Defense, 2019), accessed August 31, 2019, https://www.health.mil/Military-Health-Topics/Access-Cost-Quality-and-Safety/Health-Care-Program-Evaluation/Annual-Evaluation-of-the-TRICARE-Program.

177 **outcomes vary significantly by hospital:** *Approaches to Changing Military Health Care* (Washington, DC: Congressional Budget Office, 2017), https://www.cbo.gov/system/files/115th-congress-2017-2018/reports/53137-approachestochangingmilitaryhealthcare.pdf; *Final Report to the Secretary of Defense: Military Health System Review* (Washington, DC: Secretary of Defense, 2014), accessed August 31, 2019, https://www.health.mil/Military-Health-Topics/Access-Cost-Quality-and-Safety/MHS-Review; Defense Health Agency, *Evaluation of the TRICARE Program: Fiscal Year 2019 Report to Congress.*

177 **small military hospitals back home:** Arthur Kellermann, "Rethinking the United States' Military Health System," *Health Affairs*, April 27, 2017, doi: 10.1377/hblog20170427.059833.

177 **higher volume of a particular operation have better results:** Leon Boudourakis et al., "Evolution of the Surgeon-Volume, Patient-Outcome Relationship," *Annals of Surgery* 250, no. 1 (July 2009): 159–65, doi: 10.1097/SLA.0b013e3181a77cb3; Robert G. Hughes, Sandra S. Hunt, and Harold S. Luft, "Effects of Surgeon Volume and Hospital Volume on Quality of Care in Hospitals," *Medical Care* 25, no. 6 (June 1987): 489–503, doi: 10.1097/00005650-198706000-00004.

177 **should be allowed to operate:** Nikhil R. Sahni et al., "Surgeon Specialization and Operative Mortality in United States: Retrospective Analysis," *BMJ* 354 (July 2016): i3571, https://doi.org/10.1136/bmj.i3571; Dana M. Schwartz et al., "The Hidden Consequences of the Volume Pledge: 'No Patient Left Behind'?," *Annals of Surgery* 265, no. 2 (February 2017): 273–74, doi: 10.1097/SLA.0000000000001833.

177 **national quality improvement program:** Peter A. Learn et al., "A Collaborative to Evaluate and Improve the Quality of Surgical Care Delivered by the Military Health System," *Health Affairs* 38, no. 8 (2019): 1313–20, doi: 10.1377/hlthaff.2019.00286.

178 **over 1,000 outpatient sites:** "Find VA Locations," US Department of Veterans Affairs, accessed August 31, 2019, https://www.va.gov/directory/guide/division.asp?dnum=1.

178 **over 3,500 additional veterans were unofficially listed:** The report from the VA's audit: *Results of Access Audit Conducted May 12, 2014, through June 3, 2014* (Washington, DC: Department of Veterans Affairs, 2014), accessed August 31, 2019, https://www.va.gov/health/docs/VAAccessAuditFindingsReport.pdf.

178   **medical care from a non-VA facility:** "H.R.3230—Veterans Access, Choice, and Accountability Act of 2014," Congress.Gov, accessed August 31, 2019, https://www.congress.gov/bill/113th-congress/house-bill/3230.

178   **at a much lower cost:** Claire O'Hanlon et al., "Comparing VA and Non-VA Quality of Care: A Systematic Review," *Journal of General Internal Medicine* 32, no. 1 (January 2017): 105–21, doi: 10.1007/s11606-016-3775-2; *Comparing the Costs of the Veterans' Health Care System with Private-Sector Costs* (Washington, DC: Congressional Budget Office, 2014), accessed August 31, 2019, https://www.cbo.gov/sites/default/files/113th-congress-2013-2014/reports/49763-VA_Healthcare_Costs.pdf; *Quality of Care in VA Health System Compares Well to Other Health Settings* (Santa Monica, CA: RAND Corporation, 2016), accessed August 31, 2019, https://www.rand.org/news/press/2016/07/18.html.

179   **lower hospital-acquired blood infection and death rates:** Eddie Blay Jr. et al., "Initial Public Reporting of Quality at Veterans Affairs vs Non-Veterans Affairs Hospitals," *JAMA Internal Medicine* 177, no. 6 (June 2017): 882–85, doi: 10.1001/jamainternmed.2017.0605.

179   **$50 billion between 2012 and 2020:** *FY2020 Budget Request for the Military Health System* (Washington, DC: Congressional Research Service, 2019), accessed October 24, 2019, https://fas.org/sgp/crs/natsec/IF11206.pdf.

179   **increase of over 30% for the rest of the United States:** "NHE Fact Sheet," Centers for Medicare & Medicaid Services, accessed August 29, 2019, https://www.cms.gov/research-statistics-data-and-systems/statistics-trends-and-reports/nationalhealthexpenddata/nhe-fact-sheet.html.

179   **better outcomes and lower costs:** Defense Health Agency, *Evaluation of the TRICARE Program: Fiscal Year 2019 Report to Congress*, p. 11.

180   **Arizona Senator John McCain's last:** The NDAA is referred to each year as the John S. McCain National Defense Authorization Act: Terry Adirim, "A Military Health System for the Twenty-First Century," *Health Affairs* 38, no. 8 (August 2019), https://doi.org/10.1377/hlthaff.2019.00302.

180   **Vice Admiral Bono:** Interview of Vice Admiral Raquel Bono by the author, March 30, 2018.

180   **Navy's only brother-and-sister admiral pair:** Anthony Maddela, "She Keeps the Defense Health Agency Shipshape," *Positively Filipino*, April 6, 2016, http://www.positivelyfilipino.com/magazine/she-keeps-defense-health-agency-shipshape.

180   **readiness of active duty members:** Patricia Kime, "Services Turn Focus to Warfighters as DHA Takes Over Military Hospitals," *Military.com*, April 3, 2009, https://www.military.com/daily-news/2019/04/03/services-turn-focus-warfighters-dha-takes-over-military-hospitals.html.

180   **$1.027 billion in savings for 2019:** Adirim, "A Military Health System."

180   **discounted prices for prescription drugs:** Mike McCaughan, "Health Policy Brief #8: Veterans Health Administration," *Health Affairs*, August 10, 2017, https://www.healthaffairs.org/do/10.1377/hpb20171008.000174/full/.

181 **24% off the national sales price:** The Department of Defense (DoD) and Veterans Health Administration (VHA) got this deal only after pharmaceutical companies responded to a law that said Medicaid had to get the lowest drug prices in the market. To avoid giving Medicaid the same low prices that had been negotiated by the VHA and DoD contracts, and other large private purchasers, many manufacturers raised all their prices. The Veterans Health Care Act changed that. Now, the VHA can get even lower prices than Medicaid. As in the civilian sector, pharmaceutical manufacturers can require final prices be kept secret; published prices don't include rebates or discounts: McCaughan, "Health Policy Brief #8."

181 **Military Health System and the Veterans Health Administration:** Terri Tanielian et al., *Impact of a Uniform Formulary on Military Health System Prescribers: Baseline Survey Results* (Santa Monica, CA: RAND Corporation, 2003), accessed August 31, 2019, https://www.rand.org/content/dam/rand/pubs/monograph_reports/MR1615/MR1615.pref.pdf.

181 **cost-effectiveness research:** "Pharmacy Division," Health.mil, accessed August 31, 2019, https://health.mil/About-MHS/OASDHA/Defense-Health -Agency/Operations/Pharmacy-Division.

181 **require final prices to remain confidential:** *Prescription Drug Pricing: A Health Affairs Collection* (Bethesda, MD: Health Affairs, 2018), accessed August 31, 2019, https://www.healthaffairs.org/pb-assets/documents/Collections/Collection_CMWF_Prescription_Drug_Pricing_May_2018.pdf.

181 **dispense a prescription by mail order:** *Assessment J (Supplies)* (New York: McKinsey, 2015), accessed August 31, 2019, https://docplayer.net/13038154 -Assessment-j-supplies.html.

181 **national average of $10.50 per prescription reported in 2007:** *Cost of Dispensing Study* (Chicago: Grant Thornton, 2007), accessed August 1, 2019, http://mpi-group.com/wp-content/uploads/2012/05/CostofDispensingStudy_GT .pdf.

181 **119.7 million outpatient prescriptions:** "Pharmacy Benefits Management Services," US Department of Veterans Affairs, accessed August 31, 2019, https://www.pbm.va.gov/PBM/CMOP/VA_Mail_Order_Pharmacy.asp.

181 **have their prescriptions filled by mail:** Laura Daily, "Should You Switch to a Mail-Order Pharmacy? Here are the Factors to Consider," *Washington Post*, January 8, 2019, https://www.washingtonpost.com/lifestyle/home/should-you-switch-to-a-mail-order-pharmacy-here-are-the-factors-to -consider/2019/01/07/8b56f87a-0ede-11e9-8938-5898adc28fa2_story.html; Julie A. Schmittdiel et al., "Opportunities to Encourage Mail Order Pharmacy Delivery Service Use for Diabetes Prescriptions: A Qualitative Study," *BMC Health Services Research* 19 (2019): 422, doi: 10.1186/s12913-019-4250-7.

As an aside, one of the important features of pharmaceutical management that makes mail-order even possible came out of the Military Health System—bar-coding. In the mid 1990s, General Anderson, while serving as deputy assistant secretary of defense, worked closely with senior level colleagues in the Veterans Health Administration to solve logistic and clinical pharmacy issues. The Department of Defense had established a pharmacoeconomic center to advise on a system-wide formulary aimed at providing the best drugs at the best price. However, tracking drug stock levels worldwide, avoiding expiration of pharmaceuticals, and ensuring the best pricing were challenging. Barcodes were already routinely used in other parts of the military supply chain. Anderson and his Veterans Health Administration counterpart worked to ensure that barcodes were required on pharmaceutical purchase contracts going forward for both systems so that all drugs could be quickly identified. The barcoding was so successful that the Military Health System started requiring that all manufacturers barcode their medical equipment. The requirements were so obviously sensible that, before long, manufacturers were putting barcodes on pharmaceuticals and medical equipment, whether it was for the military or not.

182 **Commander Andrew Lin:** Interview of Commander Andrew Lin by the author, May 24, 2018.

183 **Naval Station Norfolk in Virginia:** Our first stop on the ship was the memorial in the canteen for those who died when the *USS Cole* was attacked by terrorists on October 12, 2000. While *Cole* was refueling in Yemen's Aden harbor, two suicide bombers in a small boat full of explosives approached the port side of the destroyer. They detonated and the explosion created a 40-by-60-foot hole in the ship, killing 17 navy sailors and injuring 39 more who were lining up in the canteen for lunch. Al-Qaeda claimed responsibility for the attack.

183 **14 weeks of basic training for the job:** Corpsmen are a naval invention— starting in 1898—and cousins of the army medic. Many receive extra training in laboratory medicine, optometry, radiology, pharmacy, operating rooms, and more. After the Vietnam War, the capable Navy corpsmen who returned home without a comparable professional track in the civilian sector inspired Dr. Eugene Stead at Duke University to launch the nation's first physician assistant training program. October 6, Stead's birthday, is national Physician Assistant Day ("Eugene Stead, Medical Pioneer, Dies," *Duke Today*, June 17, 2005, https://today.duke.edu/2005/06/stead.html.) The Hospital Corps is now one of the largest occupational ratings in the Navy, with 30,000 active-duty and reserve members in 39 different specialties. "In Their Own Words: Sailors Discuss What It Means to Be a U.S. Navy Hospital Corpsman," Navy Medicine Live, accessed August 31, 2019, https://navymedicine.navylive.dodlive.mil/archives/12501; "Corpsman Up," National Museum of the United States Navy, accessed August 31, 2019, https://www.history.navy.mil/content/dam/museums/nmusn/PDFs/Education/Corpsman%20Up!.pdf.

184 **the Health Professions Scholarship Program:** "HPSP Fact Sheet," Air Force Medical Service, published July 25, 2018, accessed October 24, 2019,

https://www.airforcemedicine.af.mil/Media-Center/Fact-Sheets/Display/Article/425437/hpsp-fact-sheet/.

184   **$200,000 in debt from medical school:** Association of American Medical Colleges, "An Exploration of the Recent Decline in the Percentage of U.S. Medical School Graduates with Education Debt," *Analysis in Brief* 18, no. 4 (September 2018), accessed July 10, 2019, https://www.aamc.org/system/files/reports/1/september2018anexplorationoftherecentdeclineinthepercentageofu..pdf.

184   **for the service commitments:** Beyond medical school, the Military Health System and VA train residents and fellows, which helps improve their clinical and research productivity and also serves as a pipeline for future hires. The VA health system is the largest single training system in the nation; it spends over $650 million on academic alliances and trains more than 62,000 doctors, 23,000 nurses, and 33,000 other health care professionals per year. About 70% of all physicians in the United States have received some training at a VA hospital. I am one of them.

184   **immersive virtual reality experience:** *Wide Area Virtual Environment (WAVE)* (Bethesda, MD: Val G. Hemming Simulation Center, 2014), accessed August 31, 2019, http://www.simcen.org/wave.html.

184   **"appetites for more and better medicine":** Christopher Connell, "Is War Good for Medicine?: War's Medical Legacy," *Stanford Medicine*, accessed August 31, 2019, http://sm.stanford.edu/archive/stanmed/2007summer/main.html.

185   **bleeding to death from injuries to the arms and legs:** Some reviews of battlefield injuries include Brian J. Eastridge et al., "Death on the Battlefield (2001–2011): Implications for the Future of Combat Casualty Care," *Journal of Trauma and Acute Care Surgery* 73, no. 6 (December 2012): S431–37, doi: 10.1097/TA.0b013e3182755dcc; Howard R. Champion et al., "A Profile of Combat Injury," *Journal of Trauma* 54, no. 5 (May 2003): S13–19; Caroline Lee, Keith M. Porter, and Timothy J. Hodgetts, "Tourniquet Use in the Civilian Prehospital Setting," *Emergency Medicine Journal* 24, no. 8 (August 2007): 584–87, doi: 10.1136/emj.2007.046359.

185   **causing gangrene and limb loss:** David R. Welling et al., "Historical Vignettes in Vascular Surgery," *Journal of Vascular Surgery* 55, no. 1 (January 2012): 286–90.

185   **bleeding from wounds to their extremities**: *Stopping the Bleed* (Houston: US Army Institute of Surgical Research, 2018), accessed May 26, 2019, https://www.ccems.com/wp-content/uploads/2019/10/US-Army-Institute-of-Surgical-Research-Tourniquets.pdf.

185   **reconsider their position on tourniquets:** Frank K. Butler Jr., John Hagmann, and E. George Butler, "Tactical Combat Casualty Care in Special Operations," *Military Medicine* 161, no. 1 (August 1996): 3–16, p. 5, https://doi.org/10.1093/milmed/161.suppl_1.3; US Army Institute of Surgical Research, *Stopping the Bleed*; John F. Kragh Jr. et al., "Historical Review of Emergency Tourniquet Use to Stop Bleeding," *American Journal of Surgery* 203, no. 2 (February 2012): 242–52, https://doi.org/10.1016/j.amjsurg.2011.01.028.

185   **Velcro loop to keep things secure:** US Army Institute of Surgical Research, *Stopping the Bleed.*

185   **hospital-based trauma care:** Frank K. Butler, David J. Smith, and Richard H. Carmona, "Implementing and Preserving the Advances in Combat Casualty Care from Iraq and Afghanistan throughout the US Military," *Journal of Trauma and Acute Care Surgery* 79, no. 2 (2015): 321–26; Lorne Blackbourne et al., "Military Medical Revolution: Military Trauma System," *Journal of Trauma and Acute Care Surgery* 73, no. 6 (December 2012): S388–94, doi: 10.1097/TA.0b013e31827548df.

185   **care administered, and outcomes:** Butler, Smith, and Carmona, "Implementing and Preserving the Advances in Combat Casualty Care."

185   **Basic Combat Training program:** Robert Little, "U.S. Military Widening Use of Tourniquets," *Baltimore Sun*, May 2, 2005, https://www.baltimoresun.com/news/bal-te.tourniquets02may02-story.html.

Butler credits Dr. John Kragh, a former US Army Ranger, with conducting the critical research that documented the safety of tourniquet use. Kragh signs his emails "TEGOTUS—Tourniquet Expert Geek of the United States." US Army Institute of Surgical Research, *Stopping the Bleed.*

185   **to 2.6% by 2010:** Butler, Smith, and Carmona, "Implementing and Preserving the Advances in Combat Casualty Care."

186   **in Afghanistan and Iraq:** Todd E. Rasmussen et al., "Ahead of the Curve: Sustained Innovation for Future Combat Casualty Care," *Journal of Trauma and Acute Care Surgery* 79, no. 4 (October 2015): S61–S64, doi: 10.1097/TA.0000000000000795.

186   **learnings are spilling into the civilian sector:** Pedro G. R. Teixeira et al., "Civilian Prehospital Tourniquet Use Is Associated with Improved Survival in Patients with Peripheral Vascular Injury," *Journal of the American College of Surgeons* 226, no. 5 (May 2018): 769–71, https://doi.org/10.1016/j.jamcollsurg .2018.01.047; Peter Burke, "The Return of Tourniquets: Original Research Evaluates the Effectiveness of Prehospital Tourniquets for Civilian Penetrating Extremity Injuries," *Journal of Emergency Medical Services* 33, no. 8 (July 31, 2008), https://www.jems.com/articles/print/volume-33/issue-8/patient -care/return-tourniquets-original-re.html.

186   **Vindell Washington is grateful:** Interview of Vindell Washington by the author, February 8, 2018.

186   **national coordinator for health information technology to fix them:** In that role, he says he's most proud of the work he did driving to some common standards for all 800 electronic health record vendors in the country and ensuring that patients could access the data.

186   **Nancy Dickey:** Interview of Nancy Dickey by the author, May 10, 2018. Dickey served as president of the Health Science Center at Texas A&M and president of the American Medical Association, among many leadership roles.

Chapter 12: The Long Fix

188 **Vice Admiral Raquel Bono:** Interview of Vice Admiral Raquel Bono by the author, March 30, 2018.

188 **to talk about fixing health care:** Interview of Michael Leavitt by the author, February 20, 2018.

188 **Walter Isaacson's book:** Walter Isaacson, *The Innovators: How a Group of Hackers, Geniuses, and Geeks Created the Digital Revolution* (New York: Simon & Schuster, 2014).

189 **8.5% of Americans had no health insurance:** Edward R. Berchick, Jessica C. Barnett, and Rachel D. Upton, *Health Insurance Coverage in the United States: 2018, Current Population Reports*, pp. 60–267 (Suitland, MD: US Census Bureau, 2019).

Other surveys, such as the 2018 Commonwealth Fund's Biennial Health Insurance Survey, found similar numbers, focusing just on nonelderly adults—12.4% of adults ages 19–64 were uninsured (unchanged from 2016), while the Kaiser Family Foundation survey of 2017 reported 10.2% (27.4 million) nonelderly adults were uninsured. Sara R. Collins, Herman K. Bhupal, and Michelle M. Doty, "Health Insurance Coverage Eight Years after the ACA," Commonwealth Fund, February 7, 2019, https://www.commonwealthfund .org/publications/issue-briefs/2019/feb/health-insurance-coverage-eight -years-after-aca; Rachel Garfield, Kendal Orgera, and Anthony Damico, "The Uninsured and the ACA: A Primer—Key Facts about Health Insurance and the Uninsured amidst Changes to the Affordable Care Act," Kaiser Family Foundation, January 25, 2019, https://www.kff.org/report-section/the-uninsured -and-the-aca-a-primer-key-facts-about-health-insurance-and-the-uninsured -amidst-changes-to-the-affordable-care-act-how-many-people-are-uninsured/.

189 **increasingly underinsured:** Collins, Bhipal, and Doty, "Health Insurance Coverage." The Commonwealth Fund defines "underinsured" as adults who were insured all year but experienced one of the following: out-of-pocket costs, excluding premiums, equaled 10% or more of income; out-of-pocket costs, excluding premiums, equaled 5% or more of income if low-income (<200% of poverty level); or deductibles equaled 5% or more of income.

189 **10%–12% of their economies:** By "economies," I'm referring to gross domestic product. Irene Papanicolas, Liana R. Woskie, and Ashish K. Jha, "Health Care Spending in the United States and Other High-Income Countries," *JAMA* 319, no. 10 (March 13, 2018): 1024–39, doi: 10.1001/jama.2018.1150.

190 **it is the responsibility of the federal government to make sure all Americans have health care:** "Healthcare System," *Gallup News*, accessed October 19, 2019, https://news.gallup.com/poll/4708/healthcare-system.aspx; Jocelyn Kiley, "Most Continue to Say Ensuring Health Care Coverage Is Government's Responsibility," Pew Research Center, October 3, 2018, https://

www.pewresearch.org/fact-tank/2018/10/03/most-continue-to-say-ensuring
-health-care-coverage-is-governments-responsibility/.

190 **penalize states that chose not to expand Medicaid:** National Federation of Independent Business v. Sebelius, 567 U.S. 519 (2012).

190 **14 states had not:** The Kaiser Family Foundation website maintains an up-to-date tracking of Medicaid expansion states: "Status of State Medicaid Expansion Decisions: Interactive Map," Kaiser Family Foundation, last edited September 20, 2019, https://www.kff.org/medicaid/issue-brief/status-of-state-medicaid -expansion-decisions-interactive-map/.

190 **Among all high-income nations:** Other high-income nations used in most comparative studies: UK, Germany, Switzerland, France, the Scandinavian countries, Canada, Japan, Australia, New Zealand, and Singapore, for example: Papanicolas, Woskie, and Jha, "Health Care Spending."

191 **"Is Health Care a Right?":** Atul Gawande, "Is Health Care a Right?," *New Yorker*, September 25, 2017, https://www.newyorker.com/magazine/2017/10/02/is -health-care-a-right.

191 **requirements for beneficiaries to seek employment or engage in community work:** This is being disputed in multiple courts. Centers for Medicare & Medicaid Services, "RE: Opportunities to Promote Work and Community Engagement Among Medicaid Beneficiaries" (Baltimore, MD: Department of Health and Human Services, 2018). Approximately 63% of patients are already fully or partially employed. For more details: Rachel Garfield et al., "Understanding the Intersection of Medicaid and Work: What Does the Data Say?," Kaiser Family Foundation, August 8, 2019, https://www.kff.org/medicaid/issue-brief/ understanding-the-intersection-of-medicaid-and-work-what-does-the-data-say/.

191 **Gawande interviewed a local librarian:** Gawande, "Is Health Care a Right?"

191 **even if it costs more:** From 2010–2015, Medicaid expansion increased the Medicaid budget by about 12%, although since then it has grown much more slowly than the overall health care market. Benjamin D. Sommers and Jonathan Gruber, "Federal Funding Insulated State Budgets from Increased Spending Related to Medicaid Expansion," *Health Affairs* 36, no. 5 (May 2017), https:// doi.org/10.1377/hlthaff.2016.1666.

An excellent discussion of the effects of increased preventive care can be found in this article: Aaron E. Carroll, "Preventive Care Saves Money? Sorry, It's Too Good to Be True," *New York Times*, January 29, 2018, https://www .nytimes.com/2018/01/29/upshot/preventive-health-care-costs.html.

191 **health to be significantly better:** Benjamin D. Sommers, Katherine Baicker, and Arnold M. Epstein, "Mortality and Access to Care among Adults after State Medicaid Expansions," *New England Journal of Medicine* 367 (September 2012): 1025–34, doi: 10.1056/NEJMsa1202099.

191 **several hundred published research studies:** The statistics cited come from this meta-analysis: Olena Mazurenko et al., "The Effects of Medicaid Expansion under the ACA: A Systematic Review," *Health Affairs* 37, no. 6 (June

2018), https://doi.org/10.1377/hlthaff.2017.1491. The Kaiser Family Foundation maintains this frequently updated report: Larisa Antonisse et al., "The Effects of Medicaid Expansion under the ACA: Updated Findings from a Literature Review," Kaiser Family Foundation, August 15, 2019, https://www.kff .org/medicaid/issue-brief/the-effects-of-medicaid-expansion-under-the-aca -updated-findings-from-a-literature-review-august-2019/.

192 **health systems of other high-income nations:** An excellent review of health systems of high-income nations, including the United States, can be found at the Commonwealth Fund's online Health Care System Profiles: "Country Profiles," Commonwealth Fund, accessed October 20, 2019, https://international .commonwealthfund.org/countries/.

192 **maximum wait time for nonurgent clinic visits is 18 weeks:** "Guide to NHS Waiting Times in England," National Health Service, accessed October 20, 2019, https://www.nhs.uk/using-the-nhs/nhs-services/hospitals/guide-to-nhs -waiting-times-in-england/#maximum.

193 **Unlike the US system:** There is one exception in the United States at the state level, where a major experiment in global budgeting has been underway since the 1970s. Maryland's state legislature implemented an all-payer hospital rate-setting system in which a state agency establishes the payment rates for public and private payers for all hospitals, each year. After the Affordable Care Act, the entire state of Maryland agreed to limit hospital spending growth for all payers to less than 3.58% per year, and to keep the Medicare per capita growth rate to 0.5% less than the national average, saving Medicare at least $330 million over five years. It achieved all three goals. Unfortunately, for the purposes of this discussion, hospitals still bill per admission and per service, so administrative burdens are not reduced. Rahul Rajkumar et al., "Maryland's All-Payer Approach to Delivery-System Reform," *New England Journal of Medicine* 370, no. 6 (February 2014): 493–95, doi: 10.1056/NEJMp1314868. Eric T. Roberts et al., "Changes in Health Care Use Associated with the Introduction of Hospital Global Budgets in Maryland," *JAMA Internal Medicine* 178, no. 2 (February 2018): 260–68, doi: 10.1001/jamainternmed.2017.7455; Eric T. Roberts et al., "Changes in Hospital Utilization Three Years into Maryland's Global Budget Program for Rural Hospitals," *Health Affairs* 37, no. 4 (April 2018), https://doi .org/10.1377/hlthaff.2018.0112.

193 **Take Switzerland:** Carlo De Pietro et al., "Switzerland: Health System Review," *Health Systems in Transition* 17, no. 4 (2015): 1–288, PMID: 26766626; "Who is Covered and How Is Insurance Financed?," Commonwealth Fund, accessed October 20, 2019, https://international.commonwealthfund.org/features/who_ covered/.

194 **In a 2018 Pew Center survey:** Kiley, "Ensuring Health Care Coverage Is Government's Responsibility."

195 **market-based approach:** The 1963 landmark article by Kenneth Arrow outlines the many market failures in health care: Kenneth J. Arrow, "Uncertainty

and the Welfare Economics of Medical Care," *American Economic Review* 53, no. 5 (Dec 1963): 941–73.

196 **"it's a long fix":** Interview of Clif Gaus by the author, October 4, 2019.

196 **Secretary of Health and Human Services Sylvia Burwell:** Sylvia M. Burwell, "Setting Value-Based Payment Goals—HHS Efforts to Improve U.S. Health Care," *New England Journal of Medicine* 372 (March 2015): 897–99, doi: 10.1056/NEJMp1500445.

197 **Aetna's chief executive:** Bruce Jaspen, "Value-Based Care Will Drive Aetna's Future Goals," *Forbes*, May 15, 2015, https://www.forbes.com/sites/brucejapsen/2015/05/15/value-based-care-may-drive-aetna-bid-for-cigna-or-humana/#3ec060273d70.

197 **Primary Care First initiative:** "HHS To Deliver Value-Based Transformation in Primary Care," HHS.gov, April 22, 2019, https://www.hhs.gov/about/news/2019/04/22/hhs-deliver-value-based-transformation-primary-care.html.

197 **from voluntary to mandatory:** "CMS Announces Participants in New Value-Based Bundled Payment Model," Centers for Medicare and Medicaid Services, October 9, 2018, https://www.cms.gov/newsroom/press-releases/cms-announces-participants-new-value-based-bundled-payment-model.

197 **charge $25,000 for an MRI?:** Sarah Kliff, "The Problem Is the Prices," *Vox*, October 16, 2017, https://www.vox.com/policy-and-politics/2017/10/16/16357790/health-care-prices-problem.

198 **primary care and behavioral health:** Sarah Klein, "Behavioral Health Integration: Approaches from the Field," Commonwealth Fund, August 28, 2014, https://www.commonwealthfund.org/publications/newsletter-article/2014/aug/behavioral-health-integration-approaches-field?redirect_source=/publications/newsletter/2014/aug/behavioral-health-integration-approaches-field. "Building the Business Case for Team-Based Integrated Care," AIMS Center, accessed September 1, 2019, https://aims.uw.edu/collaborative-care/building-business-case-cost-effectiveness-studies-collaborative-care; *Approaches to Integrating Physical Health Services into Behavioral Health Organizations* (Falls Church, VA: Lewin Group, 2012), accessed September 1, 2019, https://www.integration.samhsa.gov/Approaches_to_Integrating_Physical_Health_Services_into_BH_Organizations_RIC.pdf; Mark Rodgers et al., "Integrated Care to Address the Physical Health Needs of People with Severe Mental Illness: A Mapping Review of the Recent Evidence on Barriers, Facilitators and Evaluations," *International Journal of Integrated Care* 18, no. 1 (Winter 2018): 9, doi: 10.5334/ijic.2605.

198 **Patients in better mental health:** Sarah Klein and Martha Hostetter, "In Focus: Integrating Behavioral Health and Primary Care," Commonwealth Fund, August 28, 2014, https://www.commonwealthfund.org/publications/newsletter-article/2014/aug/focus-integrating-behavioral-health-and-primary-care.

198 **older adults returns more than $6 for every dollar spent:** "IMPACT Trial Results," University of Washington Department of Psychiatry & Behavioral

Sciences, last updated March 6, 2014, https://aims.uw.edu/sites/default/files/ IMPACTTrialResults_0.pdf; Jürgen Unützer et al., "Long-Term Cost Effects of Collaborative Care for Late-Life Depression," *American Journal of Managed Care* 14, no. 2 (February 2008): 95–100.

198 **Employer-sponsored health plans:** These programs are allowed to offset as much as 30% of the total costs of coverage and 50% for programs to reduce tobacco use: "Incentives for Nondiscriminatory Wellness Programs in Group Health Plans," *Federal Register,* June 3, 2013, https://www.federalregister .gov/documents/2013/06/03/2013-12916/incentives-for-nondiscrimina tory-wellness-programs-in-group-health-plans. Soeren Mattke, Christopher Schnyer, and Kristin R. Van Busum, *A Review of the U.S. Workplace Wellness Market* (Santa Monica, CA: RAND Corporation, 2012).

198 **without much success:** Mitesh S. Patel et al., "Premium-Based Financial Incentives Did Not Promote Workplace Weight Loss in a 2013–15 Study," *Health Affairs* 35, no. 1 (January 2016), https://doi.org/10.1377/hlthaff.2015.0945; Zirui Song and Katherine Baicker, "Effect of a Workplace Wellness Program on Employee Health and Economic Outcomes: A Randomized Clinical Trial," *JAMA* 321, no. 15 (April 2019): 1491–501, doi: 10.1001/jama.2019.3307.

199 **complex medical problems in Allegheny County, Pennsylvania:** Pamela Peele et al., "Advancing Value-Based Population Health Management through Payer-Provider Partnerships: Improving Outcomes for Children with Complex Conditions," *Journal for Healthcare Quality* 40, no. 2 (Spring 2018): e26–32, doi: 10.1097/JHQ.0000000000000101.

199 **Pamela Peele:** Interview of Pamela Peele by the author, February 16, 2018.

199 **Korb Matosich . . . Asserta Health:** Korb Matosich, "Bundling Direct Contracting with Risk Protection: A Win-Win for Employers, Providers & Patients," Panel, 29th Annual National Educational Conference & Expo, SIAA, San Francisco, CA, October 1, 2019.

201 **one-fifth of American adults smoke or use electronic cigarettes:** "Current Cigarette Smoking among Adults in the United States," Centers for Disease Control and Prevention, accessed October 20, 2019, https://www.cdc.gov/tobacco/ data_statistics/fact_sheets/adult_data/cig_smoking/index.htm; Katherine Schaeffer, "Before Recent Outbreak, Vaping Was on the Rise in U.S., Especially among Young People," Pew Research Center, September 26, 2019, https://www .pewresearch.org/fact-tank/2019/09/26/vaping-survey-data-roundup/.

201 **one-fifth of all children are obese:** Obesity is defined as body mass index of 30 or more. A 5-foot 9-inch person who weighs 203 pounds or more, or a 5-foot 4-inch person who weighed 175 pounds or more, would be considered obese. Overweight is defined as having a body mass index of 25–29.9. Those same two individuals, if they weighed 170 pounds or 146 pounds, respectively, would be considered overweight.

An online BMI calculator can be found at "Healthy Weight: Adult BMI Calculator," Centers for Disease Control and Prevention, accessed September 1, 2019, https://www.cdc.gov/healthyweight/assessing/bmi/adult_BMI/english_bmi_calculator/bmi_calculator.html. "Overweight & Obesity: Childhood Obesity Facts," Centers for Disease Control and Prevention, accessed September 1, 2019, https://www.cdc.gov/obesity/data/childhood.html.

201 **exercise:** "Exercise or Physical Activity," Centers for Disease Control and Prevention, accessed October 20, 2019, https://www.cdc.gov/nchs/fastats/exercise.htm.

201 **don't get enough sleep:** "1 in 3 Adults Don't Get Enough Sleep," Centers for Disease Control and Prevention, accessed October 20, 2019, https://www.cdc.gov/media/releases/2016/p0215-enough-sleep.html.

201 **partly related to health and education:** Miriam Jordan, "Recruits' Ineligibility Tests the Military," *Wall Street Journal*, June 27, 2014, https://www.wsj.com/articles/recruits-ineligibility-tests-the-military-1403909945?mod=e2tw.

201 **Vice Admiral Raquel Bono:** Interview of Vice Admiral Raquel Bono by the author, March 30, 2018.

202 **An online curriculum:** Dell Medical School's online program is available here: "Discovering Value-Based Health Care," Dell Medical School, accessed October 20, 2019, http://www.vbhc.dellmed.utexas.edu/.

202 **Stacey Chang:** Interview of Stacey Chang by the author, October 26, 2017.

202 **dean of the new Kaiser Permanente Medical School:** Interview of Mark Schuster by the author, October 20, 2019.

202 **nursing shortage:** Lisa M. Haddad and Tammy J. Toney-Butler, "Nursing Shortage," *StatPearls* (Treasure Island, FL: StatPearls, 2019), https://www.statpearls.com/kb/viewarticle/26039/; "Nursing Shortage," American Association of Colleges of Nursing, accessed October 20, 2019, https://www.aacnnursing.org/News-Information/Fact-Sheets/Nursing-Shortage.

202 **the National Health Service Corps Loan Repayment Program:** "NHSC Loan Repayment Program," Health Resources & Services Administration, accessed October 20, 2019, https://nhsc.hrsa.gov/loan-repayment/nhsc-loan-repayment-program.html.

202 **medical assistants:** Liel Blash, Catherine Dower, and Susan Chapman, *University of Utah Community Clinics—Medical Assistant Teams Enhance Patient-Centered, Physician-Efficient Care* (San Francisco: Center for the Health Professions, revised in 2011).

203 **caregivers provide over $500 billion in uncompensated care:** Stipica Mudrazija, "Work-Related Opportunity Costs of Providing Unpaid Family Care in 2013 and 2050," *Health Affairs* 38, no. 6 (June 2019), https://doi.org/10.1377/hlthaff.2019.00008.

203 **Carolyn Clancy:** Interview of Carolyn Clancy by the author, February 18, 2018. Clancy is a general internal medicine physician and health services researcher who serves as Deputy Under Secretary for Discovery, Education and Affiliate Networks, Veterans Health Administration. For ten years, she was director, Agency for Healthcare Research and Quality.

Epilogue

205 **Mariana Mazzucato:** Alisha Haridasani Gupta, "An 'Electrifying' Economist's Guide to the Recovery," *New York Times,* November 19, 2020, https://www .nytimes.com/2020/11/19/us/economist-covid-recovery-mariana-mazzucato .html.

205 **1918–1919 influenza pandemic:** The 1918–1919 influenza pandemic caused about 675,000 deaths in the United States and about 50 million deaths world-wide. "Influenza (Flu): 1918 Pandemic," Centers for Disease Control and Prevention, accessed November 27, 2020, https://www.cdc.gov/flu/pandemic -resources/1918-pandemic-h1n1.html.

205 **COVID-19:** severe acute respiratory syndrome coronavirus 2 (SARS-CoV-2)

206 **Terry Fulmer:** Interview of Terry Fulmer by the author, October 9, 2020.

206 **over 150,000 residents and staff of long-term care facilities:** "The Long-Term Care COVID Tracker," The COVID Tracking Project, *The Atlantic,* accessed January 29, 2021, https://covidtracking.com/ nursing-homes-long-term-care-facilities.

207 **about 36% of all COVID-19 deaths:** Earlier data showed that about one-quarter of all Americans die in nursing homes, assisted living facilities, or hospice, suggesting that COVID-19 was disproportionately lethal in nursing homes. "Patterns in COVID-19 Cases and Deaths in Long-Term Care Facilities in 2020," Kaiser Family Foundation, January 14, 2021, https://www.kff .org/coronavirus-covid-19/press-release/covid-19-outbreaks-in-long-term -care-facilities-were-most-severe-in-the-early-months-of-the-pandemic -but-data-show-cases-and-deaths-in-such-facilities-may-be-on-the-rise-again/.

207 **Rich Feifer:** Interview of Rich Feifer by the author, October 22, 2020.

207 **We Have Been Failing Our Frail Older Adults for Decades:** Howard Gleckman, "Why Are We so Shocked by COVID-19 Nursing Home Deaths? We Have Been Failing Our Frail Older Adults for Decades," *Forbes,* April 27, 2020, https://www.forbes.com/sites/howardgleckman/2020/04/27/why-are-we -so-shocked-by-covid-19-nursing-home-deaths-we-have-been-failing-our -frail-older-adults-for-decades/?sh=4bc0fe424aad.

207 **one in four patients sent to nursing homes:** Staffing requirements for nursing homes are far lighter than for hospitals. Most of the care is provided by certified nursing assistants (CNAs) with 1–4 months of training who work under the supervision of registered nurses and licensed practical nurses (with one year of training). A registered nurse is required to be present only eight hours a day, and a physician must be on call, but not necessarily on the premises. Vincent Mor et al., "The Revolving Door of Rehospitalization from Skilled Nursing Facilities," *Health Affairs 29,* no. 1 (January 2010), doi.org/10.1377/hlthaff.2009.0629.

207 **penalized about 11,000 nursing homes and rewarded only 4,000:** Jordan Rau, "Medicare Cuts Payments to Nursing Homes Whose Patients Keep Ending Up in Hospital," Kaiser Health News, December 3, 2018, https://khn

.org/news/medicare-cuts-payments-to-nursing-homes-whose-patients-keep
-ending-up-in-hospital/.

208 **AARP:** Ellen Stark, "5 Things You SHOULD Know about Long-Term Care Insurance," *AARP*, March 1, 2018, https://www.aarp.org/caregiving/financial -legal/info-2018/long-term-care-insurance-fd.html.

208 **an LTC fund:** Ron Lieber, "New Tax Will Help Washington Residents Pay for Long-Term Care," *New York Times*, May 13, 2019, https://www.nytimes .com/2019/05/13/business/washington-long-term-care.html.

208 **Programs like these:** Sarah Ruiz et al., "Innovative Home Visit Models Associated with Reductions in Costs, Hospitalizations, and Emergency Department Use," *Health Affairs* 36, no.3 (March 2017): 425–32, doi: 10.1377/ hlthaff.2016.1305.

208 **ChenMed:** Among those who did contract the coronavirus, ChenMed patients fared better than average; about one in five of those who contracted COVID-19 died, compared to a rate of one in three in this age group nationally. Reyan Ghany et al., "Prior Cardiovascular Risk and Screening Echocardiograms Predict Hospitalization and Severity of Coronavirus Infection among Elderly Medicare Patients," *American Journal of Preventive Cardiology* 3 (September 2020), doi.org/10.1016/j.ajpc.2020.100090.

209 **Nancy Guinn:** Interview of Nancy Guinn by the author, September 14, 2020.

209 **new technologies:** Quincy M. Samus et al., "Home Is Where the Future Is: The BrightFocus Foundation Consensus Panel on Dementia Care," *Alzheimer's & Dementia* 14, no. 1 (January 2018): 104–14, doi: 10.1016/j.jalz.2017.10.006; and Wendy Moyle, "The Promise of Technology in the Future of Dementia Care," *Nature Reviews* 15 (June 2019): 353–59, https://www.nature.com/articles/ s41582-019-0188-y.pdf?origin=ppub.

209 **in a rural or frontier community:** "Rural Health: About Rural Health," Centers for Disease Control and Prevention, accessed November 27, 2020, https:// www.cdc.gov/ruralhealth/about.html.

210 **doctors practicing in rural America:** Only one in 10 US doctors practices in rural communities. Rural areas also have shortages in dentists, physician assistants, and nurse practitioners. Emily Gudbranson, Aaron Glickman, and Ezekiel J. Emanuel, "Reassessing the Data on Whether a Physician Shortage Exists," *JAMA* 317, no. 19 (May 2017): 1945–6, doi: 10.1001/jama.2017.2609.

210 **Susan Anderson:** Interview of Susan Anderson by the author, September 22, 2020.

210 **Alaire Buysse:** Interview of Alaire Buysse by the author, October 9, 2020.

211 **Carl Lang:** Interview of Carl Lang by the author, October 6, 2020.

211 **Riley Schaap:** Interview of Riley Schaap by the author, October 9, 2020.

211 **One government report:** U.S. Government Accountability Office, *Indian Health Service: Spending Levels and Characteristics of IHS and Three Other Federal Health Care Programs*, GAO-19-74R (Washington, DC, 2018), accessed December 5, 2020, https://www.gao.gov/assets/700/695871.pdf.

211 **COVID-19 at a rate at least 3.5 times:** "COVID-19 among American Indian and Alaska Native Persons—23 States, January 31–July 3, 2020," Centers for Disease Control and Prevention, last modified August 28, 2020, https://www.cdc.gov/mmwr/volumes/69/wr/mm6934e1.htm?s_cid=mm6934e1_e&deliveryName=USCDC_921-DM35683.

212 **Scholarship and incentive programs:** Amelia Goodfellow et al., "Predictors of Primary Care Physician Practice Location in Underserved Urban or Rural Areas in the United States: A Systematic Literature Review," *Academic Medicine* 91, no. 9 (September 2016): 1313–21, doi: 10.1097/ACM.0000000000001203.

212 **10-15 rural hospitals close:** Ge Bai et al., "Varying Trends in the Financial Viability of U.S. Rural Hospitals, 2011–17," *Health Affairs* 39, no. 6 (June 2020), https://doi.org/10.1377/hlthaff.2019.01545.

212 **government payers like Medicare and Medicaid:** In 2017, Medicare and Medicaid made up 56% of rural hospitals' net revenue. "Challenges Facing Rural Communities and the Roadmap to Ensure Local Access to High-Quality, Affordable Care," Chicago: American Hospital Association, February 2019, accessed November 27, 2020, https://www.aha.org/system/files/2019-02/rural-report-2019.pdf.

212 **operate close to two-thirds empty:** In 2018, the acute bed occupancy for rural hospitals averaged 37%, which is significantly lower than urban hospitals at 62%. "Occupancy Rates in Rural and Urban Hospitals: Value and Limitations in Use as a Measure of Surge Capacity," Chapel Hill: North Carolina Rural Health Research Program, March 2020, accessed November 27, 2020, https://www.ruralhealthresearch.org/mirror/13/1302/surge-capacity.pdf.

212 **reimburses them more generously:** They receive cost basis (not DRG [diagnosis-related groups, discussed in Chapter 3]) + 1%, which means rural hospitals get paid 101% of their costs for outpatient, inpatient, laboratory, therapy and post-acute care hospital beds. They also qualify for discounted pharmaceutical pricing with 340B discounts.

212 **affiliating with a hospital or health system network:** Onyinye Oyeka et al., "The Rural Hospital and Health System Affiliation Landscape—A Brief Review," Iowa City: Rural Health Research & Policy Centers and Rural Policy Research Institute, November 2018, accessed November 27, 2020, https://rupri.public-health.uiowa.edu/publications/policypapers/Rural%20Hospital%20and%20Health%20System%20Affiliation.pdf.

212 **University of Utah:** "Neurology News: Hospital Honored for Quickly Treating Stroke Patients," University of Utah School of Medicine, February 7, 2019, https://medicine.utah.edu/neurology/news/2019/02/telestroke.php.

213 **over 90% of hospitalized COVID-19 patients:** Kalpana Thapa Bajgain et al., "Prevalence of Comorbidities among Individuals with COVID-19: A Rapid Review of Current Literature," *American Journal of Infection Control* 6553, no. 20 (July 2020), doi: 10.1016/j.ajic.2020.06.213.

213 **the rule, not the exception:** Six out of 10 adult Americans have the diagnosis of

a chronic medical condition, and the proportions rise with age. For those aged 55 and older, three out of four men, and four out of five women, have at least one chronic condition. "Chronic Diseases in America," Centers for Disease Control and Prevention, accessed November 27, 2020, https://www.cdc.gov/chronicdisease/resources/infographic/chronic-diseases.htm.

"Percent of US Adults 55 and Over with Chronic Conditions," Centers for Disease Control and Prevention, accessed November 27, 2020, https://www.cdc.gov/nchs/health_policy/adult_chronic_conditions.htm.

213 **African Americans and Hispanics:** "Disparities in Incidence of COVID-19 among Underrepresented Racial/Ethnic Groups in Counties Identified as Hotspots during June 5–18, 2020–22 States, February–June 2020," Centers for Disease Control and Prevention, accessed November 27, 2020, https://www.cdc.gov/mmwr/volumes/69/wr/mm6933e1.htm; Samantha Artiga, Bradley Corallo, and Olivia Pham, "Racial Disparities in COVID-19: Key Findings from Available Data and Analysis," Kaiser Family Foundation, August 17, 2020, https://www.kff.org/racial-equity-and-health-policy/issue-brief/racial-disparities-covid-19-key-findings-available-data-analysis/.

213 **Selwyn Vickers:** Interview of Selwyn Vickers by the author, August 27, 2020.

214 **narrowed racial and ethnic disparities:** Samantha Artiga and Kendal Orgera, "Changes in Health Coverage by Race and Ethnicity Since the ACA, 2010–2018," Kaiser Family Foundation, March 5, 2020, https://www.kff.org/racial-equity-and-health-policy/issue-brief/changes-in-health-coverage-by-race-and-ethnicity-since-the-aca-2010-2018/.

214 **Commonwealth Fund's Biennial Health Insurance Survey:** "New Survey: Two of Five Working-Age Adults Do Not Have Stable Health Coverage; More Than One-Third Have Medical Bill Problems," Commonwealth Fund, last modified August 19, 2020, https://www.commonwealthfund.org/press-release/2020/new-survey-two-of-five-working-age-adults-do-not-have-stable-health-coverage.

214 **worse outcomes:** Andreea A. Creanga et al., "Performance of Racial and Ethnic Minority-Serving Hospitals on Delivery-Related Indicators," *American Journal of Obstetrics and Gynecology* 211, no. 6 (December 2014): 647, https://doi.org/10.1016/j.ajog.2014.06.006.

214 **Ashish Jha and colleagues:** Ashish K. Jha et al., "Concentration and Quality of Hospitals That Care for Elderly Black Patients," *Archives of Internal Medicine* 167, no. 11 (June 2007): 1177–82, doi: 10.1001/archinte.167.11.1177.

215 **Willis Tower Watson survey:** Willis Towers Watson Public Limited Company, "Employees Flock to Virtual Health Care during Pandemic, Willis Towers Watson Employee Survey Finds," Arlington: GlobeNewswire, October 28, 2020, accessed November 27, 2020, https://www.globenewswire.com/news-release/2020/10/28/2116022/0/en/Employees-flock-to-virtual-health-care-during-pandemic-Willis-Towers-Watson-employee-survey-finds.html.

216 **rising rates of depression, anxiety, sleep disturbances, and other psy-**

chiatric issues: Catherine K. Ettman et al., "Prevalence of Depression Symptoms in US Adults before and during the COVID-19 Pandemic," *JAMA Network Open 3*, no. 9 (September 2020): e2019686, doi: 10.1001/jamanetworkopen.2020.19686.

216 **an estimated $80 billion:** Frank Pallone Jr., "Dividing the Country Won't Bridge the Digital Divide," *House Committee on Energy & Commerce*, January 29, 2018, https://energycommerce.house.gov/newsroom/in-the-news/dividing-the-country-won-t-bridge-the-digital-divide.

216 **Ed McGookin . . . Meryl Moss:** Interview of Ed McGookin and Meryl Moss by the author, January 15, 2021.

217 **the risk of death dropped to 7.6%:** Leora I. Horwitz et al., "Trends in COVID-19 Risk-Adjusted Mortality Rates," *Journal of Hospital Medicine* (October 2020), doi: 10.12788/jhm.3552.

217 **worldwide digital connections:** Celina Yong, "The Isolation That Has Brought Us Together," *Journal of the American College of Cardiology 75*, no. 20 (2020): 2639–41, https://doi.org/10.1016/j.jacc.2020.04.014.

217 **Bob Wachter:** Interview of Bob Wachter by the author, September 9, 2020.

218 **posting massive data sets online:** "Open-Access Data and Computational Resources to Address COVID-19," National Institutes of Health: Office of Data Science Strategy, accessed November 27, 2020, https://datascience.nih.gov/covid-19-open-access-resources.

218 **James Fallows:** James Fallows, "The 3 Weeks That Changed Everything: Imagine if the National Transportation Safety Board Investigated America's Response to the Coronavirus Pandemic," *The Atlantic*, June 29, 2020, https://www.theatlantic.com/politics/archive/2020/06/how-white-house-coronavirus-response-went-wrong/613591/.

218 **Karen Feinstein:** Karen Feinstein, "COVID-19 Has Exposed the Urgent Need for a National Patient Safety Authority," *Modern Healthcare*, September 17, 2020, https://www.modernhealthcare.com/opinion-editorial/covid-19-has-exposed-urgent-need-national-patient-safety-authority.

219 **Liz Fowler:** Interview of Liz Fowler by the author, August 26, 2020.

INDEX